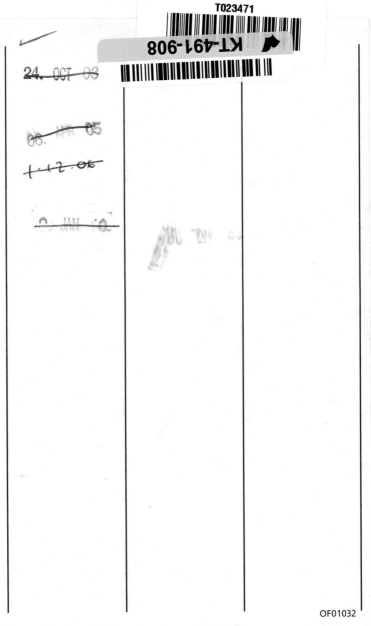

Evidence in Mental Health Care

Mental health care increasingly faces a challenge to be 'evidence based'. However, despite much policy activity in the UK, it's still not clear what sort of evidence researchers should be producing for mental health services, or what purchasers should be looking for. Stefan Priebe and Mike Slade, together with a group of contributors from different perspectives, seek to answer these questions.

Evidence in Mental Health Care evaluates a range of different research methodologies and types of 'evidence', and includes:

- a historical and conceptual analysis of what was regarded as evidence in the past, and what impact it has had in mental health care
- a presentation of different methodological approaches, and a discussion of their strengths and weaknesses in providing evidence
- how evidence is applied in different treatment and care modalities
- different angles on the way forward for providing appropriate evidence to improve current mental health care.

Evidence in Mental Health Care will prove vital for the successful extension of evidence-based evaluation to mental health services in general. It will be essential reading for researchers, students and practitioners across the range of mental health disciplines, health service managers and purchasers of services.

Stefan Priebe is Chair of Social and Community Psychiatry at St Bartholomew's and the Royal London School of Medicine, Queen Mary, University of London.

Mike Slade is Lecturer in Clinical Psychology at the Institute of Psychiatry, London.

Contributors: Nick Alderman, Simon Allard, Annie Bartlett, Derek Bolton, Tom Burns, Stuart Carney, Anthony Clare, John Cookson, Asmus Finzen, Peter Fonagy, John Geddes, David Goldberg, Howard Goldman, Peter Huxley, Peter James, Eddie Kane, Richard Laugharne, Max Marshall, Harold Pincus, Tony Roth, Heinz-Peter Shmiedebach, Terry Tanielian, Michele Tansella, Graham Thornicroft, Brian Williams.

Evidence in Mental Health Care

Edited by Stefan Priebe
and Mike Slade

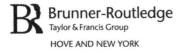
Brunner-Routledge
Taylor & Francis Group

HOVE AND NEW YORK

First published 2002 by Brunner-Routledge
27 Church Road, Hove, East Sussex BN3 2FA

Simultaneously published in the USA and Canada
by Brunner-Routledge
29 West 35th Street, New York, NY 10001

Brunner-Routledge is an imprint of the Taylor and Francis Group

Typeset in 10/12pt Times
by Graphicraft Limited, Hong Kong
Printed and bound in Great Britain by Biddles Ltd, Guildford
and King's Lynn
Cover design by Jim Wilkie

British Library Cataloguing in Publication Data
A catalogue record for this book is available
from the British Library

Library of Congress Cataloging-in-Publication Data
Evidence in mental health care / edited by Stefan Priebe
and Mike Slade.
       p. cm.
   Includes bibliographical references and index.
   ISBN 0-415-23692-4
   1. Mental health services. 2. Evidence-based medicine.
I. Priebe, Stefan, 1953–. II. Slade, Mike.

RA790.5.E844 2002
362.2–dc21   2001052545

ISBN 0-415-23692-4

Contents

Figures

Boxes

Tables

Contributors

Dr Nick Alderman, Consultant Clinical Neuropsychologist, The Kemsley Division, St Andrew's Hospital, Billing Road, Northampton NN1 5DG, UK.

Mr Simon Allard, Independent Newham Users Forum, St Alban's Centre, 157 Wakefield Street, London E6 1LG, UK.

Dr Annie Bartlett, St George's Hospital Medical School, Jenner Wing, Cranmer Terrace, London SW17 ORE, UK.

Dr Derek Bolton, Institute of Psychiatry, De Crespigny Park, Denmark Hill, London SE5 8AF, UK.

Professor Tom Burns, St George's Hospital Medical School, Jenner Wing, Cranmer Terrace, London SW17 ORE, UK.

Dr Stuart Carney, Department of Psychiatry, University of Oxford, Warneford Hospital, Oxford OX3 7JX, UK.

Professor Anthony Clare, Department of Psychiatry, Trinity Centre for Health Sciences, St James's Hospital, Dublin 8, Ireland.

Dr John Cookson, St Clement's Hospital, Bow Road, London E3 4LL, UK.

Professor Asmus Finzen, University of Basel, Psychiatrische Universitätsklinik, Wilhelm-Klein-Straße 27, CH 4025 Basel, Switzerland.

Professor Peter Fonagy, University College London, Gower Street, London WC1E 6BT, UK.

Dr John Geddes, Centre for Evidence Based Mental Health, Department of Psychiatry, University of Oxford, Warneford Hospital, Oxford OX3 7JX, UK.

Professor Sir David Goldberg, Institute of Psychiatry, De Crespigny Park, Denmark Hill, London SE5 8AF, UK.

Professor Howard Goldman, University of Pittsburgh School of Medicine, RAND Corporation, 1200 South Hayes Street, Arlington, VA 22202, USA.

Professor Peter Huxley, Institute of Psychiatry, De Crespigny Park, Denmark Hill, London SE5 8AF, UK.

Dr Peter James, Department of General Psychiatry, St George's Hospital Medical School, Jenner Wing, Cranmer Terrace, London SW17 ORE, UK.

Mr Eddie Kane, NHS Executive – London Regional Office, 40 Eastbourne Terrace, London W2 3QR, UK.

Dr Richard Laugharne, St George's Hospital Medical School, Jenner Wing, Cranmer Terrace, London SW17 ORE, UK.

Dr Max Marshall, University of Manchester, Mathematics Building, Oxford Road, Manchester M13 9PL, UK.

Dr Harold Pincus MD, University of Pittsburgh School of Medicine, RAND Corporation, 1200 South Hayes Street, Arlington, VA 22202, USA.

Professor Stefan Priebe, Unit for Social and Community Psychiatry, St Bartholomew's and the Royal London School of Medicine, Queen Mary, University of London, Mile End Road, London E1 4NS.

Dr Tony Roth, University College London, Gower Street, London WC1E 6BT, UK.

Professor Heinz-Peter Schmiedebach, University of Greifswald, W-Rathenaustr. 48, D-17487 Greifswald, Germany.

Dr Mike Slade, Institute of Psychiatry, De Crespigny Park, Denmark Hill, London SE5 8AF, UK.

Mr Terry Tanielian, University of Pittsburgh School of Medicine, RAND Corporation, 1200 South Hayes Street, Arlington, VA 22202, USA.

Professor Michele Tansella, University of Verona, Department of Medicine and Public Health, Section of Psychiatry, Hospital Policlinics, P.le A.L. Scuro, 37134 Verona, Italy.

Professor Graham Thornicroft, Institute of Psychiatry, De Crespigny Park, Denmark Hill, London SE5 8AF, UK.

Dr Brian Williams, Department of Epidemiology and Public Health, Ninewells Hospital and Medical School, University of Dundee, Dundee DD1 9SY, UK.

Foreword

From its very beginnings, psychiatry has been particularly vulnerable to swings of diagnostic and therapeutic enthusiasms. Its history is permeated by ingenious speculation and hazy guesswork, and its achievements have often been a mix of serendipitous discovery and intuitive hunch. Its disasters have contributed to the stain of stigma that smears so much of contemporary public and professional thinking about mental health and illness. Down through the years, various classificatory systems have been ingeniously elaborated and applied with a dogmatic zeal and rigidity more worthy of fundamentalist theologians than dispassionate clinicians. Treatments of the most demanding kind – one thinks of insulin coma therapy, leucotomies, regressive electro-convulsive therapy, daily psychoanalytic psychotherapy extending over many years – have been energetically peddled with scant reference to any valid and reliable information concerning their actual effectiveness.

It is something of an irony, therefore, that, along with the rest of medicine, psychiatry faces a fashion which demands that everything that doctors and other health care professionals do is done soundly and judiciously according to the best available evidence concerning its effectiveness. Evidence-based medicine, as the various contributors to this book demonstrate, has grabbed the attention of policy makers, service planners, health administrators, medical and paramedical therapists, and clinical and academic researchers, and it has done so because of the growing awareness of the shaky foundations on which so much of the expensive enterprise that is mental health care rests.

The questions raised are manifold and disquieting. *What are we as health care professionals actually doing, as distinct from what we say we do and what we think we do?* Reading the psychiatric textbooks, one would be forgiven for believing, for example, that the prescribing of a specific drug for a specific condition is the norm of everyday clinical practice. In actual fact, half of patients are receiving more than one psychotropic drug at any one time, while one in three are taking three of more. Yet, there have been few reliable studies undertaken that have examined the efficacy of such drug-taking in various combinations. *Why are we doing what we do?* Why, for example, do we place such value on the application of classificatory systems such as ICD-10 and DSM-IV when the handful of reputable studies that have been undertaken continue to demonstrate a dismal level of concordance between classifiers? *Does what we are doing make any significant difference?* Psychiatry takes great pride in and encouragement from the developments in psychopharmacology over the past fifty years yet the fact remains that one in ten patients with severe depression do not recover, while over half suffer recurrent episodes. The initial findings each time a new antidepressant is developed and tested are almost invariably highly positive – the enormous media type over fluoxetine is but one example of a misplaced therapeutic enthusiasm shared, typically, by professionals, the media and the general public. The results when such drugs are deployed in the real world of day-to-day clinical practice and never as heady. Part of the answer lies in the fact that much of the research undertaken in psychiatry is based on atypical samples. Most drugs are tested on highly artificial populations – patients free of such contaminations as co-morbidity, personality disorder, physical ill-health, pregnancy, extremes of age, serious social disadvantages – yet the great majority of the patients presenting to mental health professionals stubbornly refuse to display such clean and highly defined problem profiles. This issue of artificial selection does not just apply to studies of drug effectiveness. How many studies demonstrating the superiority of this or that psychological or social intervention fail to take account of the contribution made by the extra availability of that most precious of therapeutic commodities – time? Just as we are encouraged to place greater emphasis on establishing the usefulness of what we are doing, we are being given less and less time in which to do it.

Where should we be doing what we are doing? Should it be in general hospitals that are invariably hard-pressed; psychiatric hospitals that are frequently under-resourced; in day hospitals and day centres that are often poorly integrated within the remainder of the services; in general practice and in primary care, whose practitioners regularly complain that their role is undervalued; in what is euphemistically called the community at a time when sociologists increasingly question whether communities as we once knew them still exist; or within the family when so often the family itself is an important factor in the pathogenesis of the disorder being treated?

And does what is being done make any difference? Mental health professionals rightly, for the most part, lament the paucity of resources devoted to mental health services, yet the fact remains that recent decades have witnessed an enormous expansion of therapists, of orthodox and complimentary psychological counsellors, psychologists, community psychiatric nurses, family and marital therapists, and occupational therapists, as well as psychiatrists specialising in child psychiatry, the psychiatry of old age, forensic psychiatry, substance abuse, liaison psychiatry and the myriad of subspecialties and special interests that characterise and reflect contemporary psychiatric theory and practice. Does this proliferation of mental health care professionals make any differences to people experiencing psychological distress and disorder? *And if it does make a difference, what kind of difference does it make?* Are we as a society mentally healthier or more disturbed?

But if our enthusiasm for evidence-based psychiatry is not to go the way of earlier fashions and end up spurned and discredited, it needs to be tempered by realism. The reason these and related questions still plague psychiatry two centuries on from the dawn of the scientific revolution is that they are extraordinarily complicated – because psychiatry, of all the branches of medicine, is concerned with the most intricate and challenging questions concerning human life, namely the relationships between brain and mind, between genes and environment, between the individual and the group, between family and society, between the transcendent and the mundane. The contributors to this book reflect the fact that any consideration of the issue of mental health needs to take account of the fact that psychiatry – unlike rheumatology, obstetrics, endocrinology or even community medicine – bridges substantial domains of human thought including (in addition to biology and psychology), anthropology, philosophy, sociology, politics, epidemiology, history, law, religion and the arts. Anyone who thinks that any of the truly significant questions concerning evidence in mental health care are easy will produce simplistic answers. The history of psychiatry is replete with example of such meretricious thinking. In so far as a post-modernist perspective is helpful at this time, it is to remind us that notwithstanding the scientific value of big and macroscopic interventions and evaluations such as random controlled trials, case management policies, and consensus development conferences, there is and must be a place for the view from below and within, individual narratives, different viewpoints, the personal experience. Just as we are exhorted by the great and the good to eschew everything that has not been appropriately tried and tested, our patients are demonstrating a dissatisfaction with scientific medicine and turning to alternative therapies more congenial to their own beliefs, values and philosophical orientations. So many attempts to amass evidence involve dispensing with or minimising individual difference. So many clinical interventions are valued precisely because they emphasise the individual differences and minimise what people have in common. None of us wants to be treated as a diagnosis to which a uniform treatment response is directed. Whatever the progress made in solidifying the evidence base of contemporary psychiatry, the challenge to the mental health professional and service is how to continue to provide different treatments based on differing theoretical paradigms to different people.

This leads us to a particularly thorny question, perhaps the most difficult question, which reverberates throughout this book. *How do we decide on the relative worth of different forms of evidence?* Given the information gathered together in this book, evidence concerning theory and practice, diagnosis and treatment, services and planning, the answer has to be 'with diffi-culty'. Psychiatry is steeped in uncertainty and ambiguity. The struggle to eliminate both is urgent, compelling, essential, unavoidable. But we would do well to acknowledge that the task is a mighty one and the tools available modest. It is to the credit of the contributors to this book that to a man and woman they acknowledge this reality and shape their recommendations accordingly.

Professor Anthony Clare

Preface

Mental health care increasingly faces a challenge to be 'evidence based'. Professional journals, conferences and books aim at communicating what may rightly be regarded as 'evidence-based medicine' and 'evidence-based mental health care'. Only what is based on evidence should be practised and Mental Health Professionals are encouraged to practise only evidence-based care. As researchers, we are supposed to provide the evidence on which mental health care is to be based. However, the question arises as to what constitutes evidence and to what extent we agree on what is regarded as proper evidence. This question prompted us to ask authors from very different perspectives to contribute to this book. The book has four sections. Section 1 provides a historical and conceptual analysis of what was regarded as evidence in the past, and what impact it has had in mental health care. In the second section different methodological approaches are presented, and their strengths and weaknesses in providing evidence are discussed. How evidence is applied in different treatment and care modalities is the subject of Section 3. Chapters in Section 4 take different angles on the way forward for providing appropriate evidence to improve current mental health care.

Thus, the intention of the book is not to pile up information on what there is and is not evidence for. It rather addresses how we gain evidence, what forms of evidence there are and how they may be used and be advanced for different purposes. Inevitably, the chapters touch on historical, philosophical, epistemological, psychological and sociological issues.

We have tried to include many different perspectives without being exhaustive. Since the randomised controlled trial (RCT) is a dominant method in current evidence-based mental health care, several chapters discuss RCTs in one way or another. Yet this book is not just about RCTs, the range of approaches that are outlined and discussed is much wider and more comprehensive than that.

The contributions in this book are stylistically diverse in various ways, including their length, tone, use of jargon, and assumptions about the reader's knowledge base. This presented some challenges to us as editors. Our initial inclination was to make the chapters more homogenous, but then we realised that this very diversity is part of the message we wish to communicate. In fact, the different emphases are products of, and reflect the nature of, the different perspectives and backgrounds of the authors. Therefore we have chosen to view this diversity as a positive aspect of the book, a view which we hope will be shared by the readership.

Stefan Priebe, Mike Slade
London, 2001

Section 1

Context

Chapter 1

Knowledge in the human sciences

Derek Bolton

The paradigm of scientific knowledge belongs to the natural sciences. Its defining features include

1. objectivity of observation and evidence: based in sense-experience, and available to all
2. experiment: knowledge is based not only in observation of reality as we find it, but in the process of *intervention* and observation; here we find the idea of experiment as a 'question that we put to nature'
3. causality: the aim is to determine causal process, to find causal explanations of events, and to make predictions
4. generality: the aim is to find general laws of nature
5. mathematics: the other main epistemological method, used in conjunction with experience.

These principles were worked out in relation to physics during the Renaissance and the Enlightenment. It took a great deal of time, because the intellectual work involved was massive, moving from the previous Aristotelian-Christian theological world-view to the modern, a process sometimes known as 'the mechanisation of the world-picture' (Dijksterhuis 1961; Koyré 1968). The notion of *experiment* for example was constructed during this period, by Bacon, among others, in his *Novum Organum* (1620), and it represented an enormous intellectual achievement.

The methodology as a whole belonged to wider cultural assumptions and values of the age. For example empiricism, which based cognition in experience common to all, belonged to that great movement of the Enlightenment, the democratisation of knowledge, as opposed to revelation by authority and other forms of esoteric, privileged knowledge. Locke worked out both the general epistemology (1690a), and the theory of government by consent (1690b).

Further, all the five principles hold together intimately, each serving to define the others and each supporting the others.

1. Causality is based in generality, the connection established by Hume (1777). 'A causes B' implies that events of type A are always followed by events of type B. Knowledge of causal principles thus enables prediction.

2. This analysis leads to the need for sophisticated experimental methodology. In practice what is observed on any one occasion is not simply an event of type A being followed by an event of type B, but this conjunction in a complex of circumstances, C_i. To establish a causal link between A and B the possible confounding effects of C_i have to be determined. This involves observing the effects of C_i without A, on the one hand, and A without C_i on the other. These principles, elucidated by Mill (1843) as the 'methods of agreement and difference', underlie our modern idea of controlled experimentation.

3. In practice, particularly in the life sciences, medicine, psychology and the social sciences we rarely find universal generalisations, but rather partial ones of the form: A is followed by B in a certain proportion of observed cases. One function of a universal generalisation is to license the simple inductive inference: the next observed A will be followed by B. In the absence of a universal generalisation, the problem is to determine the *probability* of the next A being followed by B, given the proportion in the sample so far observed. This is the problem for the theory of statistical inference. Its complexity compounds, in interaction with the problem cited above, that of controlling for potentially relevant variables.

4. The fundamental importance of mathematics in natural science made its appearance right at the start, with the 'mechanisation of the world picture'. This involved the hugely successful assumption that the fundamental, or 'primary', properties of nature were essentially mathematical: mass, space and time. In fact it is more accurate to say that this was a methodological principle: whatever could not be described mathematically had to be located somewhere other than nature. This in fact was crucial to the construction of the modern idea of 'mind', which was to contain whatever could not be fitted into this scientific view of mechanised nature (Burtt, 1932). In any case, the idea was hugely successful: mathematics was integral to the formulation of general laws of nature that captured causal processes, that enabled prediction, experimentation and other forms of intervention, as in mechanical engineering and later rocket science. Its obvious and fundamental application in the human sciences is the theory of statistical inference as referred to in point 3 above.

All or most of the above principles of natural science in fact work well in the human sciences also. They define the 'scientific paradigm' in those sciences, whether economics, sociology, psychology, medicine or psychiatry, which is a relatively hard-headed approach to science, striving for

- an objective evidence base, common to all (not subjective, esoteric, un-replicable, based in intuition or some other form of uncommunicable claim to knowledge)
- knowledge of causes (not, for example, understanding meaning or reasons, if that is different – more on this below), this requires control for possibly confounding variables
- generality, requiring group studies of sufficient size for statistical power (not preoccupation with particular cases).

In terms of evidence in health care, these methodological principles point towards the randomised control trial (RCT). Measures of pre- and post-intervention states must be measured objectively and in a replicable way. The trial seeks to determine as precisely as possible the 'active' causal component of the intervention and the condition that is affected. This means that other associated factors must be controlled for, both in terms of control groups and control interventions. The scientific paradigm can countenance study of individual cases, but the pressure is always to study groups and hence generality, and groups moreover of a size sufficient to detect interesting effects according to statistical calculations. Statistical methodology has had to be adapted in order to cope with the particular demands of evaluating treatments for human beings. Much of the methodology was originally worked out in relation to events that could be controlled, for example in agriculture. In clinical trials, however, we have to countenance potential participants deciding that they do not want one arm of the choice of conditions, or participants walking out half-way through the trial. Such eventualities demand further statistical sophistication, as discussed by Marshall in this volume.

It is obvious from the way I have set this up that I believe that RCTs are here to stay. They are based on deep philosophical and cultural assumptions about nature and knowledge, assumptions that are well proven in their effectiveness.

Why such a paradigm should only now be establishing itself in mental health care, although it was established in medicine several decades ago, is a matter of recent cultural history that I will not spend time with here, though it will be addressed in other chapters. I will mention here only three social processes, the first two of which are directly linked to the points made so far

1. continued increasing democratisation of knowledge, even into medicine and psychiatry; users and society want to know what we are doing
2. continued expansion of the scientific paradigm into social policy with demands for evidence
3. increasing need for health care, or expectations of health care, inevitably demands that limited financial resources are used effectively.

These social processes are powerful and are not going to let up. There is a well-known history of quackery, and more importantly of well-intended illusion, in health care, and society, including the government, is in the position now that it wants less of it.

These social processes lock together with the broad philosophical cultural assumptions about the methodology of scientific knowledge considered earlier. The combined effect I suggest is to establish as a priority the evaluation of treatment, and the RCT as the methodological gold standard for this.

Standard practice by trained clinicians will have to be enough if no evaluation has been done, and if they believe it sometimes works and is better than doing nothing, but it has no scientific credibility. Simple audit might establish a few basic facts, some of which might by all means seem crucial. Single case studies begin the process of scientific evaluation, then open uncontrolled group studies, but these leave open questions of specificity in cause and effect, that only the RCT can answer.

This completes my brief account of the philosophy of science (or epistemology) of treatment evaluation and the RCT in particular, and of its recommendations.

There is, however, something else in history and currently, which makes the picture more complicated, and the truth (if I may use that expression) more subtle.

The end of the nineteenth century saw the appearance of a new kind of science called, in German, the *Geisteswissenschaften*. These sciences included particularly history and social science, and had as their subject matter the expression of mind in society, and the *meaning* that permeates human activity. With the appearance of these sciences there arose a fundamentally new problem, which remains ours today, namely, that knowledge of mind and its expression in meaningful activity does not conform readily to the methodological assumptions and rules of the natural sciences, it requires instead a distinctive hermeneutic methodology. The tension found expression in the celebrated distinctions between *meaning* and *causality*, and between *understanding* and *explaining* (von Wright 1971, for an historical, critical review). Points of tension included the following

- first, natural science deals (mostly) with repeated and/or repeatable phenomena; however historical events such as the decline and fall of the Roman Empire, or a cultural practice such as a particular system of government, are singular, or even unique events
- second, natural science seeks and uses general causal laws in its explanations, however history and social science construct and use diverse ways of understanding a whole variety of events
- third, the contrast is more explicitly epistemological; understanding seems to be subjective, to draw on empathic abilities which vary from person to person, or from culture to culture, while the methods of observation

in the natural sciences are objective, and the results are meant to be the same for all.

The whole problematic hit psychiatry harder than most disciplines, mainly because it never had a choice but to embrace *both* hard, causal science, *and* the need to understand, so far as is possible, abnormal states of mind and the person who has them. Jaspers was the first to grasp the relevance of the new problematic to psychiatry, and perhaps the last to be able to hold on, even-handedly, to both methodologies. Jaspers (1923) emphasised the importance of both the science of psychopathology and the indispensable need to understand meaning by empathy. However, he had no coherent account of how these two methodologies could be coherent together and both valid (Bolton 1984).

Another pioneer in psychiatry, less of a phenomenologist and more of a scientist than Jaspers, came across the same problem in another way, and indeed pointed the way ahead to a solution. Freud saw that some apparently senseless mental states and behaviour could be understood as meaningful, and that intervention in the meaningful processes could effect change, i.e. would be causal (Breuer and Freud 1895). Freud, the neurologist, recognised that if this were so, then the mental, meaningful processes would somehow have to be mapped onto, and realised in, brain processes. However Freud recognised that the current state of cognitive neuroscience could not explain how this would be so, or what the architecture and functional characteristics of the brain would have to be like for it to be so, and he left his 'project' unfinished (Freud 1895; Spitzer 1998).

Integration was, in fact, half a century away, and the intervening decades were taken up with the more primitive way of dealing with conflict by splitting

- causality as opposed to meaning
- explanation as opposed to understanding
- behavioural science as opposed to hermeneutic non-science.

These splits reached their most violent in the 1960s, with vehement attacks on Freud for being unscientific, albeit preoccupied with meaning (Popper 1962), and equally ferocious attacks on mainstream psychiatry for systematically stripping madness of its meaning, for dehumanising madness, albeit scientifically (Foucault 1961; Laing 1960; Szasz 1961).

One major sign of the integration between scientific methodology and the phenomena of mind and meaning also began to appear in the 1960s, in the so-called cognitive revolution in psychology (Baars 1986). Since then cognitive states figure centre stage in the best behavioural science that we have. To what extent there really is an integration here remains by all means a matter of current controversy. Outstanding issues include whether the 'information processing' studied in cognitive psychology really is the same kind of thing as *meaning*, and whether *meaning* can really be encoded in the brain, and hence causal (Bolton and Hill 1996; Thornton 1997; Widdershoven 1999).

In practice, on the other hand, the contemporary science of psychopathology relatively rarely has any problem with principles, for example that meaning (or information) is encoded in the brain, that behaviour is multi-determined, including by the meaning of events, as well as by disturbance of neural structures – and if necessary putting all such various factors in the same statistical regression model. There is nothing here about meaning being immeasurable, unscientific and non-causal, or about individual differences being so great that generalisation, or study of groups, is misconceived. Examples of the current methodologies used to measure meaning are the Life Event and Difficulty Schedule (Brown and Harris 1978), and the Adult Attachment Interview Schedule (Main and Hesse 1990), both of which are explicitly used to identify causal processes (Brown and Harris, 1986; Main and Hesse 1990).

On the other hand, there is undoubted pressure to keep alive something like the old science/hermeneutics distinction, basically involving repetitions of what is familiar in the old paradigms. These include statements to the effect that the most important (basic, fundamental) science consists of studying the brain and brain–behaviour relationships *as opposed to* mind and meaning. This attitude has no problem with RCTs, though it may indeed have a problem with psychological therapies, suspecting that they deal in epiphenomena only. The problem with this old way of looking at things, however, is that it cannot account for the fact that meaning (causally) regulates behaviour, and that any causal model of the behaviour that omits this fact will be drastically inadequate. On the other side of the same coin, there are the claims that personal, family and social meanings are a matter for hermeneutics *as opposed to* causal science, are out of reach of scientific theory and investigation, are fundamentally a matter of relating, and so on. One sign of the problem in this kind of account of knowledge in the human sciences is that the study of meanings, or the individual's interpretation of events, is left stranded apart from causal science. In particular, there can be no coherent account of why therapy should make any difference, in so far as it is not involved with causal processes. Then the appropriateness and need for evaluation at all – let alone randomised controlled trials – will also be rejected on principle.

These extreme positions are, however, in my view, on the way out. There was indeed a genuine tension within the human sciences, and in psychiatry in particular, between the hermeneutic study of meaning and scientific method. However, during the closing decades of the last century, and continuing still, the tension is being creatively resolved. As was remarked at the beginning of this paper, the methodology of the natural sciences had to be constructed over a long period. So far as our time is concerned, it was only a few decades ago that meaning was seen as nothing to do with causation of behaviour, and it was only a few decades before that that mental states were considered irrelevant to science. The present task is to accommodate mind and meaning within a transformed scientific paradigm. Scientific enquiry has to adapt to increase its sensitivity to mental states and meanings, and hermeneutics (or semiotics) will have to get used to be becoming more scientific, to thinking how it might answer questions about measurement and causality, concerning for example risk factors, and to the evaluation of treatment interventions.

This is not to say that scientific methodology can answer all questions that arise in the provision of health care.[1] In particular, science is neutral to morality. It cannot say, for example, whether it is better to devote limited financial or staffing resources to the relief of current extreme suffering of the few, or to a public health preventative programme for the many. Science can contribute to an estimation of the outcome of each policy, but is neutral to the further question as to which is morally right. Scientific methodology is also limited by internal considerations, by its own nature. As outlined above, the methodology depends essentially on the occurrence of repeated, and preferably repeatable, events in order to determine which among the various factors involved are causal, and to what extent; and in order to make predictions. Scientific methodology is therefore not a good fit with relatively rare events involving many potentially causal factors. One kind of case familiar in health-care provision that is jeopardised in this way is the question of relative effectiveness of different models of health-care delivery. In mental health care, for example, questions arise as to the relative effectiveness of in-patient and community care, or of two kinds of community care, as discussed by James and Burns in Chapter 4 of this volume. In this kind of case, the phenomena being compared are so complex, involving many potentially causal factors, while at the same time, and connected, the capacity to observe repeated phenomena is so limited, that scientific evaluation, and RCTs in particular, are likely to be problematic. This is not to say that science has no role in comparisons of this kind, but it depends on breaking up very large questions into smaller, more manageable ones, where the requirements of repeatability and control over the number of potentially relevant variables can more easily be met. In evaluating a whole system of community care, for example, it might be possible to conduct trials evaluating particular components, such as team care as opposed to care provided continuously by a particular member of staff.

The point that traditional scientific methodology is not a good fit with relatively rare events involving many potentially causal factors was of course

1 I am grateful to Dr Mike Slade for discussions that led to the inclusion of this paragraph.

precisely the insight of early theorists in the *Geisteswissenschaften*. Social systems and revolutions do not readily lend themselves to repeated observations, and they certainly involve many factors. The question of the scientific study of human beings has always been ambiguous in this respect. It is possible to argue on the one hand that each human being is unique, and complex, and on the other that we have much in common, and there are many of us, so that repeated observation is quite possible. One side of this argument points to hermeneutics as the appropriate methodology for understanding human beings, the other leads to the psychological and behavioural sciences.

Chapter 2

Evidence in mental health: a historical analysis

Heinz-Peter Schmiedebach

In the 1980s the notion of 'evidence' came to occupy a dominant position in medicine and mental health care (Geddes *et al.* 1997). Terms such as 'evidence-based medicine' have been used to underline and to legitimise new types of therapy in a rapidly changing field of medicine (Sackett *et al.* 1997). But 'evidence' was always an integral part of human reasoning and even of religious faith. Nevertheless, the answer to the question 'what is evidence?' has changed over the course of time. The nature of 'evidence' is not only historically shaped. It also depends on cultural circumstances, on philosophical and epistemological reflections (Feldman 1993), and on disciplinary boundaries. In law, 'evidence' includes physical objects and events, such as weapons or footprints; for a deeply devout Christian a miracle can be 'evidence' for the existence of God.

I will confine my further exposition to the question 'what was evidence in mental health?' In Europe, the rise of systematically pursued mental health care under the supervision of physicians began in the second half of the eighteenth century. At the beginning of the nineteenth century the notion 'psychiatry' emerged, and at the same time a scientifically based medicine took shape and influenced the comprehension of 'evidence'. Thus, the development of modern research skills and scientific methods (Coleman 1987) in medicine and psychiatry must be considered in the context of the historically different forms of 'evidence' in mental health.

The changing nature of 'evidence' depends on additional different historical issues. I would like to emphasise only the following

1. the cultural and social function of emerging psychiatry
2. the professional side of the field.

The physicians in mental health care attempted to enhance their own reputation by developing a strategy to become accepted as truly scientifically based physicians. I would also like to underline that the changing nature of 'evidence' is linked to the changing concepts of madness. Over the course of time we can discern different concepts, sometimes following one another, but sometimes also coexisting with one concept in a dominant position to another. It is therefore necessary to refer to all of these concepts.

My thesis on the changing nature of evidence runs as follows. Around the middle of the nineteenth century when the scientifically based concepts of mental illness emerged, physicians' research activities aimed to understand madness fully. The doctors expected that finding somatic causes of madness would lead to successful treatment. Yet the main purpose of their endeavour was the understanding rather than the healing of madness. Evidence at this time, including evidence with regard to therapy, was primarily derived from the scientifically based understanding of madness.

Over the course of time it became obvious that there was no sole obligatory concept of madness (Porter 1993), and in the 1930s and 1940s in particular, new types of treatment were implemented. Clinical treatment evidence became more and more linked to clinical trials, avoiding reflections on the nature of mental illness. This led to a narrow type of evidence strongly connected to the therapeutic side of mental health care.

Evidence and social, political and cultural beliefs

From the seventeenth century onwards in Europe enormous houses of confinement became numerous. The great majority of mad individuals were found among the populations of workhouses, prisons and other institutions. Because of the Enlightenment's esteem of reason, education and work, lunatics and socially abnormal people were confined in order to punish and correct them, and to force them to work. This confinement (Foucault 1967) was the first example of mad and mentally ill people being segregated from society, though certainly not as a group of ill persons and not within a hospital-like institution.

However the reasoning about the nature of unreason initiated a widespread discussion which challenged the physicians (Dörner 1993). If people are tormented by delusions, might it be possible to correct and to educate them by awakening reason and the power of volition? For physicians this seemed to be a situation in which they could extend their social and administrative power. There was a chance to demonstrate their competence in an improvement of the mad people and to turn them into useful members of society. In order to conduct this great social experiment with insane people for the first time in history it was necessary to segregate this group from all other imprisoned people. It was necessary to declare insane people to be ill persons belonging under the care of physicians. Insanity was transformed from a vague, culturally defined phenomenon into a condition which could only be diagnosed, certified and dealt with by a group of legally recognised experts, as the English medical historian Andrew Scull described the situation (Scull 1979).

A particular presupposition for this transformation had to be accomplished. If the insane were to be accepted as ill persons, then they could no longer be dealt with in the same way as murderers and other criminals. If the insane were to be seen as ill then there must have been a means of curing them – or at least a certain number of them. The best way to have demonstrated this newly recognised view on the insane would have been the liberation of mad people from their chains. At the end of the eighteenth century we find these gestures in Italy as well as in France: Chiarugi (1759–1820) in Florence (Guarnieri 1994) and Pinel's assistant, Jean Baptiste Pussin (1745–1811), who on his own initiative first freed the insane men at Bicêtre in Paris from their fetters (Weiner 1994). This liberation was the first act in recognising that madness is a mental illness that belongs to the field of medicine.

Of course, at the end of the eighteenth century physicians could only refer to a small number of experiences regarding successful cure of the insane. These few records did not provide sufficiently accepted empirical 'evidence' for any curability of madness. The more relevant motives for this reform came from the widespread argument about human rights, the equality of men and religious faith. Also the model of the 'Retreat', first created by Samuel Tuke (1784–1857) in York, was rooted in religious motivation. 'Evidence' that initiated the emergence and establishment of modern psychiatry came from social, political and religious beliefs, and personal convictions.

Looking for a suitable means of handling the problem of insanity in a medical manner, the physicians referred to methods used in other scientific disciplines. The scientific origins of psychiatry can be studied in the case of Pinel (1801). The first step consisted of differentiating insane people within the increasing number of specialised institutions for the insane (Castel 1976). Pinel intended to offer society assurance that mental illness is treatable and sometimes curable. When he was appointed as physician to the infirmaries at Bicêtre in 1793, the ward for madmen attracted his special attention. He looked upon this establishment as a source of new enlightenment and instruction, and a most welcome opportunity to contribute to public usefulness.

As Dora B. Weiner (1994) summarised, the important new ingredient was the empirical approach, meaning the systematic observation of human behaviour. With his method of observation, description, comparison and classification Pinel approached each inmate's illness from different points of view

1. the precipating event
2. the specific types of madness
3. the general varieties in the behavioural characteristics of madness.

He gathered his information by talking and listening to deranged patients at length.

The focus on the specific types of madness yielded a crucial criterion: that of regularity, recurrence and hence periodicity of violent bouts. Pinel recognised the new concept of periodic madness. All his life Pinel rejected the theory that the size and shape of the skull or the anatomy of the brain yielded firm evidence of normality or pathology in a person. Pinel explained madness as a disturbance of mental faculties, as a disorder of psychological processes. He adhered to the central importance of observation of living patients as the key to an understanding of mental alienation (Weiner 1993).

Regarding the therapeutic practice of Pinel and his successors it becomes obvious that there was no conclusive therapy that resulted from his approach. Pinel was shaped by his early studies in theology and his Catholic faith, and he brought the humane aspect of Catholic charity to clinical medicine. He developed a special type of psychological treatment, consisting of repeated, probing, personal conversations with his mental patients. His rejection of physical violence against patients, the attention he paid to the complaints of the poor as well as the rich, and his prohibition of drastic treatment measures were motivated by his religious and humane attitude. But the reform which had been initiated by him provided the requirements for a long-term observation of the patients and for a perception of the different forms of insanity.

A similar situation existed at the York Retreat. The 'moral treatment', established by Samuel Tuke, began by rejecting existing responses as worse than useless, and not legitimised by a systematically performed evaluation of different therapeutic measures. According to Andrew Scull, the new approach of 'moral treatment' was little more than an application of common sense and humanity (Scull 1979). But the employment of terms borrowed from medicine, such as 'patient', 'mental illness' and 'treatment', implied a medical problem. A new atmosphere of systematic observation, division and classification of mental illness easily occupied the field of mental health care. The main assignment of the newly emerging psychiatry was to create an order that structured the chaotic and manifold shapes of insanity. Treatment played a minor role. The moral or psychological treatment as discussed above was not accepted in general. The gap between research and practice in mental health care, which still exists today, became a characteristic label for psychiatry.

Evidence and madness as a disease of the brain

In 1822 A.J. Bayle (1799–1858) described a chronic arachnitis in six patients, and claimed that the alteration was the cause of a symptomatic mental alienation. He provided the first widely accepted evidence for mental alienation caused by detectable pathological modification of the brain. The hypothesis that the brain is the seat of mental illness created a new concept which made a strong impact on further discussion about the nature of madness. The new approach was conducive to creating a new type of evidence: a perceptible somatic alteration as a cause for a mental illness.

The hypothesis that the brain is the seat of mental illness was strongly supported in the following years by increasing research activities in the field of pathological brain anatomy and histology. The technical improvement of the microscope, and the development of special extirpation methods of brain tissue, rendered a large body of new facts that have been seen as evidence for the above-mentioned hypothesis. Single functions of brain physiology as well as particular anatomical alterations of tissue could now be deciphered.

The emancipation of the insane from any kind of bodily restraint was another inevitable consequence derived from this new approach. Of course, there was the fear of madness that hampered a vast and widespread consent to these demands. Despite these reservations, the concept of madness as a brain disease fostered the definite integration of mental health care into the sphere of medicine. Moreover, the concept also supported equality between mentally ill patients and those who were physically ill.

The sole somatic brain alteration did not provide sufficient evidence for the thesis that madness was a brain disease. The new concept required the link between the pathologically altered substance and the symptoms produced by the living patient. The painstaking observation of patients and their shapes of insanity, introduced by Pinel, remained now, as before, a crucial method of research. Only the combination of observation of the living patient and post-mortem analysis of brain alteration provided evidence for the new concept of madness. Based on this concept, psychiatry set itself the task of explaining the causes of mental illness and of contributing to the demystification of madness.

Despite the expansion of anatomically oriented research in the field of mental illness, even self-observation was still used in order to find ways of explaining several psychological phenomena, such as hallucination, illusion and obsessional neurosis. In 1867 Wilhelm Griesinger (1817–1868) read a paper on 'Physical-psychological self-observations'. He described the phenomenon of 'rapid eye movement', shortly before one falls asleep. In a speculative manner he linked his observation with reasoning about the connection of eye movement with the emergence of ideas within the brain (Griesinger 1868–69). Until the middle of the 1870s such articles based on a careful self-observation did not cause objections by the fellow psychiatrists. Yet descriptive self-referential evidence lost credit during the following decades when the experimental method occupied research on mental disorders (Schmiedebach 1986).

In the beginning of the 1920s a similar self-referential approach to research played a role for about 10 years. After the discovery of the hallucinogenic drug mescaline, several doctors undertook experiments on themselves using the drug (Forster 1930). Mescaline was regarded as a hallucinogenic drug that did not dim consciousness (Zucker and Zador 1930). Thus the doctors thought they had found an ideal drug that produced hallucinations but the individual maintained the ability to perceive and to describe their personal experience. Through that method they expected to understand their patient's sensation (Zucker 1928). But this type of construction of self-referential evidence did not play a major role in mental health care.

The therapeutic practice during the second half of the nineteenth century was characterised by the abolition of bodily restraints. In 1869 chloralhydrate was developed by Oscar Liebreich (1839–1908) and introduced into mental health care. Chloralhydrate sedated patients and calmed their furious shouting, making the use of strait-jackets unnecessary. The indication for the application of other remedies was derived from pathological brain findings. If at post-mortem there was inflammation of the brain that was seen to have produced certain symptoms, a patient with similar symptoms was thought to suffer from brain inflammation and was prescribed antipyretic remedies. However, the main purpose of psychiatric research at that time was to find explanations for mental disturbances based on detectable alterations in brain tissue. The research activities of psychiatrists were aimed primarily at a full understanding of madness. Evidence with regard to treatment was derived from that understanding.

At the end of the nineteenth century this undertaking had reached an impasse. Despite the fact that numerous functions of the brain had been deciphered, it remained impossible to construct evidential support for most phenomena of mental disturbances by referring to pathologic alterations of circumscribed regions of the brain. To overcome the stagnation psychiatrists and neurologists followed different courses.

Freud (1856–1939) started the great enterprise of deciphering the subconscious and invented the psychoanalytic method. Emil Kraepelin (1856–1920) constructed a new classification system of mental illness which soon became a widely accepted guideline (Engstrom 1997; Roelcke 1999). Others emphasised new approaches, now looking for hereditary or endocrinological correlations beyond the anatomical and physiological context. At the beginning of the twentieth century hereditary explanations reached a peak although convincing evidence was not present. However, numerous doctors were so occupied with that topic that sterilisation was widely seen as a suitable approach to prevent mental illness. The call for corresponding laws in several countries was not ignored.

In Nazi Germany the most far reaching law was enacted in July 1933. According to that law, patients with schizophrenia, hereditary epilepsy, manic-depressive cyclothyme or severe alcoholism, could be forced into compulsory sterilisation. Some German psychiatrists, such as Bonhoeffer (1868–1948), complained about missing evidence for hereditary genesis of these diseases, but nevertheless, the hereditary concept reached a wide level of acceptance. Psychiatry was looked upon as a discipline that could provide the medical measures to solve a large number of problems which emerged from these 'inconvenient' people. And the psychiatrists used any chance to present themselves as the competent experts in order to solve these social problems.

Evidence and newly developed methods of treatment

Towards the end of the nineteenth century – according to contemporary psychiatrists – almost all European countries experienced a rise in the incidence of insanity. The allegedly growing number of insane people is not easy to explain. At the same time, the number of large asylums mounted as well. Probably the increase in the rate of insanity was due to a more exact identification of mentally ill patients as a result of newly developed diagnostic methods, or it was the accumulation of chronic long-term cases, sent to the newly erected asylums. Andrew Scull (1979) offered an explanation which seems more plausible. He emphasised the fact that beyond the initial hard core of easily recognisable mental disturbance, the boundary between the normal and the pathological was left extraordinarily vague and undetermined.

Moreover, the existence of the asylum made available a culturally legitimate alternative, for both the community as a whole and the separate family, which delivered the intolerable individual to the asylums. The existence of that institution not only provided a place for all sorts of 'inconvenient' people, it also affected the degree to which people were prepared to put up with inconvenience. Thus the increasing number of asylums all over Europe inevitably reduced family and community tolerance, and in so doing, induced a wider concept of the nature of insanity (Scull 1979).

Those mounting numbers of mad and 'inconvenient' people expanded the realm of psychiatric competence; it also put considerable pressure on psychiatrists, who were forced to legitimise their competence by providing various types of cures. These were the conditions around the turn of the century that made the therapeutic side of mental illness more relevant. As early as the nineteenth century, treatment methods which referred to an artificially initiated febrility had been performed, particularly in cases of progressive paralysis. Evidence was derived from literary sources, some of which dated back to antiquity. With the help of ointments, the physicians maintained a suppurating inflammation which sometimes led to a necrotic destruction of the skull. During the last two decades of the nineteenth century such drastic cures became obsolete despite the fact that an improvement concerning the mental state had been reported in some cases. Looking for the reason for such successful treatments, psychiatrists declared the febrile disease to be the effective cause.

In 1887 Julius Wagner-Jauregg (1857–1940) published a basic article on that problem and dedicated part of his research activities to the investigation of the relationship between febrile infection and psychosis. Influenced by the impressive results of modern bacteriology, he also used germ matter to provoke fever in order to cure chronic mentally ill people.

In the summer of 1917, based on this experience, Wagner-Jauregg infected nine patients suffering from progressive paralysis, with blood that had been taken from a patient with malaria tertiana (Wagner-Jauregg 1918/19).

Three of the nine patients showed good results: even 10 years later they remained totally recovered with an enduring ability to work (Gerstmann 1928). The method rapidly spread all over the world and investigations on that topic were undertaken in several countries. Most of these studies examined groups of 10 to 300 patients and developed a study design embracing three to five categories of improvement reaching to full recovery. Systematically performed randomised controlled trials did not take place.

In October 1926 the *British Medical Journal* published a statistical account of patients from six asylums located in the London area (Alexander *et al.* 1926). The authors compared two different groups of patients: 227 paralytic patients who had been admitted to the asylums during the period from August 1920 to July 1923 and who did not receive treatment, and 191 non-selected patients suffering from the same disease who were treated with malaria between February 1923 and August 1925. The two groups revealed a quite distinct course of the disease. By August 1925 33.5 per cent of the malaria-treated group were ready for discharge compared with only 2.6 per cent of the untreated group. The authors reported a similar difference in the mortality rates of the two groups: 62.1 per cent of the non-treated patients died, compared with only 20.9 per cent of the treated patients. Even those patients who could not be discharged despite receiving treatment showed a considerable improvement in their general condition. Wagner-Jauregg was awarded the Nobel prize in 1927 for the development of the malaria therapy.

A number of other somatic treatments, generally based upon a very different logic, came into the foreground in the 1930s and early 1940s. At that time such innovations as insulin coma therapy, cardiazol, and electrically induced convulsions, together with various forms of lobotomy (Crossley 1993), were widely hailed. The term 'convulsive therapies' refers to a group of medical cures that treat certain mental disorders by means of a provoked fit. These convulsive therapies were based on the hypothesis that there was a negative correlation between schizophrenia and epilepsy. That view was derived from both epidemiological and neuropathological work. Berrios has noted that by the early twentieth century the relationship between epilepsy and schizophrenia had been discussed in some detail, and psychiatrists believed in either a positive or a negative correlation, or no association at all. The dominating view was determined by research, fashion and changes in the definitions of illness (Berrios 1996). Despite the lack of evidence a rapid advance in electroconvulsive therapy occurred, particularly during the early 1940s, when it was shown that it worked sufficiently well in the treatment of depression.

In contrast to the nineteenth century approach, psychiatrists did not legitimise their treatment methods with regard to their understanding of madness. The concept of madness did not play any role with respect to the evidential legitimisation of the treatment. The empirically experienced treatment method stood for itself and had to provide its own evidence. To meet that challenge, psychiatrists had to look for new statistically based methods of evidential support.

The modern, somewhat narrow notion of evidence, nearly always linked to the therapeutic efficacy of remedies, took shape simultaneously with the improvement of statistical methods during the second half of the twentieth century. Around 1950 the statistical techniques of analysis of variance became implemented into clinical research (Danziger 1987). In 1952 chlorpromazine was used in a French hospital for treating psychiatric disorders, and with the development of chlorpromazine and other neuroleptic medications a new era of treatment came into being. Three years later the first congress in Paris to discuss the neuroleptic remedies took place. At that meeting Linford Rees presented three papers in which strict double-blind control methods had been used (Rees 1997). Within the next years the methodological discussion of all the different methods used in controlled trials expanded enormously.

In the context of an increasing number of remedies, it became more and more necessary to discern *real* clinical success from *apparent* clinical success. The medical profession that monitors therapies for efficacy defined what was to be counted as adequate proof of efficacy. Therefore therapies were tested rigorously by randomised controlled trials. But Mark D. Sullivan emphasised that much is generally left unsaid about the context within which that occurs. 'What is being treated, what is the treatment, and what is the criterion of successful treatment are all specified prior to the randomised controlled trial and not tested by it' (Sullivan 1993).

The goals of medical intervention are more variable than the model of a straightforward cure of an infection would lead us to believe. This is particularly relevant for mental health care. With regard to the opening of doors in British mental hospitals in the 1950s it is obvious that some medical superintendents followed a broader approach of mental health care. According to Liam Clarke, the open door pioneers 'were infused with a kind of evangelical conviction in their desire to treat their fellow man as equal' (Clarke 1993). This improvement was motivated by a rediscovery of the humanitarianism of the past, and evidence was derived from personal conviction linked to several examples of successful historical practice in different times.

Conclusion

This historical account has revealed the rich variety and the different nature of evidence. I have tried to describe this change in the context of mental health care over the course of time. At first glance it looks like a step-by-step process mounting from low, impressionistic and empirical levels to the higher methodologically legitimised evidence of the present day. But this impression is very deceptive. The historical perspective shows that

1. there was a change in what has been accepted as evidence at different times, according to the scientific state of medicine, and the concept of madness
2. that different notions of evidence have always coexisted within the same academic community.

We can discern at least three different types of evidence. First, a type which is rooted in social, religious, philosophical, cultural, or political contents and attitudes, or convictions in society at a certain time. Second, a type derived from the scientifically oriented research methods, which was concerned with understanding mental illness. This type embraced evidence of treatment, hoping that treatment would become obvious once the illness has been fully understood. Finally, a modern type which focuses on treatment only, leaving aside all reflections on the nature of mental illness and eliminating all social, and cultural aspects of mental health care.

It is not easy to make a substantial statement, or to formulate something like a historical law on the relationship of these different types of evidence in mental health care. In a simplified manner it looks as if the more society discussed the role of insanity, unreason and mental health care, the more the non-medical evidence occupied a more dominant position. Then the public demanded answers from the experts and forced them to include the cultural and social aspects into their considerations. The modern notion of evidence came to play a major role when new treatment methods emerged and psychiatrists became optimistic about abolishing insanity, without necessarily having understood madness. Then evidence focused on treatment only and created the modern narrow term.

Chapter 3

Influence of evidence on mental health care over the last 200 years

Asmus Finzen

The title of this chapter implies that there has been an influence of evidence on mental health care during the past 200 years. It is a statement. Shouldn't it rather be a question? Has there been any influence of evidence on mental health care in past and recent history? And if there has been, what kind was it? When did it begin?

If I were a professional historian, I believe I would not dare attempt to answer this question. Being a psychiatrist with modest historical interests, I am less scrupulous. I will try to look back on the works of our forefathers, on the development of psychiatric care and mental health institutions. I will also try to have a critical look at the professional basis of these developments, as well as at their ideological, philosophical and, in the early times, in part religious foundations, and last but not least, the political and philanthropic motivations they were driven by. In doing so I am deeply indebted to the works of Ackerknecht (1957) and Porter and Micale (1994).

There is a certain consensus that 'modern' psychiatry and mental health care are a result of enlightenment, that they started with Philippe Pinel's legendary act of liberating the insane from their chains at Bicêtre Hospice in Paris in 1793 at the time of French Revolution. This *geste de Pinel* seems to be a psychiatric myth; historical facts do not support it (Müller 1998). Nevertheless, it's a good date and a good event to remember on one end of the rainbow of psychiatric care:

> The story in its broad outlines is familiar and dramatic. . . . After the tortures and the judical murders of the middle ages . . . there were the cruelties and degradation of the madhouses of the seventeenth and eighteenth centuries, in which authority used chains and whips as its instruments. Humanitarian effort put an end to these abuses. Pinel in France, Charughi in Italy, Tuke in England inaugurated an era of kindness and medical care which prepared the way for a rational humane approach to the mastery of mental illness.
>
> (Lewis 1967, p. 3)

The founding fathers inaugurated the era of moral treatment, which is considered to be the first rationally founded way of treating and caring for the mentally ill. Whether or not moral treatment was evidence based is a totally different question. And I am afraid it was not. There are strong arguments that Pinel's act, or rather the myth of it, is to be seen in the context of the French Revolution as a matter of *Liberté, Egalité et Fraternité*, and not as the beginning of evidence-based psychiatry. Yet, I believe that evidence from different contexts and with different meanings is of importance for its development. In German philosophy there is the term of *Evidenz*, which incidentally causes some confusion when we discuss evidence based medicine in our language. This is especially true because *Evidenz* is also used in certain branches of alternative medicine. *Evidenz* means no more and no less than that you do not need 'evidence' to prove your point because a fact is self-evident.

You may remember the beginning of the American Declaration of Independence 'We hold these truths to be self-evident: That all men are created equal, that their creator has endowed them with certain unalienable rights, that among these are life, liberty and the pursuit of happiness.' On this background a development of moral treatment was not evidence based but self-evident, because these rights were claimed for the insane as well.

I shall not deal with the religious aspects of moral treatment in England, nor with aspects of idealistic philosophy in German psychiatry at the beginning of the nineteenth century. But I cannot refrain from mentioning and quoting Goethe's novel *Wilhelm Meister* which appeared between 1792 and 1796. In this novel Goethe develops some basic principles of moral treatment, which Henry Maudsley in his book *Physiology and Psychology of the Soul* describes as remarkable and enlightening.

> The means to prevent and to heal madness are the same as to prevent healthy humans getting mad. The ill persons have to be activated. They have to become used to a certain order. They have to be convinced that they are equal to other people. They have to be shown that extraordinary talents, fullfilling happiness and fortune and extreme misery are just small deviations from the common. When these principles are observed, madness won't get rooted in the soul, and even if it does it will eventually vanish.
>
> (Maudsley 1868, p. 468)

It is not by chance that it is a clergyman to whom Goethe assigns the role of the successful moral psychotherapist – or is it rather sociotherapist? Psychiatry – the term was coined in 1808 by Johann Christian Reil – at this time oscillates between philosophy, theology and practical medicine. It is definitely not a branch of scientific medicine. I have some doubts, though, that any medicine might rightly be called scientific at that time.

In central Europe the first half of the nineteenth century was the age of romantic medicine and romantic psychiatry. The protagonists of these disciplines, such as Heinroth, believed that all diseases were a consequence of sin. To Heinroth and his followers, madness was definitely an illness of the soul, a punishment from god. Their secular colleagues, such as Ideler, considered mental illness as an extreme form of individualism – pathological individualism (Ackerknecht 1957).

Treatment and care of the mentally ill, in consequence, took place in moral or religious institutions. In this period more than thirty asylums for the mentally ill were founded in Germany, eighteen in France, and thirty-eight in Britain. Between 1830 and 1860 German psychiatry was dominated by the medical chiefs of the asylums – in practice as well as in theory. Ideologically their orientation was that of a philosophical anthropology (Ackerknecht 1957).

Psychiatry took a more medical approach when Wilhelm Griesinger entered the scene in the middle of the century. For him mental illnesses were diseases of the brain and as a consequence psychiatry became brain psychiatry, which, incidentally, was linked to the developing university departments of psychiatry. It is more than remarkable that this first era of brain psychiatry had no consequences on either mental health care or on therapy (Finzen 1998).

Caring for the mentally ill continues to be the monopoly of public and private asylums. A second wave of construction of large mental hospitals, most of them in the countryside of European countries and the USA, lasted from 1880 to 1910.

Let us have a look at the nineteenth century treatment methods. Throughout the century these were hot and cold water, revolving chairs, 'aversion' and 'pain' therapies, and many other treatments that we can rightly consider as torture. We find eras of restraint and non-restraint, of work for all residents in the asylums and of putting all residents to bed. Henry Maudsley (1868) lists a large number of drugs, or rather poisons, that were employed, opium and later morphine being the most harmless and the most efficient of them.

Therefore, if we look at the first century of psychiatry and specific mental health care, we have to conclude, sadly, that there is no trace of evidence-based medicine. There is no evidence at all that any of the chemical treatments did anything good for the mentally ill. There is hardly any evidence that the manifold physical treatments were of some use. Most of them were based on speculation, the more rational ones on observation.

Looking back on mental health care and psychiatric therapy, the nineteenth century turns out to have been the age of sociotherapy. The normalising principals of moral treatment, the non-restraint policy of John Conolly and his followers in many countries, the therapeutic use of work in moral treatment, and the rediscovery of work as therapeutic in the last decades of the twentieth century. But overall practical psychiatry in the nineteenth century was a matter of belief, of ideology, of philosophy, of policies and politics, at times a matter of humanism and, at its best, a matter of common sense. But it was not scientifically based medicine.

Looking back on nineteenth-century psychiatry Daniel Hack Tuke in his *Chapters on the History of the Insane in the British Isles* concludes

> If the success of the treatment of insanity bore any considerable proportion to the number of the remedies which have been brought forward, it would be my easy and agreeable duty to record the triumphs of medicine in the distressing malady which they are employed to combat. But this, unhappily, is not the case.
>
> (Tuke 1882, pp. 484–5)

Now did we do any better in the twentieth century? Yes we did. Did we really? Let me skip the first half of the century by quoting Richard Hunter and Ida Macalpine (1963). They are considered to be the two leading British historians of psychiatry at the time by Roy Porter and Mark Micale (1994). I quote from 'Reflections on Psychiatry and its Histories'

> [In psychiatry] there is not even an objective method of describing or communicating clinical findings without subjective interpretation and no exact and uniform terminology which conveys precisely the same to all. In consequence there is wide divergence of diagnosis, even of diagnoses, a steady flow of new terms and an everchanging nomenclature, as well as a surfeit of hypotheses which tend to be presented as fact. Furthermore, etiology remains speculative, pathogenesis largely obscure, classifications predominantly symptomatic and hence arbitrary and possibly ephemeral: physical treatments are empirical and subject to fashion, and psychotherapies still only in their infancy and doctrinaire.
>
> (Porter and Micale 1994, pp. 6–7)

Of course there is no consensus on Hunter and Macalpine's conclusions. There never is in psychiatry. So let me quote Sir Aubrey Lewis again

> In the twentieth century psychopathology has been elucidated and psychological treatment given ever widening scope and sanction. Revolutionary changes have occured in physical methods of treatment, the regime in mental hospitals has been further liberalized, and the varieties of care articulated into one another, individualized, and made elements in a continuous therapeutic process that extends well into the general community, beginning with the phase of onset, Stadium incrementi, and proceeding to the ultimate phase of rehabilitation and social settlement

... This is the conventional picture, one of progress and enlightenment
... [and] it is not far out.

(Lewis 1967, p. 3)

Porter and Micale (1994) offer an explanation for such completely different views of the achievements of psychiatry in the past

Psychiatry boasts no stable and consensual theoretical vantage point from
which to construct itself historically. From its earliest days, psychiatric
medicine has been marked by the persistence of competing, if not bit-
terly opposing schools. Most noticeably, the field since the eighteenth
century has been convulsed by a deep, dichotomous debate between the
somatic and mentalist philosophies of mind. The historiographical
effects of this division have been great. From generation to generation,
as the perceived cognitive content of the discipline has changed, the
projected disciplinary past of psychiatry has changed with it. Moreover,
for professional purposes, each generation of practitioners has written a
history that highlights those past ideas and practices that anticipate its
own formation and consigns to marginal status competing ideas and
their heritages. In this process, individual figures and texts – indeed,
entire historical periods and bodies of knowledge – have at times been
omitted from the historical record. With an intensely subjective matter,
complex multidisciplinary origins, and insecure and shifting epistemological base, porous disciplinary boundaries, and a sectarian and dialectical dynamic of development, it has thus far proved impossible to
produce anything like an enduring, comprehensive, authoritative history of psychiatry.

(Porter and Micale 1994, pp. 5–6)

So who am I to produce one? I shall confine myself to a few remarks on
the developments in the past century. We have watched – and some of us
lived with or suffered from – the rise and fall of psychoanalysis. We have
witnessed the doubtful consequences of degeneration theory, eugenics,
and the early age of genetics ending in the Nazi mass murders and mass
sterilisations of mentally ill and mentally handicapped fellow human beings.
We have witnessed the era of insulin treatment and electroconvulsive treatment, of the heroic (heroic for the patients) malaria treatment of third-stage
syphilis by Wagner-Jauregg (rewarded with the Nobel Prize) and the muti-
lations of the brains of hundreds of thousands of human beings introduced
by E. Moniz (also rewarded with the Nobel Prize). And all of us wish
something like an evidence-based medicine had existed in the first half of the
twentieth century.

And then the 'golden age' of psychiatry arose. The change from custodial
care to therapeutic and rehabilitational care (beginning in Britain in the

1940s) the development of group therapy, milieu therapy and therapeutic community, the age of deinstitutionalisation, the discovery of the first psychotropic drug and later the development of dozens of psychotropic drugs, mostly in the 1950s, the introduction of controlled clinical trials (not much later than in internal medicine and other medical disciplines), the reconstruction of psychiatric diagnostics by inventing the DSM-II,-III and -IV (American Psychiatric Association 1994) and the ICD-8,-9 and-10 (World Health Organisation 1992), the splendid renaissance of brain psychiatry, including the suggestion that we should drop the term psychiatry altogether in favour of 'clinical neurosciences' (Detre 1997), the age of Prozac (Shorter 1997) and the promotion of the new atypical neuroleptics.

From the way I phrase my words you can easily conclude that I am not a hundred per cent convinced. Let me put it like this: Was mental health care in the 1960s, 1970s, 1980s and 1990s evidence based? Is it acceptable to conduct controlled clinical trials that are financed mostly by industry? Is it acceptable to use clinical studies lasting only 6 weeks to gather evidence for the treatment of an illness that lasts a lifetime (e.g. schizophrenia that may last 60 years)?

Couldn't it be that controlled clinical trials in psychiatry and mental health care only secure evidence when they are complemented by biographical lifetime studies that include all the annoying side, and social factors which are purposefully excluded by the design of the controlled clinical trial? I don't have a final answer to this but I want to point out two things.

First, ICD-10 and DSM-IV are neither the result nor the expression of evidence-based scientific logic. They claim to be a theoretic, but they are not. Jim Birley commented as early as 1990, they are 'essentialist wolves in nominalist sheep skins'. ICD-10 claims to exclude social factors as primary diagnostic criteria, but this is not true. DSM-IV includes a huge amount of social values and devaluations rooted in American society and culture. We have to think about the consequences. And if we compare diagnoses made on the bases of DSM-IV and ICD-10 as Andrews and colleagues (1999) did, we get a concordance of 33 to 66 per cent in seven of twelve disorders compared; in only five disorders the concordance was above 66 per cent. This really cannot make us very trustful in the reliability of research and the validity of the established diagnostic systems. We are right to distrust them because neither of the systems is the result of scientific work that matches the criteria of evidence-based medicine. It is true they were worked out by expert committees. But in the end they were agreed on by vote, the ICD by delegates from 130 different countries in the WHO, the DSM-IV by a number of committees and boards of the American Society of Psychiatry. And all of us know that the multiplication of diagnoses from DSM-II (229) to DSM-IV (395) has no scientific reason in the first place. It is last but not least a reflection of the fight between different medical disciplines in the US about who is to be allowed to treat and be paid for which disorder.

Second, treatment in psychiatry is, even more then in general medicine, a continous interaction between patients, carers and caretakers, on different social and cultural levels and backgrounds. The effectiveness of a thera-peutic agent, be it a drug, some psychotherapy or sociotherapy, is one thing. But the complexity of its interaction in a particular social surrounding is another. So we shall definitely have a long way to go in order to base psychiatric diagnoses and treatment on true evidence.

Chapter 4

The influence of evidence on mental health care developments in the UK since 1980

Peter James and Tom Burns

Introduction

Humans have always used 'evidence' to influence their understanding about the world and hence their subsequent behaviour. To some extent we are all amateur scientists. However, the use of a scientific model or paradigm by experts in various fields of knowledge is a fairly recent development. Woolgar (1988) divides the development of science into three broad phases.

1. the *amateur* phase (1600–1800), in which financially independent men investigated their own particular area of interest
2. the *academic* phase (1800–1940), which saw the advent of universities to cope with increased scientific knowledge and literature
3. the *professional* phase (post 1940), which witnessed research being increasingly judged in terms of its ability to improve economic prosperity and the quality of life.

The burgeoning cost of good scientific research has resulted in the need for central government funds and the involvement of industrial interests. Research and the use of evidence within mental health care follows a similar pattern, although lagging behind the harder sciences, not least because healthcare systems are in the early stages of development.

The use of evidence in mental health care prior to 1980 was fairly limited and advancements in practice were based on clinical experience. The 1950s saw the discovery of the beneficial effects of psychotropic drugs such as chlorpromazine for psychosis, lithium for mania and imipramine for depression. The 1960s and 1970s saw an explosion in neuroscience and psychopharmacology research driven by research funds from the drug industry. This led to the development of a plethora of antipsychotic oral and depot drugs, tricyclic antidepressants and benzodiazepines, all of which had a great influence on the practice of psychiatry. An early controlled trial of modified insulin coma treatment was a powerful call to scientific rigor in psychiatric practice. The practice of modified insulin treatment had hitherto been widespread and was considered to be a highly effective, though risky, treatment for severe mental disorders. However the trial showed that patients who received a placebo drug together with the same intensive nursing care as that required by the patients receiving insulin, responded equally well to the treatment. The hegemony of clinical experience was no longer absolute. The scientific methods that had been developed within psychopharmacological research were required across all areas of clinical practice.

Apart from a handful of isolated studies (Hargreaves *et al.* 1977; Mattes *et al.* 1977; Pasamanick *et al.* 1966) there was very little research into the mental health services prior to 1980. The past two decades have seen a massive increase in the quantity of research published in every field of mental health care. A number of interconnected forces are at play. First, the process of deinstitutionalisation that began in the 1960s accelerated in the 1980s under its new label 'care in the community'. Although the 1990s saw the introduction of legislation and practice guidelines to support this change, interest in treating people with serious mental illness in the community as an alternative to hospitalisation generated much research throughout the 1980s and 1990s. Many commentators were cynical about this new direction, claiming the reduction in psychiatric beds was purely a cost-cutting measure. Since 1980 greater attention has been paid to cost effectiveness of mental health services. In the UK this manifested itself in attention to managerial aspects and human resources issues, such as the recommendations of the Griffiths Report (1988). The creation of the 'internal market' at the beginning of the 1990s meant that providers of health care had to render evidence of the effectiveness and efficiency of services. Clinical audit and evidence-based practice have become essential components of any service. Academic departments, particularly within psychiatry, have dramatically expanded in order both to disseminate existing knowledge through teaching and consultation and to further the knowledge base through good quality, relevant research.

There has been a vast quantity of methodologically sophisticated psychopharmacological research in the past 20 years, which has greatly influenced psychiatric practice. Other research can be crudely divided into two parallel strands and it is on these that this chapter will focus. First, there are specific psychological and psychosocial interventions. For the most part these have used highly sophisticated methodologies but they have had a relatively modest influence on mental health-care practice. The second group – research into mental health-care systems – has exerted considerable influence on mental health services in the UK, despite being methodologically more simplistic. The broad groupings of these research areas will be outlined and their influence on practice explored.

Psychological and psychosocial interventions

Psychodynamic psychotherapy

Developed from the beginning of the twentieth century, psychoanalysis was the first of the talking therapies. Psychodynamic psychotherapy originated from the various schools of psychoanalysis and was distinguished from them by a reduction in the frequency of sessions and by limitation of the goals of treatment. From the 1960s practitioners attempted to shorten the length of treatment leading to a number of brief or time-limited models of psychodynamic psychotherapy (Davanloo 1980; Malan 1976; Mann 1973; Sifneos 1979). It is this type of psychodynamic therapy that is most commonly practised in UK mental health services.

Up until the 1960s, psychoanalysis and psychodynamic psychotherapy overvalued their contribution to mental health care, with little discrimination about what they could achieve. A lack of alternative psychological models and therapies consolidated their position, and this retains some influence today. The development of behavioural, interpersonal and cognitive therapy required psychodynamic psychotherapy to demonstrate its effectiveness. This proved difficult for a number of reasons. Malan (1963), for example, distinguished between the 'symptomatic' and the 'real' improvement, which psychodynamic psychotherapy would achieve. Attempts to develop suitable psychodynamic outcome measures have had little success.

Psychodynamic psychotherapies have used randomised controlled trials (RCTs) to demonstrate their value in the treatment of depression (Shapiro *et al.* 1994), and some personality disorders (Winston *et al.* 1991, 1994). There is no evidence that psychodynamic psychotherapy is superior to other psychological treatments or, to antidepressants for depression, and it may be harmful in schizophrenia (Drake and Sederer 1986; Mueser and Berenbaum 1990). This general lack of evidence has influenced the provision of services, and psychodynamic therapy, especially in its pure form, has lost influence despite the bibliography produced by the Association for Psychoanalytic Psychotherapy in the NHS (Milton 1993).

Interpersonal therapy

Interpersonal therapy (IPT) is based on the interpersonal school of psychology founded by Harry Stack Sullivan (1953), and the form used in most studies is derived from the work of Gerald Klerman and colleagues (Klerman *et al.* 1984). The emphasis of the intervention is on the onset of symptoms and current problems with interpersonal relationships rather than enduring aspects of personality. Interpersonal therapy is generally used as a short-term therapy for 8 to 30 sessions.

A number of well-designed RCTs have investigated IPT in major depression. DiMascio *et al.* (1979) and Weissman *et al.* (1979) found no significant differences between IPT and amitriptyline when compared with controls and that a combination of the two treatments was more effective than either one alone. The most convincing evidence of the efficacy of IPT for depression came from the National Institute of Mental Health (NIMH) Treatment of Depression Collaborative Research Programme (Elkin *et al.* 1989), which randomised 250 patients to 16 weeks of imipramine, IPT, cognitive-behavioural therapy (CBT) or placebo. Interpersonal therapy was found to be comparable to imipramine even for the most severely depressed patients and somewhat superior for this group than CBT.

Interpersonal therapy, originally intended for adult depression, has been investigated for the treatment of other disorders (Weissman and Markowitz 1994). It may be a useful therapy for depressed adolescents (Mufson *et al.* 1994), older adults (Sloane *et al.* 1985) and those who are HIV positive (Markowitz *et al.* 1992). Not surprisingly, given its emphasis on interpersonal relationships, it benefits depressed patients with marital problems (Foley *et al.* 1989). Further controlled trials with adequate sample sizes are still needed in these areas.

Interpersonal therapy has had relatively little uptake in UK mental health services. This may have been initially because the largely American interpersonal school was competing with a well-established psychoanalytic establishment and was then overshadowed by advances in behavioural and cognitive therapies.

Behavioural and cognitive-behavioural therapy

Behaviour therapy evolved from the theories of classical and operant learning. It revolutionised the treatment of obsessive-compulsive disorder through the use of exposure and response prevention, and phobias through systematic desensitisation (Emmelkamp 1982). These disorders had been considered either intractable or they have been treated ineffectively with psychoanalysis. Learning theory has also informed the assessment and intervention of challenging behaviours exhibited by persons with learning disabilities (Sturmey 1996).

The role of cognitions in psychopathology was developed into models of therapy by Meichenbaum (1974), Ellis (1962) and, most prominently, by Beck (Beck 1976; Beck *et al.* 1979). Initially the emphasis was on thoughts that maintained dysfunctional emotions and behaviour, but more recently the role of underlying beliefs or schemas has received attention (Young 1990). Cognitive-behavioural therapy (CBT) integrates the two theories.

Cognitive and cognitive-behavioural therapy have been widely researched for a range of psychiatric problems, particularly depression. However, the findings have not been unequivocal. In his meta-analysis of twenty-eight studies Dobson (1989) concluded that CBT produced greater change than waiting-list controls or other treatments such as pharmacotherapy or behaviour therapy. Cognitive-behavioural therapy, either alone or with medication reduced relapses (Evans *et al.* 1992; Kovacs *et al.* 1981). This generally positive view of CBT was shaken by the NIMH depression study (Elkin *et al.* 1989, 1995). With equal effectiveness in the less depressed group, CBT was no better than placebo, and significantly less effective than imipramine for the more severely depressed patients. However, in a study of similar methodology to the NIMH trial (Hollon *et al.* 1992), CBT fared equally to imipramine, and twenty sessions of CBT over a 12-week period had a greater prophylactic effect than imipramine taken for the same period. The Sheffield Psychotherapy Project in Britain (Shapiro *et al.* 1994; Shapiro and Firth 1987) compared CBT to psychodynamic psychotherapy in a well-designed study and, in general, found no differences between the treatments. For the most severely depressed patients, 16 weeks of therapy of any kind was significantly better than 8 weeks.

Cognitive-behavioural therapy has been shown to be successful with some anxiety disorders (Chambless and Gillis 1993). A meta-analysis of studies investigating CBT for generalised anxiety disorder, panic disorder with and without agoraphobia, and social phobia, indicated that CBT is consistently more effective than waiting-list and placebo control groups. What has been less clear is the differential effect of the various components of CBT.

The behavioural treatment of exposure and response prevention (ERP) for obsessive-compulsive disorder has been shown to be effective by a number of studies (Fals-Stewart *et al.* 1993; Foa *et al.* 1984) and has become the treatment of choice for this disorder. More recently cognitive techniques have been used as an adjunct to ERP (Salkovskis *et al.* 1998), although as yet the effectiveness of this remains debatable. Cognitive-behavioural therapy has also had some success in the treatment of bulimia nervosa (Wilson and Fairburn 1993), although there have been relatively few controlled trials. This view was supported by a recent Cochrane systematic review (Hay 2000), though the authors emphasise an approach based on individual needs.

In the past 10 years there has been growing interest in CBT for psychosis, particularly for alleviating medication-resistant positive symptoms. Initial evidence came from individual case reports and small, uncontrolled studies (Chadwick and Lowe 1990; Fowler and Morley 1989; Garety *et al.* 1994; Kingdon and Turkington 1991). Larger RCTs (Kuipers *et al.* 1997; Tarrier *et al.* 1998) have also demonstrated its potential usefulness, although currently enthusiasm surpasses the evidence of its effectiveness. Cognitive-behavioural therapy has been studied in early psychosis (Haddock *et al.* 1998) often in inpatient settings, where it may reduce symptoms and speed recovery (Drury *et al.* 1996a, 1996b; Jackson *et al.* 1998).

Behavioural family management

As a direct result of experimental evidence, clinicians now accept a combination of medication and psychosocial intervention as standard treatment for psychoses. Schizophrenia has been the subject of extensive psychosocial research. In the 1950s Brown and colleagues investigated the relationship between relapse rates in schizophrenia and the home environment to which patients were discharged (Brown *et al.* 1962). This work led to the concept of 'expressed emotion' and the 1980s and 1990s saw research into interventions, often referred to as 'behavioural family management'. These were designed to reduce high expressed emotion in families, thereby reducing relapse rates (Falloon *et al.* 1982; Falloon and Pederson 1985; Hogarty *et al.* 1986; Kottgen *et al.* 1984; Leff *et al.* 1982; Leff *et al.* 1985; Tarrier *et al.* 1988). The studies differed but most contained three components

1. education about schizophrenia
2. general support and problem solving
3. family therapy to modify dysfunctional interactions between family members.

A recent review (Pharoah *et al.* 2000) concluded that behavioural family management can decrease relapse frequency and may decrease hospitalisation and encourage medication compliance.

Impact of psychological therapies

Research into psychological therapies has had a mixed influence on mental health services in the UK. Overall, services have moved away from psychodynamic towards cognitive-behavioural therapies. Cognitive-behavioural therapy techniques are adapted for various disorders so that core training can provide versatile clinicians. This has profoundly influenced training courses, despite little evidence on how to tailor CBT to particular clients. In Goldfried and Wolfe's (1996) review of the changes in psychotherapy research methods, they identify a 'third generation' of research methods from around 1980. These strive for internal validity by the investigation of two variables, the diagnosis and the type of therapy. Other 'confounding' factors were controlled for by the randomisation of patients and the use of strictly defined, manualised therapy. This approach has been criticised as detrimental to external validity, i.e. how well the findings of the studies generalise to what is happening in clinical practice. In particular the use of diagnosis as a defining variable excludes other crucial patient variables, so adherence to one therapy modality is ineffective and unsound.

Without such external validity the evidence on psychological therapies may continue to have only a limited influence on clinicians' practice. Instead, type of therapy and the duration of treatment will be influenced by other factors such as the interest and skills of the clinician, training school, and clinical experience about patient factors (other than diagnosis) that affect the outcome. The challenge of the next generation of research is to attempt to strike a better balance between internal and external validity.

In contrast to this classical psychotherapy research, a strength of the behavioural family management studies generating a high level of external validity is that they have used 'real' clinicians working with 'real' patients and families. While to the detriment of internal validity, it was deemed impractical or unethical to control variables such as medication or other aspects of routine care. Although there has been debate over which elements of the interventions are the active ones, there is abundant evidence of their efficacy in reducing relapse rates in high-risk patients (Pharoah *et al.* 2000). Despite this, the use of behavioural family management in the UK is scarce in routine services. Anderson and Adams (1996) suggest possible reasons for this. The intervention is highly labour intensive, and current evidence suggests the need to treat seven families for a year to prevent one relapse. Without economic analyses, services may be reluctant to direct already limited resources into this area. Certainly setting up such a service is, in the short term, likely to be more of a cost than a benefit.

An unexplored area around the provision of psychological therapies has been that of motivation – who wants the therapy? This has been understandable with classical psychodynamic approaches as it has seemed self-evident – patients seek out the treatment and often show conspicuously high levels of motivation to get it (tolerating long waiting lists, paying fees even for missed appointments, etc.). With the introduction of psychotherapies within the British National Health Service there has been no replication of the fee-for-service relationship (whether private or through insurance schemes) that demonstrates the patients' commitment and may also help support the therapists' motivation. The targeting on the severely mentally ill means that it is usually the therapist, rather than the patient, who suggests the psychological treatment. This is especially so in some of the behavioural treatments and in behavioural family management in schizophrenia where the patient and family may be resistant to exploring painful issues where compromises have been won over time.

Mental health-care systems research

The balance between research and implementation in UK mental health care since 1980 demonstrated in the psychotherapies, is reversed in mental health-care systems research. Here there has been a furious pace of change while much of the evidence base is still questionable. In part this reflects the socially determined changes in mental health care which derive from major shifts, both nationally and internationally, in how the mentally ill are viewed and how industrialised societies think they should be treated. It is not simply a mental health issue either – the last two decades have witnessed a fundamental re-evaluation of social structures and the role of the welfare state. The development of more flexible, non-institutional, support systems has gone hand in hand with a more libertarian approach to individuals' needs. Personal choice and determination are emphasised more than comfort and basic security (perhaps because the latter have become taken for granted).

Deinstitutionalisation of mentally ill people has also been an attractive option in times of financial stringency when the possibility of running down and selling off large institutions became evident. This has been referred to as 'an unholy alliance between mental health liberals and fiscal conservatives'. The move to community care has been associated with an unprecedented volume of health-care systems research. Mueser's extensive review (Mueser *et al.* 1998) contains over seventy-five published studies of different forms of community support systems. Similarly, since the Programme of Assertive Community Treatment (Stein and Test 1980) approach to assertive outreach was published there have been over twenty replication studies worldwide. Randomised controlled trials within these studies have been subject to systematic review (Marshall and Lockwood 1998) as have other case management services (Marshall *et al.* 1997). Despite the sheer volume of studies, controversy still reigns around the therapeutic value and cost benefits of these approaches (Burns 1997; Marshall 1996).

Over a decade ago, Mosher (1983) suggested that continuing research in this field constituted displacement activity by psychiatrists who simply wanted to hold back the tide of progress. Mosher's claim might have been difficult to refute had research stopped when he recommended it. However continuing research in this area has altered the picture. Most strikingly the results from Europe, and in particular the UK, failed to replicate the substantial advantages in terms of reduced hospitalisation (and sometimes also in improved clinical and social functioning) demonstrated in the US. While the first major UK study did find a marginal benefit to the community case managed patients (Marks *et al.* 1994; Muijen *et al.* 1992), later studies, often with larger samples, have stubbornly failed to do so (Burns *et al.* 1999b, Holloway and Carson 1998; Thornicroft *et al.* 1998).

Why these differences should exist between countries is open to debate. It has been suggested that UK studies fail to find US-sized differences because of poor clinical implementation – that we simply don't 'do' case management as well as our US counterparts (McGovern and Owen 1999). This is an important consideration. A study of case management services for dual diagnosis patients in New Hampshire found that teams which drifted from the prescribed model of practice performed significantly less well than those who adhered to it (McHugo *et al.* 1999). Not only did two of the intensive teams stray from the model sufficiently to compromise their patients' outcomes but one of the control teams 'overtook' the intensive model and its procedures and outcomes paralleled them. Despite these concerns there is extraordinarily little published about the content of the experimental care in such studies, and even less about the control care (Burns and Priebe 1996). Teague and colleagues have made a start by developing an instrument to measure 'treatment fidelity' in assertive community treatment (Teague et al. 1998). Also systems of classifying services have been described (Johnson et al. 1998). While these may help in ensuring that like is compared with like, they will not resolve the treatment fidelity issue. Prospective process recording is one possible approach to the problem but this is labour intense (Burns et al. 2000) and the likelihood of getting agreement that one has measured the 'right' ingredients is low.

Attention to treatment fidelity is one approach to understanding differing results in assertive community treatment where there is some consensus about the active ingredients (McGrew and Bond 1995). Unfortunately this consensus is not evidence based nor is there anything like as much consensus for understanding trials of other forms of community intervention (e.g. crisis teams, home-care teams). What of the controls? It may be that there is more to be learnt from understanding the variation in control services than there is in treatment fidelity in the experimental teams.

There are long-standing differences in European and North American services for the severely mentally ill, which arise more from the availability of universal health cover and evolved social welfare provision than from service ideology. Freely available comprehensive medical and social care, even with minimal co-ordination, may have a profound impact on functioning in patients with long-standing psychotic illnesses (Tyrer 1998, 2000). It is also quite possible that a significant proportion of the 'assertive community treatment' package is redundant – irrelevant to outcomes. The study of process in the UK700 trial confirms that there were substantial differences in rates of contact and focus of contact between the two arms despite the absence of an outcome difference (Burns et al. 2000). However there were also important similarities such as multi-disciplinary reviews and outreach in both teams. Head-to-head comparisons of health-care systems can only inform on their difference in effectiveness. Before importing the results of such studies from one health care culture to another it is essential to compare both the control and the experimental service with that which is available locally. This has not been done with respect to assertive outreach in the UK where it has been endorsed as an essential component of the modernisation agenda (Department of Health 1999). Those currently establishing assertive outreach teams in the UK may anticipate unrealistic impacts on hospital usage.

Even if variation in the controls were not a problem, the context in which a service is delivered is likely to modify its impact (Burns and Priebe 1996; Creed et al. 1999). It is unlikely, for example, that intensive case management will significantly improve the care of the long-term psychotic patient unless there are social-care provisions with which to integrate it (Creed *et al.* 1999). Context is a crucial consideration when using evidence to drive policy formation (Pelosi and Jackson 2000).

The context of community psychiatry evidence can also be historical and personal. Why is such a study being conducted in this service at this time? The presence of enthusiasts advocating a service model is an essential pre-requisite for any study taking place at all. In mental health research such 'product champions' (now officially endorsed as a component for taking the National Service Framework forward) have a prominent place. Interpreting their work can be difficult – the benefits of the service configuration need to be disentangled from the charisma and drive of the figurehead (Coid 1994). In addition to drawing attention to the Hawthorne effect that is common to such studies, Coid highlights the ungeneralisability of many experimental teams. These often have enhanced resources and stringent patient entry criteria that do not reflect normal practice. Once attention is paid to these short-comings and more routine practice is tested (Creed *et al.* 1999; Thornicroft *et al.* 1998) then less spectacular outcome differences are reported.

Although there has been attention to some of the more glaring inadequacies of the earlier trials there is little evidence of an evolution of sophistication in community psychiatry studies. Two significant steps have been taken in the UK700 study (Creed *et al.* 1999), one of the few sufficiently large studies to confirm a negative result. First, the study reduces confounding from a 'charisma' effect by being multi-site so that there was no obvious emotional investment in the experimental teams. Being multi-site it was also likely to be more generalisable. Second, it is the first such study to examine the impact of varying only one service characteristic between the two treatments. In this trial it was caseload size, 12 to 15 patients per case manager in the intensive care group, and 30 to 35 per case manager in the standard care group.

This is one of the first attempts to unpack the 'black box' of a care system in a controlled experiment. Given the number of head-to-head studies in this area it is unlikely that much more can be learnt from them. Yet they are still being conducted. The consensus about the essential components of assertive community treatment (McGrew and Bond 1995) is simply the opinions of experts. Evidence of equal strength to that provided about caseload size by the UK700 trial is required for each of these major components if the current UK policy is to be truly evidence based.

Why such vigorous endorsement?

We have highlighted serious limitations of the evidence in areas such as intensive case management and assertive community treatment. In other areas of community psychiatry (e.g. day care, substance abuse, vocational placements) the evidence is often too thin even to support the debate that has taken place in case management. Why then is there such support from the government for the movement towards community psychiatry in practice despite public pronouncements to the contrary?

Community psychiatry needs to be understood as part of a wider social movement. It may be supported because it reflects the *Zeitgeist* of the postwar developed world. As the emphasis on human self-determination and actualisation has grown, the place for enormous, monolithic, paternalistic mental hospitals has shrunk. Aided by the scandals of the 1960s and the influential writings of social theorists such as Goffman (1961) and antipsychiatrists such as R.D. Laing (1960), hospitals had simply come to be viewed as 'a bad thing'. Social inclusion is only the latest expression for a process which has been gaining momentum since the end of the Second World War. The rundown of mental hospitals was initiated by clinicians but the potential financial savings (or more often 'cost shifting') were soon recognised by politicians. As mental health economics has become more sophisticated the cost–benefit advantages of community care are less self-evident.

As research has been imported from one context to another the opportunity arises for using developments for different needs. Policy can build on the research but subtly alter the agenda. With assertive outreach most of the early findings emphasised the reduction in hospitalisation and consequent increase in 'community tenure'. Citing this research UK policy has mandated assertive outreach but the primary goal is to increase engagement (Department of Health 1999), despite little evidence to link this approach with increased engagement.

It is also possible that there are purely political motivations for fostering such changes, ostensibly driven by the evidence base. Governments need to be seen to be doing something about improving public mental health services. While it can be argued that the negative public perception of these services may have more to do with media presentation and an unrealistic inflation of expectations (Burns and Priebe 1999), the need for 'innovation' can be pressing. Change in care structures also offers the possibility of transferring power from one profession to another, or from the professions to health-care managers and politicians. Changing the language associated with the process of care can subtly shift the balance of power.

Conclusions

Mental health practice in the UK has become increasingly evidence based in the last two decades. The pace of change has been increasing and is likely to continue to do so. Despite concerns that it may usher in dehumanised or mechanistic care (Laugharne 1999) there is little real pressure to return to the inconsistency of practice that preceded these developments. The public awareness of the previous widespread use of useless and potentially damaging treatments (whether unnecessary ENT operations on children or insulin treatment for schizophrenia) has made society more sceptical of professional endorsements. 'Evidence-based medicine' is here to stay in modern UK psychiatry.

The relationship between evidence and change in practice, however, is neither direct nor predictable. In the psychological therapies change in practice has been slower than the evidence suggests, although there have not been any surprises. In care-systems research it has been more mixed. We have used as an example the complications of deriving practice change in assertive outreach from the evidence base – how the strength of conviction embodied in the policy exceeds the firmness of the evidence. Equally intriguing is why some evidence is not picked up at all in service development and policy. The work on acute day hospitals as an alternative to in-patient care is a striking example (Creed *et al.* 1990, 1991). Creed and colleagues have conducted their research within the context where it could be generalised without translational problems. It may be that their willingness to explore the difficulties of implementation (rather than gloss over them as enthusiasts do) has restricted a fuller endorsement of their model.

The evidence for what is actually happening in care systems is very thin. Studies in this area, even more than those in psychological therapies, need to take seriously the unpacking of the black box of treatment. Despite the problems with RCTs (the cost, time, narrowness of the question, etc.) there is little excuse for not investing more energy in larger multi-site studies that can give firm answers to more precise questions. Without this we are unlikely to realise the potential of evidence-based mental health practice. We run the risk of discrediting the approach and losing control of the development of our services.

Chapter 5

The influence and role of evidence in the United States

Terri L Tanielian, Harold Alan Pincus and Howard Goldman

This chapter aims to describe the role of evidence-based medicine (EBM) in mental health in the United States (US) by highlighting the development and implementation of EBM in American psychiatry during the past 20 years. In this chapter we describe the ideological shift in American psychiatry, the changes in mental health practice and policy, and the role of the US federal government in ensuring quality medical care. We also describe several strategies and tools designed to foster the dissemination and use of evidence-based psychiatry. Finally, we discuss the challenges and lessons learned from the 'real world' of mental health practice in the US.

Historical perspective

For most of its history, US public mental health policy has been focused at the state level. Alternately rocked with scandal and reform, budgets for largely state-run public institutions were generally inadequate to move beyond custodialism. What passed for 'reform', whether the expectations for moral treatment or the advocacy of Dorothea Dix, was based on humanitarian values, or anecdote. Even as medicine, in general, advanced to a more academic perspective with the Flexner Report (Flexner 1910), American psychiatry remained in the throes of competing ideologies. Following the Second World War, Federal involvement in mental health research and training and, ultimately, clinical care steadily increased.

In 1946 the National Mental Health Act (Public Law 79-487) authorized the establishment of a National Institute of Mental Health (NIMH), which was charged with

1. conducting research into the causes, diagnosis, and treatment of mental illness
2. training personnel in matters related to mental health
3. assisting states in developing community-based services.

With the assumption that the treatment of mental illness would be furthered most effectively through a strong program of research and personnel training, the NIMH was placed under the auspices of the National Institutes of Health (NIH).

The NIMH research budget grew from $0.8 million in 1948 to $7.8 million in 1956. In the late 1950s, however, with the initial promise of psychopharmacology, NIMH research began to take off, growing to $50 million in 1962 (Pardes *et al.* 1985).

President Kennedy's initiatives in mental health helped to increase the research budget to over $80 million by 1965; however, this planted the seeds for later problems as the increased focus on community mental health services diverted attention from research issues. The NIMH was removed from the NIH and placed in a series of continually reorganized health and social service bureaucratic entities.

Following the movement to deinstitutionalise psychiatric patients in the 1950s and 1960s, it was hoped that the community mental health centers would meet the needs of their patients, and legislation developing these centers became a focal point for development in the 1960s. However, resources were inadequate and centers did not concentrate their efforts sufficiently on severely ill individuals (Sabshin 1990).

During this time of community and social services focus, mental health research support stabilized and then declined. Grants from the NIMH dropped 15 per cent during the 1980s, while NIH grants rose by 85 per cent. Importantly, just at the time that the research programs at NIMH were de-emphasized, the importance of science and especially the conduct of rigorous clinical trials was attaining a central role in medicine. The Kefhauver Amendment passed by Congress in the early 1960s required that the Food and Drug Administration (FDA) determine the safety and efficacy of medications by systematic evidence-based methods. While biological psychiatry began to make significant inroads during this time, competing social, behavioral, and psychodynamic approaches vied for pre-eminence, but more on an ideological than empirical basis. As a result, empirically demonstrated treatments such as lithium carbonate, discovered by Cade to be effective for the treatment of bipolar disorder in 1949, were not prescribed widely in the US for more than two decades.

The past 15 years, however, have seen a major reversal in the fortunes of science and the importance of empirical data. The NIMH moved back into the NIH. The NIH funding to academic departments of psychiatry grew from $80 million in 1984 to over $400 million in 1998, with psychiatry moving from the tenth-ranked department in medical schools to the second. This growth was more than paralleled by the expansion of the pharmaceutical industry, CNS research, and the resultant development (and marketing) of new products. At the same time there were revolutionary changes in payment for medical services and an increased demand for cost-effective services based on objective data.

Changes in mental health practices

Vast changes in health-care systems in general, the mental health system in particular and in the practice of psychiatry have emerged as a result of several scientific, political, administrative, and economic developments during the past 20 years (Mechanic 1998; Pincus *et al.* 1996, 1998). These rapid changes have produced an increasing need to understand the nature of psychiatric practice. Enormous changes in the structure, financing, and delivery of care in American psychiatry have been documented during the past 20 years (US Department of Health and Human Services 1999). For example, with regard to the provision of care, several national studies have revealed an increase in the treatment of psychiatric patients by non-psychiatrist providers as well as a shift in how providers treat these patients (e.g. they became more oriented toward a pharmacologic treatment) over the past two decades (Kessler *et al.* 1994; Olfson and Pincus 1994; Pincus *et al.* 1999).

Under the structure of managed care, patients with less complex and more common mental conditions are likely to be treated by their primary care physician or to be referred to non-psychiatric mental health providers (Olfson and Pincus 1996). In addition, how psychiatrists (as well as non-psychiatrist physicians) treat these patients has also shifted. In 1974, an American Psychiatric Association study revealed that non-analyst psychiatrists in private practice provided medication to only 29 per cent of their patients (Marmor 1975). The 1989 Professional Activities Survey found that 54.5 per cent of outpatients received pharmacologic treatment alone or combined with psychotherapy (Olfson *et al.* 1994). More recently, 1997 data show that approximately 90 per cent of psychiatric patients were receiving medication for their mental disorders (Pincus *et al.* 1999). It is important to note that more than half (55.4 per cent) of the outpatients in the same study were receiving both medication and psychotherapy, either with both services provided by the psychiatrist or in conjunction with another mental health professional. Several explanations for the increased use of pharmacologic agents have been suggested, including the increase in the evidence base in clinical psychopharmacology and the growing armamentarium of new and safer medications to support the shift toward the provision of medication to most psychiatric patients. (Pincus *et al.* 1999).

Over the same time as we witnessed these enormous changes in mental health policy and practice, increased demands for accountability and objective data became paramount. While the scientific funding increased and the evidence base expanded, so did the call for the translation of the new research into practice.

Definitional evolution of evidence-based medicine

Many working definitions of EBM have been generated, but the basic concepts remain the same. Sackett *et al.* (1996 p. 71) define EBM as the conscientious and judicious use of current best evidence from clinical care research in the management of individual patients. Haynes *et al.* (1996) lay out a simple model for evidence-based clinical decision making that includes three components

1. clinical expertise
2. patient preferences
3. evidence from research.

According to Geddes (1996), the practice and teaching of EBM focuses on five linked activities.

1. formulating the precise clinical question; this involves three main steps
    *   defining the patient's problem
    *   defining the manoeuvre
    *   specifying the clinical outcomes of interest
2. finding the evidence to answer the clinical question
3. appraising the evidence for its validity and relevance
4. integrating the evidence with clinical expertise and patient values and applying the results to the clinical problem
5. evaluating the clinician's performance.

Evidence construction and interpretation

Inherent in the definition and practice of EBM is the ability to find the best available evidence from research. Biomedical and clinical research has relied heavily on the process of finding and verifying clinically useful information. However, finding the information can be the most daunting task. Haynes *et al.* (1997), in a review of internal medicine journals, found the percentage of original studies and systematic review articles that provided reasonably strong signals that were ready for application in clinical practice to be about 10 per cent.

Once a clinician navigates the literature and tries to understand its meaning, he or she must ask 'how good is the evidence?' and 'how does this apply to my patients?' Such critical appraisal skills and an understanding of the rules of evidence are essential to the application or implementation of EBM. In determining its applicability and clinical relevance, the clinician is forced to understand the nuances of the research design and protocol. The majority of studies with treatment relevance follow the randomised clinical trial (RCT) design (case studies provide interesting lessons but often do not form the basis of treatment recommendations). Otherwise known as the gold standard, RCTs apply random allocation of patient groups into comparison groups to measure the outcomes of the 'intervention'. Most of the evidence concerning safety and efficacy is based on RCTs that use limited study populations (specific diagnostic codes, age, etc.) receiving a single medication. It has been argued that these studies do not reflect the real-world patient population where comorbidity is common and the use of polypharmacy frequent (Pincus *et al.* 1999; Schmidt *et al.* 1996). Few clinical trials examine multiple drug regimens (American Psychiatric Association 1996; Nayak 1998).

The implementation of EBM (and in particular the physician's ability to understand the evidence) is additionally plagued by associated problems with the construction and publication of evidence. These include the absence of evidence and evidence insufficiency. Just because there hasn't been a published finding indicating the efficacy of a treatment approach does not mean that there is evidence that such treatment is not efficacious. A considerable proportion of medical research never gets published, often because of the bias against publishing 'negative results', and just because a study has been published does not guarantee its quality. In a 1994 article, Altman noted the poor quality of much medical research and further pointed out that many responsible doctors do not appreciate the principles underlying scientific research.

Further complicating the ability to sort out, digest and interpret the evidence is when evidence is incomplete or even contradictory. In these cases, EBM offers little help (Schmidt *et al.* 1996). Even after reviewing the evidence, clinicians must integrate this information (Geddes step 4 1996) with their own previous experience or their own evidence, making the clinical decision still a very personal one. However, as Naylor (1995, p. 841) argues, the 'prudent application of evaluative sciences will affirm rather than obviate the need for the art of medicine'.

The role of evidence-based medicine

Depending on your perspective, EBM is employed to serve several purposes. Stated goals of EBM that have been applied to development strategies for tools in the US, include the following.

- To enhance the quality of care by providing clinicians with information on which to base their clinical decisions.
- To ensure that individual patient care is based on the most up-to-date evidence and results in the best possible outcomes (Geddes 1996).
- To minimize the gap between knowledge and practice (Tonelli 1998). Initially, an apparent goal of EBM was to minimize the use of non-evidentiary knowledge and reasoning in clinical practice. More recently,

the focus has shifted to integrating clinical expertise, pathophysiologic knowledge and patient prefences in making decisions regarding the care of individual patients (Ellrodt *et al.* 1997; Sackett *et al.* 1996).
- To encourage physicians to maximize the likelihood of positive outcomes over many patients, rather than just the patient at hand (Tonelli 1998).
- EBM does not promise the best decision in a particular situation (Asch and Hershey 1995).

Strategies, tools and applications in US mental health services

As we have already stated, during the past 20 years enormous changes in the delivery and financing of health-care services in the US have brought increased attention to system and provider accountability and to the quality of care. To enhance the quality of care, several evidence-based tools and strategies have been developed and subsequently disseminated for application in clinical practice. In turn, research into mental health services has focused on bringing accountability to the delivery of care by measuring the impact of these strategies and tools on practice.

Pushed by the expansion of the evidence base and pulled by greater public demands for accountability, the mental health field during the past two decades has witnessed a firm and systematic move in the direction of evidence-based psychiatry. Beginning with the evolution of a criteria-based nomenclature to the development of practice guidelines and methods to measure real-world practice, several tools are now available, providing the ability for practitioners to assess and practise evidence-based psychiatry.

Diagnostic and Statistical Manual for the Classification of Mental Disorders (DSM)

According to Sabshin (1990), one of the best symbols of late-century American psychiatry has been the increasing centrality of nosology in our scientific and clinical work. The purpose being to provide a common language and system for classifying and understanding mental disorders. During the 1950s, nosology was perceived by many as an esoteric nonentity, but DSM-III and DSM-III-R influenced American psychiatry profoundly. Amongst criticism about the unreliability of psychiatric diagnosis, DSM-III committees and task forces at the American Psychiatric Association produced documents that changed the shape of American psychiatry, influenced by the need for objectivity in American psychiatry. Psychiatry needed to prove that psychiatric disorders could be diagnosed and that a rational basis for determining how to deal with psychiatric patients could be developed. Between DSM-III-R (1987) and DSM-IV (1994) there were increased calls for accountability, an increased reliance on evidence, and the increased availability of empirical data, to inform the clinical decision making process. Therefore in the development of DSM-IV, the APA made an explicit commitment to a 'formal evidence based process' (American Psychiatric Association 1994). For DSM-IV, the definition of EBM was taken beyond individual patients and applied systematically in a broader clinical/policy-making process. The development process has been described and fully documented in the four-volume DSM-IV sourcebook. With the release of DSM-IV, clinicians have been provided with an effective and reliable means of diagnosing mental disorders.

Guidelines for treatment

In response to growing calls to make its research relevant to clinical practice, the NIH began a series of 'consensus development conferences' in the 1970s. Intended to guide clinicians in making the best use of available research, the statements emanating from these conferences were widely publicized and influential. The NIMH initiated a series of these in the 1980s, which formed the initial infrastructure for more extensive development of mental health practice guidelines (Pincus *et al.* 1983).

As such, clinical practice guidelines have been formulated to assist the clinician in devising treatment strategies based on evidence for a particular diagnosis. Practice guidelines are systematically developed strategies of patient care that assist clinicians and patients in clinical decision-making. Guidelines are meant to be recommendations for treatment that should be followed in the large majority of cases (Institute of Medicine 1992).

Within the US during the last decade, there has been an explosion in the development of practice guidelines throughout medicine. Guidelines have been drawn up by professional associations, insurance companies, health-maintenance organizations, provider groups, state governments and the federal government. They have become essential to accreditation processes and are beginning to influence educational programs.

Many different development approaches have been employed to develop practice guidelines. These range from consensus statements (using an 'expert panel' to build consensus around specified objectives and recommendations based on clinical experience or knowledge) to the collection and weighting of available evidence in the development of treatment recommendations. In 1990 the American Medical Association described five 'attributes' that guidelines should have (American Medical Association 1990)

1. guidelines should be developed by or in conjunction with physician organizations
2. they should use reliable methodologies that integrate relevant research findings and clinical expertise
3. they should be as comprehensive and specific as possible

4. they should be based upon current information
5. they should be widely disseminated.

In 1996 a sixth attribute was added to include outcomes research, goals and measures. In addition, the Institute of Medicine identified eight attributes of good guidelines (Institute of Medicine 1992)

1. validity
2. reproducibility
3. clinical applicability
4. clinical flexibility
5. clarity
6. multidisciplinary process
7. scheduled review
8. documentation.

   Guidelines related to mental health have been developed by federal agencies, primary care specialties, industry sponsored groups and mental health specialty groups such as the American Academy of Child and Adolescent Psychiatry and the American Psychiatric Association. For example, beginning in 1989, the APA established a process and committee to oversee the development of practice guidelines for psychiatry (Zarin et al. 1993). To date, ten guidelines have been developed and disseminated in such areas as

- Alzheimer's disease and other dementias of late life
- bipolar disorder
- major depressive disorder in adults
- schizophrenia and alcohol
- cocaine
- opioid use disorder, etc.

These guidelines have been widely disseminated through publication in the American Journal of Psychiatry and can be purchased from the American Psychiatric Press. In addition, many of the national guidelines have been adopted for use by insurance companies or local agencies.

Obstacles and challenges to implementing guidelines

The major opposition to guidelines has been the notion of 'cookbook' medicine and the potential for their misuse. There are also concerns that guidelines limit innovations in practice and increase professional liability exposure. However, a process that is evidence based and open and that has involved a large number of clinicians is intended to decrease some of these concerns. At the same time, the democratization of the development process may result in guidelines that are overly flexible and/or general and not closely tied to rigorous evidence. However, there remains a valid concern that the guidelines process might diminish clinical innovation and the development of novel approaches to patient care.

Research has demonstrated, however, that just because guidelines are available and are disseminated does not mean that clinicians will use them (Asaph *et al.* 1991; Greco and Eisenberg 1993). Such provider-level obstacles can include their own bias toward guidelines and the lack of time to read and adapt their clinical decision-making to the guidelines. Efforts to encourage use and compliance with guidelines have been tested, including the use of 'opinion leaders' (recognized excellent clinicians highly regarded by their peers) who lead special sessions to review and discuss the guidelines and their implementation. These approaches have had mixed results. For example, one study of the use of 'opinion leaders' demonstrated a change in the direction encouraged by the guideline (Lomas *et al.* 1991). Another major dissemination strategy in the US has been to incorporate guidelines into teaching programs at all levels: medical students, residency and continuing education. For example, the APA guidelines have been sources of questions on re-certification exams and the Psychiatric Residents in Training Examination (PRITE). However, there is limited evidence as to the effectiveness of these and other strategies in changing provider behavior and more importantly in improving patient outcomes.

Recently, efforts have been taken to increase the 'user friendliness' of practice guidelines to include easy-to-follow treatment algorithms and quick reference guides. Companion pieces to inform and activate patients as 'informed consumers' have also been developed. Over time in the US, we have learned that change is not linear and that intervention is needed at multiple levels to include the patient, provider, practice system and purchaser of care. New models of and tools for evidence-based decision making are being developed that combine strategies for all of these dimensions to effect change and improve quality (Wagner *et al.* 1996, 1999).

Federal and private initiatives

The Agency for Healthcare Research and Quality (AHRQ), formerly known as the Agency for Health Care Policy and Research (or AHCPR), as part of the US Department of Health and Human Services is the lead agency charged with supporting research designed to improve the quality of health care, reduce its cost, improve patient safety, decrease medical errors and broaden access to essential services. The AHRQ sponsors and conducts research that provides evidence-based information on health-care outcomes, quality and cost, use and access. The information is meant to help health-care decision makers – patients and clinicians, health-system leaders and policy makers – make more informed decisions and improve the quality of health-care services. The agency was originally created in December 1989 and re-authorized in December 1999. The AHRQ was an early leader in developing evidence-based tools such as clinical practice guidelines (or evidence reports) for clinicians and patients. It should be noted, however, that with the re-authorization in 1999, the legislation eliminates the requirement that the AHRQ support the development of clinical practice guidelines. The AHRQ now supports the development of evidence reports through its twelve evidence-based practice centers and the dissemination of evidence-based guidelines through a National Guideline Clearinghouse (which assembles and provides access to existing evidence-based guidelines).

As part of its renewed mission to improve the quality of health care, the AHRQ disseminates scientific findings about what works best in health care. Through the evidence-based practice centers, they conduct systematic, comprehensive analyses and syntheses of the scientific literature to develop evidence reports and technology assessments on clinical topics that are common, expensive and present challenges to decision makers. Three of the eleven reports released to date focus on mental disorders (depression, alcohol dependence and attention-deficit/hyperactivity disorder). In addition, AHRQ recently began its Translating Research into Practice initiative aimed at implementing evidence-based tools and information in diverse health-care settings among practitioners caring for diverse populations (see the AHRQ website www.ahrq.gov).

Outcomes research initiatives, such as the Patient Outcomes Research Teams (PORTs) funded by the NIMH and the AHRQ, help to build the science base by testing clinical practice guidelines in real-life settings. In turn, findings from these studies influence and support policy decision making. For example, the AHRQ updated their guidelines for treating major depression in primary care and the National Committee on Quality Assurance used these treatment guidelines to define its Health Plan Employer Data and Information Set (HEDIS) measure for treating depression. The RAND Corporation conducted an AHRQ funded PORT, the Partners in Care Study, documenting the effectiveness of a moderately intense intervention designed to provide training and resources in managed primary care practices to improve treatment for depression (Wells et al. 2000). The schizophrenia PORT developed a set of treatment recommendations and demonstrated the gap between those recommendations and actual practice (Lehman et al. 1998). In addition, the Veterans Affairs Administration and the Department of Defense have developed depression guidelines and tool kits for implementation in their treatment facilities. Similarly, the National Alliance for the Mentally III developed a pamphlet, *Treatment Works*, based on the treatment recommendations developed by the schizophrenia PORT. Various organizations have established initiatives in performance measurement and quality assurance, including the National Association of State Mental Health Program Directors, the American College of Mental Health

Administrators, and the Joint Commission on Accreditation for Health Care Organizations. Increasingly payers and managed-care organisations are concerned about measuring performance.

Lessons from the 'Real World' where are we today: problems and issues

> Common sense remains a central paradigm in modern US evidence-based medicine. Common sense approaches, or educational guesses, continue to guide everyday clinical decision-making. Given remaining gaps in our knowledge base, we may question the soundness of some of the educational guesses made, but when it comes right down to making a clinical decision, the clinician must rely on his or her own knowledge of the existing evidence or lack of evidence, previous experience, and clinical intuition. Much of the clinical intuition defines the 'art of medicine'.
>
> (Tonelli 1998)

Philosophical underpinnings for the Diagnostic and Statistical Manual: what is the right role of evidence?

While evidence-based approaches to psychiatric classification are essential to the credibility of the field, it has important limitations and is not without its implicit and explicit set of values (Pincus and McQueen in press). The goals of DSM-IV are fourfold

1. clinical
2. research
3. educational
4. information management.

Within each category, DSM-IV provides enhancement of the evidence-based process, but limitations are noted. For example, the application of criteria enhance the reliability of communication and assessment by providers, but the provision of a diagnosis does not provide the full spectrum of knowledge needed for treatment planning (as stated in the DSM-IV introduction). Also, while the DSM-IV helps to categorize information from different clinical sources and practitioners for information management, it was not designed to be a reimbursement manual for psychiatry. Rather the International Classification of Diseases, Ninth Revision, Clinical Modification (ICD-9-CM), maintained by the federal government, is the official reimbursement classification system in the US. ICD-9-CM codes are required for reimbursement from Medicare, Medicaid and most third-party payors. While the DSM-IV selected and attached appropriate codes from ICD-9-CM to DSM definitions, the primary purpose of DSM-IV remains as a communication tool for use among clinicians, and between clinicians and researchers.

Though DSM-IV represented the successful use of an evidence-based process, there are some problems in applying strict evidence-based approaches to psychiatric nosology (Kendler 1990). For example, in an evidence deterministic model, there would be a very limited role for historical tradition, clinical evidence, clinical experience, and common sense. In particular, some areas of the DSM-IV are less amenable to investigation and testing such as the utility of the multi-axial system. While its incorporation allowed clinicians the opportunity to capture and document relevant information across several domains, testing the hypothesis 'there should be a multi-axial system' has been difficult. In addition, if a very high standard of evidence is applied, only a very small number of conditions would be validated and these would not meet administrative or clinical needs.

Throughout the application of EBM, clinicians must apply their own experience, knowledge and intuition. As stated in the introduction of DSM-IV, the evidence, often derived from more rarified tertiary care settings, should not be taken too literally in applying it to individual patients; providers must use common sense to combine the various components of knowledge.

Examples from polypharmacy

Studies of real-world practice in American psychiatry have indicated that the evidence available does not always reflect what is actually happening. In a survey of psychiatrists, Pincus et al. (1999) documented that of the patients being treated by psychiatrists, 58.4 per cent were receiving more than one psychotherapeutic medication and 31.2 per cent were receiving three or more. The overwhelming use of polypharmacy has raised concern regarding the increase in the potential for drug–drug interactions, side effects and non-compliance. However, it is unclear whether this polypharmacy or co-pharmacy (the simultaneous use of different classes of medications) found in routine practice represents less than optimal care or should be thought of as a divergence from the evidence (Reus 1993; Post et al. 1996). Good reasons may exist for the use of polypharmacy. Possible explanations for this practice include the complexity and severity of the patients' conditions, as well as patient preferences (Pincus et al. 1999). For example, patients in typical practice settings may be systematically different from those seen in clinical trials. Data from the Pincus et al. (1999) study demonstrated significant comorbidity and heterogeneity among the patient population treated by psychiatrists, which may necessitate the use of several medications. In addition, under the structure of managed care, it is possible that those patients that are referred to and treated by psychiatrists are 'further down on the algorithm' and earlier treatments may have failed, thus requiring more complicated treatment regimens. It is also possible that patients prefer to receive an additional medication after only experiencing a partial response to a single medication rather than risk relapse by substitution (by giving up their current medication).

US Surgeon General's report on mental health

The release of *Mental Health: a Report of the Surgeon General* in 1999 (US Department of Health and Human Services 1999) marked the end of a decade of accumulating evidence about the efficacy and effectiveness of mental health services. The landmark report emphasized the gap between the opportunities offered by scientific advances and the realities of practice. It called for increased access and widespread improvements to mental health services in the US. The report underscores the importance of EBM for mental health services in the new century.

Conclusions

During the past 20 years, there has been an enormous expansion in the scientific base of mental health. The extent to which mental health practice in the US has become more evidence based is debatable however. The adoption of evidenced-based approaches has been led in part by the tremendous growth in NIH and pharmaceutical industry funding as well as by efforts taken within American psychiatry to develop an evidence-based system for classifying mental disorders. These efforts have been greatly influenced by national changes in the structure, financing, and provision of mental health services. Various activities, such as health-care reform, continue to evolve as a driving force to refocus the agenda for EBM. Therefore, the strategies and tools developed to promote EBM have also evolved to incorporate strategies at multiple levels (provider, health plan, patient/consumer, practice/ delivery system, purchaser) to improve their implementation and compliance, as well as mechanisms and tools for measuring their success. As studies continue to be conducted, the true test of their utility will be determined as we evaluate whether the evidence in fact influences clinician behavior and/or improves the quality of the care provided.

Chapter 6

Evidence – the postmodern perspective

Richard Laugharne

Modernism and scientific evidence

Scientific evidence can be viewed as a highly modernist concept. Modernism is the philosophical movement emerging from the enlightenment and is characterised by rationalism, materialism and reductionism. Nature follows rules that are reasonable and found by measuring features of the material world. If the material world is complex it can be understood by breaking it down by its component parts and measuring how these parts work and how they interact. In practice this philosophy results in the observation and meas-urement of the universe. The non-material world is regarded as of dubious validity, such as belief systems which are impossible to verify through observation. From many different observations general rules are looked for, with an underlying assumption that the fragments of observation can lead to the discovery of universal laws that will then predict future observations. The observers are assumed not to affect the system being observed and to be impartial in interpreting their measurements. This distance between observer and observed leads to the objectivity of the truth which is found.

Scientific evidence in mental health has endeavoured to utilize this model despite some inherent difficulties. Many of the phenomena of mental illness are hard to locate in a material world and scientists have tried to measure subjective experience through the patient's own reports instead. Nevertheless a quantification of reductionist components of mental experience has been the mainstay of mental health research.

Evidence-based medicine has its roots in the modernist paradigm and this model has a remarkable track record in its effects on our lives. The consequences of science and technology have provided human beings with greater efficiency in production, greater prosperity (for some) and improved health through medicine. Few would argue that there have been huge benefits. However, the other side of the coin has included the capacity and reality of military destruction on a truly devastating scale and the possibility of ecological disaster leading to destruction of life on a similar if not greater scale. At a more intimate level people feel dehumanized by the scientific world view. They are reduced to a complex machine by medics, a means of production by industrialists and businessmen, and a means to power by politicians.

The postmodern challenge to a scientific world view

The postmodern challenge to modernist scientific thinking is difficult to summarize, and indeed avoids easy definition. The most straightforward summary is in what it rejects – the modern paradigm. First it rejects the idea of meta-narratives, big stories explaining reality, and hence the concept of universality. Science can be seen as a meta-narrative, tyrannical in its assumption that the truths it establishes are superior to other world views (Lyotard 1984). Instead micro-narratives relevant to certain people at a certain time and place are acceptable without demanding relevance to all.

Second the concept of objectivity is rejected. Many in our society question the idea of a scientific community disinterested in the results of its observations. Scientists seek knowledge not for pursuit of truth but for power, whether that power is through status or commercial interest. Does a pharamaceutical company honestly claim objectivity when financing a scientist? Has the scientific community effectively created a climate in which negative findings have equal status to positive findings? In mental health the relationships between knowledge and power have a special relevance as psychiatrists have to balance their role of advancing the medical science of treating the mentally ill with the social role given to the profession of depriving certain citizens of their liberty on the grounds of mental illness.

Third postmodern thought asserts there are different views of truth. In mental health different viewpoints have consistently been put forward by patients, carers, clinicians (with differing views from each profession), purchasers of care and the public. Each cites different evidence to support their viewpoints. There is evidence from biological, psychological and social research with differing methodologies. Psychoanalytic models cite forms of evidence that are different to the research given by behavioural or biological models. In a modernist world a single universal group of laws would be sought from all this data. In a postmodern world this is not only futile but also unacceptable. And an acceptance of uncertainty should underline the differing views present.

Conflicts with scientific evidence-based medicine

The postmodern viewpoint can seem a nihilistic rejection of enlightenment values, the consequences of which could lead to chaos. However, postmodern thinking is already having an impact on mental health care and on society as a whole. The rise of the user movement in mental health care has many postmodern features (Laugharne 1999). The user movement challenges the objectivity of scientific medicine, arguing that the selected evidence supports the power of clinicians and the use of medication, creating wealth for the pharmaceutical industry (Perkins 2000). The evidence of patients, clearly subjective, is given more validity than observations from non-patients. Another challenge is to the application of research on groups of patients to individual patients. Each person wants to be treated as an individual and not as a member of a diagnostic group on whom a uniform treatment is applied. This is a fundamental challenge to the concept of treatment guidelines, when effectively people are reduced to a diagnosis. In other words, in a postmodern world different people require different treatments according to different truths.

The increase in influence of evidence-based medicine has been enhanced by the need to keep health costs under control. It is quite reasonable to try to control costs by insisting that treatments are backed up by evidence. However there are two problems with this approach. First it assumes there is enough evidence to make a judgement on the options available and that this evidence is objective. Second the evidence is often interpreted by a panel of professionals and is therefore paternalistic in nature. As patients have increased access to information and evidence through the internet, why can not they make their own interpretation of the evidence? Here we come to the externally vexed question of how much health care can be influenced by consumerism. When most aspects of commercial life are governed by consumerism, the expensive business of health-care delivery will not continue as a process of experts telling consumers what they can and cannot have, especially when the consumers have access to the evidence, and can criticize its inadequacy and observe its lack of objectivity. The professional cry for the need for more and better research to come to a final objective reality is a demand for utopia as naïve as any religious cult. An unarguable and objective truth through scientific research in mental health is, according to postmodern thought, impossible.

Despite the increasing importance given to evidence-based medicine in health, the public is refusing to reject treatments that are argued to have a lack of evidence base. A recent piece of qualitative research, carried out by users on users, found one of the greatest demands by patients was for increased access to complementary medicine (Mental Health Foundation 2000). Another study on the use of alternative medicine reported that 'the majority of alternative medicine users appear to be doing so not so much as a result of being dissatisfied with conventional medicine but largely because they find these health care alternatives to be more congruent with their own values, beliefs and philosophical orientations towards health and life' (Astin 1998, p. 1548). It appears that 'in the modern era, the effectiveness of health-care interventions has increased, but has also been accompanied by an increase in alienation and dissatisfaction' (Gray 1999, p. 1552).

Spiritual belief and moral frameworks have always had an uneasy relationship with the modernist philosophy because of their non-material foundations.

Whilst many scientists have had strong religious faith and seen evidence for the existence of God in the natural world, the scientific model has worked without need for a spiritual or moral explanation. But the importance of spiritual belief has been repeatedly found when patients have been asked what helps them most with living with mental health problems (Mental Health Foundation 1997, 2000).

Evidence in a postmodern society

The modernist model of scientific evidence is robust. It has a clear philosophy and a track record of some remarkable successes that have benefited humankind enormously. Any philosophy that has survived and thrived for about 400 years can cope with some strong challenges. But these challenges will not go away and must be met. Science in the past has looked at other ways of viewing reality as inferior.

> The scientist questions the validity of narrative statements and concludes that they are never subject to argumentation or proof. He classifies them as belonging to a different mentality: savage, primitive, underdeveloped, backward, alienated, composed of opinions, customs, authority, prejudice, ignorance, ideology. Narratives are fables, myths, legends, fit only for women and children. At best, attempts are made to throw some rays of light into this obscurantism, to civilize, educate, develop.
>
> (Lyotard 1984)

The future must surely be not to reject scientific evidence in mental health care but first to acknowledge its strengths and limitations and learn to present it as a valuable source of information that can co-exist with other forms of evidence. Practitioners of scientific viewpoints can accept the validity of other positions such as users, carers, purchasers and the public. Whilst an acceptance of the doubtfulness of objectivity of scientific evidence is needed, the acceptability of openly subjective evidence from sufferers of mental illness needs to be acknowledged by the scientific community.

The practice of mental health care should not be a scientific exercise but an exercise in humanity, informed by ethical and moral choices. We as clinicians are educated in the scientific method and should advocate for its inclusion in the overall narrative of mental health care provision. We should not expect this evidence to be supreme over other evidence or 'trump' evidence from other sources. Different forms of evidence from different people with different viewpoints may not create chaos but enrich the decisions that are made and lead to an ethical service acceptable to the people who matter most, the recipients of mental health care.

Section 2

Methodological approaches

Chapter 7

Randomised controlled trials – misunderstanding, fraud and spin

Max Marshall

Overview

The purpose of this chapter is to draw attention to some of the limitations of randomised controlled trials (RCTs) in psychiatry. I will illustrate these limitations using examples drawn from my experience of conducting systematic reviews of non-pharmacological interventions for schizophrenia. I will conclude the chapter with some thoughts on how psychiatric trials could be improved.

Advantages and limitations of the randomised controlled trial in psychiatry

The RCT is notable simply because it is randomised (there is no other essential difference between the RCT and other quasi-experimental ways of evaluating treatment) (Kleijnen *et al.* 1997). Randomisation is important because it is the only sure way of abolishing bias at the point of patient assignment. I do not intend to review the considerable evidence for the importance of randomisation, but some idea of the extent of this evidence is given in a recent paper in the *British Medical Journal* (Kunz and Oxman 1998). This paper is a systematic review of systematic reviews that had compared the size of effect in randomised versus non-randomised trials. The review found that of eight systematic reviews (covering 280 trials), five showed a gross overestimation of size of effect by non-randomised trials, one showed an accurate estimation and two showed a gross underestimation. Thus non-randomised trials rarely give an estimate of effect size that is close to the true value. The review concluded that failure to use adequately concealed random allocation can distort the apparent effects of care in either direction, though usually in overestimation, causing effects to seem larger or smaller than they really are. The bottom line is that if you want to know whether a treatment works there is no alternative to the RCT.

Much of this chapter will be spent outlining the special pitfalls in psychiatric RCTs, but these criticisms are not intended to imply that the RCT should be abandoned. There is no doubt that it remains our best available method for evaluating the effectiveness of a treatment. However, being the best available method is not the same as being the perfect method, and there is no doubt that RCTs have limitations. Randomised controlled trials do not tell us how treatments work or why they fail to work. They have great difficulty in dealing with rare outcomes; for example no randomised control trial is ever going to tell us whether assertive outreach teams or 'risk assessment' reduces homicide. There are problems with generalisability – just because a treatment works in a trial does not mean it will work in everyday practice. But perhaps the biggest problem, at least for psychiatry, is that RCTs are not free from bias: they are just free from bias at the point of assignment. In fact RCTs are not the perfect way of evaluating a treatment, they are just the least unsatisfactory way.

The general problems with RCTs are well known, and although I have alluded to some of them above, I do not intend to deal with them at length in this chapter. Instead I am going to focus on three special problems, two of which are common in psychiatric trials. The first problem I have called 'misunderstanding' – misunderstanding of what a treatment is and how it has changed over time. The second problem, fraud, is defined as deliberate falsification of results. The third problem, which I call 'spin', is an attempt to mislead that falls short of actual falsification.

Misunderstanding

A good example of the 'misunderstanding' of data from RCTs is the introduction of the care programme approach in the UK. The care programme approach has been described as the 'cornerstone' of English community care policy (Shepherd 1990). It is based on an American idea known as case management which holds that every patient should have a key worker who is responsible for assessing their needs, constructing a care plan to meet these needs, making sure the care is delivered and maintaining contact with the patient. Case management has been described as a key way of reducing rates of re-admission to hospital, as well as improving outcome (Solomon 1992), but there is evidence to suggest that it does not work well.

The Cochrane plot in Figure 7.1 summarises the evidence for the effectiveness of case management at reducing admission rates in England. The relevant trials are listed on the left-hand side of the figure. Each trial is associated with two fractions in the next two columns from the left. The numerators in each fraction represent the numbers of people in the treatment (first fraction) and control groups (second fraction) admitted to hospital during the trial, whilst the denominators represent the total number in the treatment and control groups. In the fourth column each trial is represented by a square pierced by a horizontal line. The size of the square represents the size of the trial, and the centre of the square indicates the

Comparison: case management versus standard care
Outcome: number admitted to hospital

Study	Case management n/N	Control n/N	RR (95% CI fixed)	Weight %	RR (95% CI fixed)
Audini et al. 1994	9/33	9/33		2.8	1.00 [0.45, 2.20]
Marshall et al. 1995	17/40	10/40		3.2	1.70 [0.89, 3.25]
Ford et al. 1995	17/39	14/38		4.5	1.18 [0.68, 2.05]
Tyrer et al. 1995	58/196	35/197		11.0	1.67 [1.15, 2.41]
Holloway and Carson 1998	15/35	11/35		3.5	1.36 [0.73, 2.54]
Burns et al. 1999	219/353	238/355		75.0	0.93 [0.83, 1.03]
Total (95% CI)	335/696	317/698		100.0	1.06 [0.96, 1.18]

Chi-square 14.52 (df = 6) P = 0.01 Z = 1.10 P < 0.00001

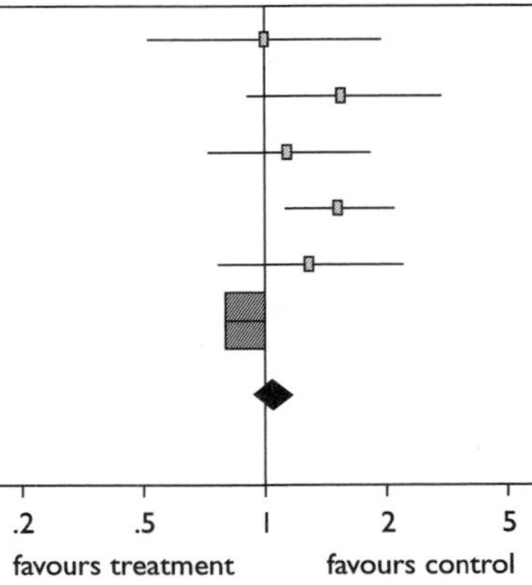

.2   .5   1   2   5

favours treatment   favours control

Figure 7.1 Effect of case management on admission rates in the UK

relative risk of being admitted to hospital for participants in the trial. The horizontal line piercing the square represents the 95 per cent confidence intervals for the relative risk. The squares are distributed about a vertical line called 'the line of no effect', which represents a relative risk of one (i.e. no difference in risk between treatment and control groups). When the centre of a square falls to the left of the line of no effect, by convention this indicates that the trial represented by the square found that the experimental treatment was superior to the control treatment. Similarly, when the centre of a square falls to the right this indicates that the control treatment was superior. When the line piercing the square intersects with the line of no effect, this indicates that the difference between treatment and control groups was not significant, whereas if it fails to intersect with the line this indicates that the difference was significant. The combined data from all the trials represented in Figure 7.1 is represented by a summary diamond at the bottom of column four, the centre of the diamond represents the summary relative risk, whilst the horizontal points of the diamond are the confidence intervals for the summary relative risk.

Figure 7.1 shows that case management has no clinically significant effect on admission rates in the UK. Case management does improve engagement in care a little (the number needed to treat for the studies shown in Figure 7.1 is 11, 95 per cent CI 8–19, this means that for every 11 people who receive case management one fewer is lost to follow up than if they had all received standard care), but it does not affect the duration of admission or any other clinical variable. Costs to the NHS tend not to be increased (Marshall *et al.* 1999). Looking at this data it seems hard to understand why psychiatric services in the UK have spent so much energy implementing such an ineffectual intervention. This misunderstanding is reflected in the long list of synonyms that are applied to case management in the scientific literature: case management, care management, intensive case management, intensive care management, clinical case management, home-based care, intensive outreach, assertive outreach, the Madison Model, assertive case management, care programme approach, etc. This confused terminology obscures the fundamental point that there are basically two different approaches to case management. The first, 'assertive community treatment', is a highly specified team-based approach, defined by treatment manuals and fidelity scales. The second, 'case management', is a more individualistic approach that is not tightly specified.

Trials from the US suggest that assertive community treatment is an effective way of reducing admission rates and that it can reduce costs when applied to high users of in-patient care. On the other hand US trials of case management are not promising (Marshall and Lockwood 1999; Marshall *et al.* 1999). Yet when one looks back at policy documents justifying the introduction of case management into the UK, they generally refer to US trials of assertive community treatment, not to US trials of case management. Thus an ineffectual intervention was promoted as a result of a misunderstanding that arose from the confusing nature of 'case management' terminology – assertive community treatment was mistaken for ordinary case management. By the time that UK trials had confirmed that case management was ineffective it was too late; the care programme approach had arrived.

Another form of misunderstanding arises because psychiatric treatments (including control treatments) have a tendency to evolve. This problem is illustrated in Figure 7.2a, which shows a Cochrane plot from a review in progress (Marshall et al. 2000). This review is concerned with the use of day-hospital treatment as an alternative to in-patient care, and the variable in question is number of patients lost to follow up. At first sight the trials on the Cochrane plot seem inconsistent in their findings – some trials seem to show the day hospital doing well on this variable, whereas others show it doing badly. This variation in effect size between trials is known as heterogeneity. Heterogeneity, when present at a statistically significant level (as in this trial, see the chi-squared test at the bottom of the plot) suggests that the difference in effect size between trials is caused by something more than random variation. The probable cause of the heterogeneity becomes clear when the trials are ordered by year (see Figure 7.2b). From this figure it appears that early day-hospital trials tend to lose more patients to follow up than control treatments, whereas more recent trials tend to lose about the same or less. This suggests that clinical practice in day-hospital trials has been evolving, and this supposition is supported by the descriptions of the day hospitals provided in the trial reports. The more recent trials (e.g. Creed 1990; Wiersma 1991; Sledge 1998) all involved day hospitals that were equipped with some form of respite or outreach care, whilst the later trials did not. Thus day-hospital treatment has evolved in line with the general tendency for psychiatric services to put more emphasis on engaging and retaining contact with their patients. This finding may also explain why early day-hospitals researchers believed that day-hospital treatment was reducing re-admission rates, perhaps patients who would have been re-admitted were simply being lost to follow up.

Another apparent example of the evolution of a treatment can be found on the Cochrane Library review of family intervention for schizophrenia (Pharoah et al. 2000). This review discovered a marked tendency for the difference in relapse rates favouring family intervention to decrease steadily over the years. This effect is particularly evident at a 7- to 12-month and a 19- to 24-month follow up. The reviewers concluded that 'the pioneering clinicians who first evaluated family interventions do seem to get better results than those who came later'. The reasons for this curious finding are unclear.

Study	Treatment n/N	Control n/N	RR (95% CI fixed)	Weight %	RR (95% CI fixed)
Creed et al. 1990 (UK)	19/51	13/51		11.0	1.46 [0.81, 2.63]
Creed et al. 1997 (UK)	23/94	23/93		19.6	0.99 [0.60, 1.63]
Dick et al. 1985 (UK)	5/43	3/48		2.4	1.86 [0.47, 7.33]
Herz et al. 1971 (US)	11/45	7/45		5.9	1.57 [0.67, 3.69]
Sledge et al. 1996 (US)	19/93	37/104		29.5	0.57 [0.36, 0.93]
Wiersma et al. 1991 (NL)	36/103	29/57		31.6	0.69 [0.48, 0.99]
Total (95% CI)	113/429	112/398		100.0	0.88 [0.71, 1.09]

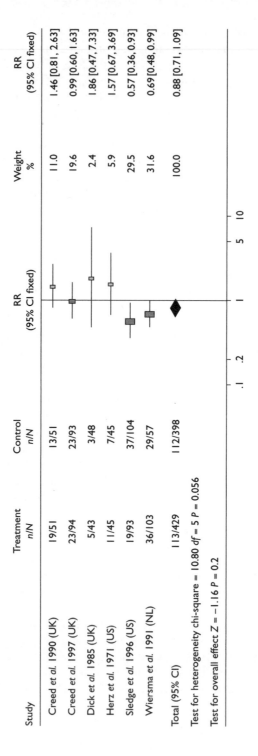

Test for heterogeneity chi-square = 10.80 df = 5 P = 0.056

Test for overall effect Z = –1.16 P = 0.2

Figure 7.2 Day hospital versus admission to hospital
a) Numbers lost to follow-up at the end of the study

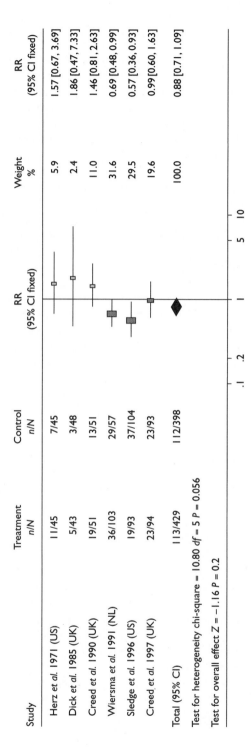

Study	Treatment n/N	Control n/N	RR (95% CI fixed)	Weight %	RR (95% CI fixed)
Herz et al. 1971 (US)	11/45	7/45		5.9	1.57 [0.67, 3.69]
Dick et al. 1985 (UK)	5/43	3/48		2.4	1.86 [0.47, 7.33]
Creed et al. 1990 (UK)	19/51	13/51		11.0	1.46 [0.81, 2.63]
Wiersma et al. 1991 (NL)	36/103	29/57		31.6	0.69 [0.48, 0.99]
Sledge et al. 1996 (US)	19/93	37/104		29.5	0.57 [0.36, 0.93]
Creed et al. 1997 (UK)	23/94	23/93		19.6	0.99 [0.60, 1.63]
Total (95% CI)	113/429	112/398		100.0	0.88 [0.71, 1.09]

Test for heterogeneity chi-square = 10.80 df = 5 P = 0.056

Test for overall effect Z = −1.16 P = 0.2

Figure 7.2b numbers lost to follow-up at the end of the study, trials ordered by year

Fraud

Fraud occurs when researchers make up results, whereas 'spin' occurs when they deliberately misrepresent or misinterpret real results. The purpose of both fraud and spin is usually to increase the chances of publication in a peer-reviewed journal, by making a treatment seem more effective than it actually is. It is hard to be certain that fraud has occurred unless someone confesses to it, but it is not unusual in the course of a systematic review to come across anomalies that raise questions about the veracity of the data. One such indicator is an 'outlier', a phenomenon that is hard to spot when reading trial reports, but quite obvious from a Cochrane plot. Outliers are by no means a sure sign of fraud, but fraudulent studies will tend to be outliers, because it is difficult for those who are creating fraudulent data to guess the true effect size. Figure 7.3 illustrates an outlier using anonymised data from a Cochrane plot. The summary diamond and all the trials, bar one, are centred to the right of the line of no effect, strongly suggesting that on this variable the intervention is not effective. However one study (study D) shows a substantial effect, even though the intervention and the patient population were similar to those used in the other trials. Note that the summary diamond does not fall within the study D's very wide confidence intervals, suggesting that effect is unlikely to be caused by the small size of the study.

I am aware of two other anomalies that suggest, but do not prove, that something may be amiss with a trial. The first anomaly concerns data with an unexpectedly normal distribution. For example, studies that involve interventions that affect admission rates are notorious for producing skewed economic data. This is because in-patient care is so expensive relative to other types of care that there tends to be a long 'tail' in the cost data, representing those patients who have spent time in hospital (Gray et al. 1997). Typically, in a trial of this kind, the standard deviation of summary cost data will be of about the same magnitude as the mean (or larger), indicating that the data are skewed. However, there are rare examples of data of this kind where the standard deviation indicates that the data are normally or near-normally distributed. This is a phenomenon that I am unable to explain.

The second anomaly is related to the observation that when several rating scales are used in the same trial they tend to obtain different completion rates (for reasons such as patients tiring with the procedure or disliking the format of a particular scale). Occasionally, the systematic reviewer will come across a trial where the follow-up rate on all instruments is the same. This may be coincidence, but one's suspicions are deepened in situations when one or more of the rating scales requires the co-operation of family members to complete. It is an odd coincidence if all the patients followed up in a schizophrenia trial (other than a trial of a family intervention) happen to live with co-operative families.

Comparison: intervention versus standard care
Outcome: admitted to hospital

Study	Experimental n/N	Control n/N	Peto odds ratio (95% CI fixed)	Weight %	Peto odds ratio (95% CI fixed)
Study A	48/147	22/145		22.0	2.60 [1.52, 4.45]
Study B	17/39	14/38		7.7	1.32 [0.53, 3.26]
Study C	62/213	38/204		31.4	1.77 [1.13, 2.78]
Study D	0/20	6/21		2.2	0.11 [0.02, 0.59]
Study E	17/40	10/40		7.5	2.17 [0.86, 5.44]
Study F	58/196	35/197		29.3	1.92 [1.21, 3.06]
Total (95% CI)	202/655	125/645		100.0	1.84 [1.43, 2.37]

Chi-square 12.88 (df = 5) P = 0.04 Z = 4.77 P < 0.00001

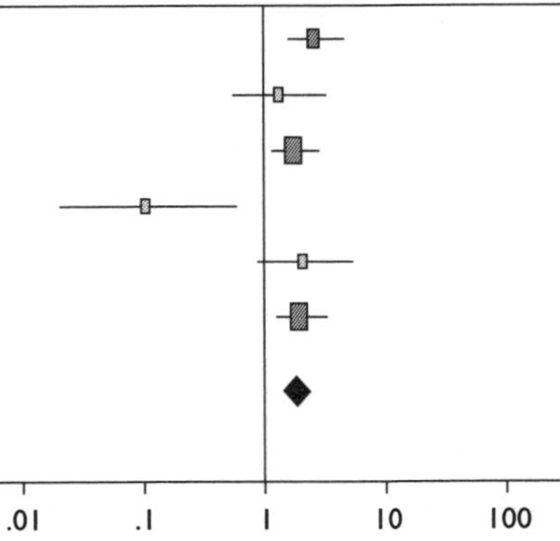

.01   .1   1   10   100

Figure 7.3 Example of an outlier

It is not possible at present to make an accurate estimate of the frequency of the anomalies discussed above. From my own experience of systematic reviews in schizophrenia I would guess that they occur at frequencies of about one in forty to one in one hundred trials.

Spin

Fraud in non-pharmacological schizophrenia trials is probably rare, whereas 'spin' is endemic. Three common types of 'spin' can be identified

1. spinning by selective reporting
2. spinning using rating scales
3. meta-spinning.

Spinning by selective reporting

Selective reporting most commonly occurs when a researcher decides not to report a disappointingly negative finding. This is easier in psychiatry than in other areas of medicine because psychiatric trials tend to use many different outcome measures. An example of possible selective reporting is apparent in a soon-to-be-published systematic review of trials of different approaches to vocational rehabilitation (Crowther *et al.* 2000). The review considers two different approaches to helping severely mentally ill people obtain employment, the first approach is pre-vocational training to gradually prepare clients for work, whilst the second is supported employment, helping clients to find a job as quickly as possible and then offering on-the-job support. Both approaches have been reasonably well studied in RCTs. The review identified five RCTs of pre-vocational training versus standard care, involving about 1,000 patients in total. The review also identified five RCTs of supported employment versus pre-vocational training, involving about 500 patients in total. The main point of vocational rehabilitation is to help people with severe mental disorders to obtain competitive employment, but curiously the number of people obtaining competitive employment was only reported in two of the five trials of pre-vocational training versus standard care (and in both cases there was no significant difference). The trials of supported employment versus pre-vocational training shed some light on this omission. They found that supported employment was significantly more effective than pre-vocational training in helping people to obtain competitive employment, whereas the success rate of pre-vocational training in absolute terms was low, at best about 14 per cent. It would be interesting to know whether the three trials of pre-vocational training versus standard care that failed to report rates of competitive employment actually collected data on this outcome.

Spinning using rating scales

Two other opportunities for 'spinning' arise from the psychiatric tradition of evaluating outcome using multiple rating scales. These opportunities involve either multiple testing or the use of unpublished scales. Some idea of the scale of these types of 'spinning' can be seen in a recent study from the Cochrane Schizophrenia Group (Marshall *et al.* 2000). In this study two teams of raters examined a randomly selected sample of 300 trials from the Schizophrenia Group's register of randomised controlled trials of treatments for schizophrenia. One hundred and fifty of the trials were of pharmacological treatments and 150 were of non-pharmacological treatments. The teams identified all comparisons between experimental and control groups that were made using rating scales. The teams identified each occasion on which the authors of the paper claimed that there was a significant difference between treatment and control groups in favour of treatment, based on data from a rating scale. These claims were then classified according to whether they were based on

1. a summary score before the end-point of the trial
2. a score on a scale sub-factor or constituent item
3. the summary score on the scale at the end-point of the trial.

The study found that 205 of 456 comparisons between experimental and control groups resulted in the researchers claiming a significant difference in favour of the experimental treatment. However only 90 of the 205 claims of a significant difference were based on summary scores at the end point of the trial. In other words, 56 per cent of the claims of significance arising from rating-scale data were based on some form of multiple testing; either separate testing of scale items or sub-factors, or testing at follow-up points other than the end point of the trial.

However, the 'spinning' did not end with multiple testing. In the second part of the study, the teams established the publication status of each scale used in the trials, whilst blind to the outcome of any comparisons made using the scale. Subsequent analysis showed that researchers were more likely to claim that a treatment was superior to control when the comparison was made using an unpublished scale (relative risk 1.94, 95 per cent CI 1.35–2.79). Without invoking bias, it is hard to explain why unpublished scales are twice as good as published scales at detecting significant differences in trials. The most plausible explanation is that there has been some *post hoc* adjustment of the constituent items of unpublished scales. This would involve dropping items from the scale in order to create or enlarge a difference on the overall score in favour of the experimental treatment. Unpublished scales are particularly amenable to this kind of 'adjustment', as they tend to belong to the researchers themselves or their colleagues, making protests unlikely.

In summary, in a random sample of 300 schizophrenia trials, only 50 out of 205 claims of treatment superiority, based on rating-scale data, could be considered safe. 'Spinning' in schizophrenia trials was not the exception but the rule.

Meta-spin

The pervasiveness of misunderstanding and 'spin' in psychiatric trials has important consequences for reviews. As I have shown, psychiatric interventions tend to be poorly defined and even within trials our means of assessing outcome tend to be prone to bias. Consequently, psychiatric trials, particularly of social psychiatric interventions, tend to show inconsistent results, especially on variables where outcome is measured by rating scales. Reviewers, who have to evaluate these inconsistent results, tend to end up in disarray. An example of this phenomenon can be seen in reviews of the effectiveness of case management from the early 1990s, see Box 7.1. The problem that these reviewers faced was how to deal with studies producing utterly inconsistent results on measurements of mental state, social functioning and quality of life. As you can see in Box 7.1, experts A and B concluded that the evidence was inconclusive whereas experts C and D, working from the same trials, concluded that the data were favourable. In the end the reviewers' conclusions were primarily determined by whether they were pessimists or optimists, the former looking on inconsistent results with suspicion, and the latter welcoming the 'broad range' of positive findings

---

Box 7.1   Reviewers' conclusions about case management

Expert A, 1990   'much of the evidence is inconclusive and somewhat contradictory'
Expert B, 1991   'inconsistent results fall short of providing conclusive evidence that any case management models are effective'
Expert C, 1992   'overall . . . favourable findings in relation to a wide range of clinical, social and economic variables'
Expert D, 1992   'the evidence seems to indicate that case management is most effective in reducing the number of rehospitalizations and . . . reducing the length of stay'
Expert E, 1991   'a great deal more research is required'
Expert E, 1995   'despite the extensive research available, only tentative and qualified conclusions can be made'

(even though most 'positive' findings were outnumbered by negative findings on the same variable). This is not a problem that can be solved by more research as expert E discovered. In a review in 1991 (Holloway 1991) he/she concluded that a great deal more research was needed, but 4 years later, after a great deal more research, he/she concluded that the inconsistencies in the data permitted only tentative conclusions.

Improving randomised controlled trials in psychiatry

The introduction of systematic review techniques has done much to clarify the problems caused by the inadequacies of psychiatric trials, but there is still much that could be done. Based on the information presented in this chapter there are four obvious reforms that could clear up much misunderstanding and spin. First, researchers who develop new non-physical treatments should be expected to provide treatment manuals and fidelity scales that can be employed by the researchers who follow in their footsteps. Second, researchers, and especially policy makers, should be more careful with terminology, in particular avoiding synonyms (such as 'care management' for 'case management') and 'sounds-like' terms (such as 'assertive outreach' for 'assertive community treatment'), except in cases where there is a clearly explained and overriding justification for the new term. Third, editors should not permit researchers or reviewers to draw conclusions about the effectiveness of treatment based on rating-scale data, unless that data consists of a summary score at the end point of the trial. Fourth, editors should not accept trial reports that contain outcomes based on data from unpublished scales.

Chapter 8

Systematic reviews and meta-analyses

John Geddes and Stuart Carney

Introduction

Over two million articles are published each year in 20,000 biomedical journals (Mulrow 1994). Some form of summary of this information is clearly essential. Even if a clinician or researcher restricted their reading to high-yield clinical psychiatry journals, they would need to read over 5,000 articles a year (Geddes *et al.* 1999a). This is clearly impossible for the majority of clinicians who have around 30 minutes a week to keep up to date with the latest developments (Sackett *et al.* 1997). There is an obvious need, with such a wealth of information, for reliable reviews of the literature. Systematic reviews attempt to address this need for reliable summaries of primary research.

The terms *systematic review*, *overview* and *meta-analysis* are often used interchangeably but actually refer to different things. In this chapter we will use these terms according to the following definitions.

- *Systematic review (synonym overview)* a review of primary research studies in which specific methodological strategies that limit bias are used and clearly described in the systematic identification, assembly, critical appraisal and synthesis of all relevant studies on a specific topic.
- *Meta-analysis (synonym quantitative overview)* a systematic review that employs statistical methods to combine and summarise the results of several studies (Cook *et al.* 1995).

Systematic reviews can be contrasted with traditional narrative reviews, which often have no method section and a number of methodological flaws (Mulrow 1987). There is a specific, rapidly developing, methodology for systematic reviews. It is worth emphasising that meta-analyses should only be undertaken following systematic review and they are not an essential part of a systematic review because it may be inappropriate to proceed to statistical summary of the individual studies (see pp. 78–80). A meta-analysis that is performed in the absence of a systematic review of the literature can be particularly misleading because it can lead to a biased estimate of effect. The mental health worker may be interested to know that the first use of the term 'meta-analysis' was by Smith and Glass in their systematic review of the effects of psychotherapy (Smith and Glass 1977).

As a research tool, a systematic review of the literature can be applied to any form of research question. A methodologically sound systematic review helps to avoid *systematic error* and bias. The statistical techniques of meta-analysis, however, should not be used indiscriminately. Nevertheless, when used appropriately meta-analysis provides a method of pooling research data from more than one study to provide an estimate of effect size, which has greater power and precision than any of the constituent studies. This has obvious advantages for clinical research and practice because it provides a method of minimising *random error* and producing more precise, and potentially more generalisable, results.

In this chapter we will discuss the benefits of conducting systematic reviews of the literature and the circumstances in which it is appropriate to perform a meta-analysis. Our view is that the results of systematic reviews, with or without meta-analyses, can reliably and efficiently provide the information needed for rational clinical decision making (Mulrow 1994). However, in our experience the results of a review are rarely unequivocal and require careful appraisal and interpretation. When using reviews, clinicians therefore need to integrate the results with clinical expertise and the patient's preferences.

Systematic reviews

Why do reviews need to be systematic?

The literature is littered with unsystematic reviews, where the methods for identifying and appraising relevant studies are not explicit and it cannot be assumed that the methodology is adequate. The conclusions of such reviews must be viewed with suspicion as they may be misleading, though the extent to which they are unreliable is usually difficult to judge. In contrast, systematic reviews use explicit, and therefore reproducible, methods to limit bias and improve the reliability and accuracy of the conclusions (Mulrow 1994).

The first stage in conducting a systematic review is the formulation of a clear question. The nature of the question determines the type of research evidence to be reviewed and allows for the *a priori* specification of inclusion and exclusion criteria. For instance, to answer a question such as 'in the treatment of depressive disorder, are dual action drugs more effective than selective serotonin reuptake inhibitors?' the most reliable study design would be a randomised controlled trial (RCT). Randomisation avoids any systematic tendency to produce an unequal distribution of prognostic factors between the experimental and control treatments that could influence the outcome (Altman and Bland 1999). However, RCTs are not the most appropriate research design for all questions (Sackett and Wennberg 1997). A question such as 'do obstetric complications predispose to schizophrenia?' could not feasibly be answered by a RCT because it would neither be possible or ethical to randomise subjects to be exposed to obstetric complications. This is a form of *aetiological* question that would be best addressed by primary cohort and case controlled studies. Likewise, a *diagnostic* question such as 'how well can brief screening questions identify patients with depressive disorder?' would be best answered by a cross-sectional study of patients at risk of being depressed. The rationale for systematic review is the same for all questions – the avoidance of random error and systematic bias. Systematic reviews have been useful in synthesising primary research results in both aetiology (see, for example, the review of the association between obstetric complications and schizophrenia by Geddes and Lawrie 1996) and diagnosis (see, for example, the review of case-finding instruments for depression by Mulrow and her colleagues 1995). Systematic reviews of these other study designs have their own methodological problems, and guidelines exist for undertaking reviews and meta-analyses of diagnostic tests (Irwig *et al.* 1994) and the observational epidemiological designs used in aetiological research (Stroup *et al.* 2000).

The Cochrane Collaboration

The recognition of the need for systematic reviews of RCTs, and the development of the scientific methodology of reviews has been one of the most striking developments in health services research over the last decade (Chalmers *et al.* 1992). The first UK Cochrane Centre was established in Oxford in 1992 as part of the information systems strategy developed to support the National Health Service Research and Development Programme; centres have since been established in several other countries. Within the Cochrane Collaboration, there are several collaborative review groups in areas of practice relevant to mental health clinicians. There are active collaborative review groups in the field of mental health including the Cochrane Schizophrenia Review Group and the Cochrane Depression, Anxiety and Neurosis Group. Within psychiatry there are now over 100 Cochrane reviews.

The sources of bias in systematic reviews

Despite their potential to avoid bias, a number of factors can adversely affect the conclusions of a systematic review. When conducting a primary study it is important to ensure that the sample recruited is representative of the target population, otherwise the results may be misleading (selection bias). The most significant form of bias in systematic reviews is analogous to selection bias in primary studies, but applies to the selection of primary studies, rather than participants. There are various forms of selection bias including publication bias, language of publication bias and biases introduced by an over-reliance on electronic databases.

Publication bias

Publication bias is the tendency of investigators, reviewers and editors to differentially submit or accept manuscripts for publication based on the direction or strength of the study findings (Gottesman and Bertelsen 1989). The conclusions of systematic reviews can be significantly affected by publication bias. The potential pitfalls of publication bias are obvious: if only studies that demonstrate a treatment benefit are published, the conclusions may be misleading if the true effect is neutral or even harmful. As early as 1959 it was noted that 97.3 per cent of articles published in four major journals had statistically significant results (Sterling 1959) although it is likely that many studies were conducted which produced non-significant results and these were less likely to be published.

Various strategies have been proposed to counter publication bias (Gilbody and Song 2000). These include methods aimed at detecting its presence and preventing its occurrence. It is generally accepted that prevention is likely to be the most effective strategy and it has been proposed that the most effective method would be to establish trial registries of all studies (Simes 1986). This would mean that a record of the trial or study would exist regardless of whether or not it was published and should reduce the risk of 'negative' studies disappearing. It should also facilitate the work of systematic reviewers. Although registries of ongoing research have been slow to become established – perhaps because it is not clear who should take a lead or fund them – some have been created, for example a registry of trials (see, for example, http://www.controlled-trials.com/) and the register of studies performed under the auspices of the UK National Health Service (http://www.doh.gov.uk/research/nrr.htm/). While such registries may be useful prospectively, they do not solve the problem of retrospectively identifying primary studies. There are a number of methods for estimating the likelihood of the presence of publication bias in a sample of studies. One commonly used way of investigating publication bias is the *funnel plot* (Egger *et al.* 1997). In a funnel plot, the study-specific odds ratios are plotted against a measure of the study's precision (such as the inverse of the standard error or the number of cases in each study). There will be more variation in the results of small studies because of their greater susceptibility to random error and hence the results of the larger studies, with less random error, should cluster more closely around the 'true value'. If publication bias is not present, the graphical distribution of odds ratios should resemble an inverted funnel. If there is a gap in the region of the funnel where the results of small negative studies would be expected, then

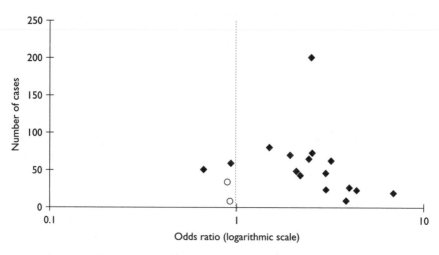

Figure 8.1 Funnel plot. The study-specific odds ratios have been plotted against a measure of the study's power (in this example, the number of cases). The diamonds represent case-control studies and the circles cohort studies. There is an absence of small case-control studies with odds ratios close to (or less than) 1. By chance, such studies should exist and their absence implies a degree of publication bias (from Geddes and Lawrie, 1996).

this would imply that the results of these studies are missing. This could be because of publication bias or it could mean that the search failed to find small negative studies. An example of a funnel plot from the meta-analysis of the association between obstetric complications and schizophrenia is shown in Figure 8.1. In this example it is clear that there is a gap in the distribution of odds ratios in the region of small negative studies. This would imply the presence of publication bias (Geddes and Lawrie 1996).

Strenuous attempts to avoid publication bias can cause other problems because it may require the incorporation of unpublished data which may not have been subject to peer review in systematic reviews and this has been controversial. Cook studied attitudes amongst meta-analysts and journal editors and found that meta-analysts were more inclined to use unpublished data than journal editors (Cook *et al.* 1993). Indeed 30 per cent of editors questioned would not publish overviews that included unpublished data. The journal editors argued that unpublished data was more likely to be subject to fraud or distortion and was less scientifically rigorous. It is, however, becoming increasingly recognised that publication in a peer-review journal, even a prestigious one, is no guarantee of scientific quality (Oxman *et al.* 1991). Unpublished data, however, can be problematic as the data supplied may not be a full or representative sample (Cook *et al.* 1993). Reliance only on published data may also be problematic and, in many situations, it is useful to obtain the disaggregated original data – though this dramatically increases the size of the task of reviewing (Clarke and Stewart 1994; Geddes *et al.* 1999b).

Nowhere is the impact of publication bias more obvious than in a meta-analysis. Using the 'trim and fill' method to evaluate bias in funnel plots, Sutton *et al.* found that in 8 per cent of reviews in the Cochrane Database of Systematic Reviews, the statistical inferences regarding the effect of the intervention were changed (Sutton *et al.* 2000). The 'trim and fill' method adjusts for any asymmetry in a funnel plot in calculating the pooled estimate of effect. Although this method is controversial, the study does demonstrate the potential impact of publication bias on the estimate of effect size.

Language of publication bias (Tower of Babel bias)

Restricting a search to one language (for example searching only for English-language papers) can be hazardous. It has been shown that studies that find a treatment effect are more likely to be published in English-language journals, whilst opposing studies may be published in non-English-language journals (Egger and Smith 1998). Language of publication bias has also been called the 'Tower of Babel' bias (Gregoire *et al.* 1995).

Uncritical use of electronic databases

With the increasing availability of convenient electronic bibliographic databases, there is a danger that reviewers may rely on them unduly. This can cause bias because electronic databases do not offer comprehensive or unbiased coverage of the relevant primary literature. Adams investigated the adequacy of Medline searches for RCTs in mental health care and found that the optimal Medline search had a sensitivity of only 52 per cent (CI 48–56 per cent) (Adams *et al.* 1994). Sensitivity can be improved by searching other databases in addition to Medline, for example Embase, PsycLit, Psyndex, CINAHL and Lilacs.

To avoid the limitations of relying on electronic databases – or any other resource – for the identification of primary studies, reviews undertaken under the auspices of the Cochrane Collaboration seek to use optimally sensitive, over-inclusive searches to identify as many studies as possible with a combination of electronic searching, handsearching, reference checking and personal communications (Cochrane Collaboration 1995).

Meta-analysis

While a meta-analysis is not an essential part of a systematic review, a meta-analysis should only be performed in the context of a systematic review. The technique of meta-analysis has been controversial and this is perhaps because it is potentially so powerful, but it is also particularly susceptible to abuse. Here, we review a number of key issues in meta-analysis.

Increasing statistical power by pooling the results of individual studies

Many trials, especially in psychiatry, are small (Johnson 1983; Thornley and Adams 1998). There are many difficulties in recruiting patients to randomised trials, although some of these difficulties have been minimised in other areas of medicine by simplification of trial procedures, allowing large scale, definitive trials (Peto et al. 1993).

Although there is a need for larger randomised trials in psychiatry, it is also important to make the most efficient use of the trials that have been completed. Meta-analysis is a tool that can increase sample size, and consequently statistical power, by pooling the results of individual trials. Increasing the sample size also allows for more precision (i.e. a more precise estimate of the size of the effect with narrower confidence intervals).

Assessing variation between studies

Combining studies, however attractive, may not always be appropriate. As Eysenck and others have pointed out, the inappropriate pooling of disparate studies can be likened to combining oranges and apples – the result is meaningless (Eysenck 1994). There are two main approaches to dealing with variations in the primary studies. First, it is necessary to ensure that the individual studies are really looking at the same clinical or research question. Individual studies might vary with respect to study participants, intervention, duration of follow up and outcome measures. Such a decision will usually require a measure of judgement, and for this reason a reviewer should always pre-specify the main criteria for including primary studies in the review. In Cochrane reviews, a protocol is first developed, and the inclusion criteria, outcomes of interest and proposed methods of analysis are described. This is peer reviewed before the review can go ahead (Cochrane Collaboration 1995). Having decided that the primary studies are investigating the same, or a close enough, question, an important role of meta-analysis is to investigate variations between the results of individual studies (*heterogeneity*). When such variation exists, it is useful to estimate if more heterogeneity exists than can be reasonably explained by the play of chance alone. If so, attempts should be made to identify the reasons for such heterogeneity, and it may then be decided that it is not reasonable to combine the studies, or that it is, but that the overall pooled estimate needs to take the variation into account (Thompson 1994).

Investigating the impact of study quality

Individual studies vary in their methodological quality. Most has been written about the factors that impact on the quality of randomised trials. It has been shown that allocation, concealment and randomisation, blinding or masking and whether or not an intention-to-treat analysis was performed (i.e. all participants are considered and they are analysed in the groups to which they were randomly allocated), can all affect the direction of the results (Schulz *et al.* 1995). Studies that are deficient in any of these areas tend to overestimate the effect of the intervention. This presents a dilemma to the meta-analyst, who must determine to what extent the variations in methodological quality threaten the combinability of the data.

Many scales have been developed to assess the methodological quality of randomised trials. The scores on these quality assessment scales may be incorporated into the design of a meta-analysis with a 'quality weight' applied to the study-specific effect estimate. Although a huge number of quality scales are available, the current consensus is that their use is problematic because of uncertain validity. It has also been shown that the results of using different scales leads to substantial differences in the pooled estimate (Juni *et al.* 1999). The optimal approach at present is to assess qualitatively those aspects of trial design that affect its internal validity (allocation concealment, blinding, study attrition and method of analysis). Sensitivity analyses can then be conducted to investigate the effect of excluding poor quality trials.

Investigating patient subgroups

The main treatment effect of a trial gives an indication of the average response for an average patient meeting the inclusion criteria. Individual patients in real-life clinical practice deviate from the average to greater or lesser degrees. To tailor the results of a trial to an individual patient it is tempting to perform a sub-analysis of the trial participants with a specific characteristic or set of characteristics.

As we have already discussed many trials conducted in psychiatry are small. Further division of these trials into subgroups reduces the sample size even more and consequently the statistical power of the results. Inevitably, estimates of the treatment in subgroups of patients are more susceptible to random error – and therefore imprecision, than the estimate of the average effect for all patients overall (Counsell *et al.* 1994). Furthermore, unless the randomisation was initially stratified according to the important subgroups, the protection from confounding afforded by randomisation will not apply and any observed subgroup difference in treatment effect may be caused by confounding. Meta-analysis pools data from individual studies, with a consequent increase in power, and this may make subgroup analyses more reliable. However, it should be emphasised that meta-analysis on its own cannot prevent systematic error in the analysis of subgroups. Subgroup analyses should therefore always be viewed cautiously. Clearly, dredging the results of a meta-analysis to identify *post-hoc* subgroups can still lead to erroneous results though random error.

Conclusion

Systematic reviews that seek to synthesise all relevant studies in response to a clearly defined clinical question, are an invaluable resource for both clinicians and researchers. Not all reviews, however, are systematic, and even those that are described as 'systematic' may be deficient methodologically. Strategies have been developed to reduce bias in systematic reviews, especially publication bias and the biases introduced through the over-reliance on electronic databases. A high quality systematic review, by definition, provides the best available evidence on a specific topic.

The usefulness of a systematic review can be further enhanced by the calculation of a statistical summary of the results by the techniques of meta-analysis. By pooling the results of the studies, the risk of random error is reduced, increasing both statistical power and allowing for a more accurate estimate of effect size. It must not be forgotten, however, that whilst pooling the results reduces random error, it is not eliminated. Consequently, meta-analyses are still susceptible to both type I and II errors. When critically appraising a meta-analysis it is not only necessary to assess whether statistical combination was appropriate, but the significance and robustness of the results must be investigated.

Chapter 9

Mental health services research

Graham Thornicroft and Michele Tansella

Introduction

This chapter describes the types and applications of research that are relevant to mental health services, it includes, in the widest sense, evaluations designed to create evidence about which treatments and services do and do not offer benefits to patients. The term 'evaluation' is both widely and imprecisely used. This is especially the case when evaluation is applied to health services rather than to specific treatments. Our first task in discussing the evaluation of mental health services is therefore to *define terms*. In this chapter we shall proceed to consider *why* mental health services should be evaluated, especially because the clarification about the purpose of a particular evaluation is likely to bring into sharper focus subsequent decisions about research design. We shall next respond to the question of *what* needs to be evaluated, at the different levels of the mental health service, to produce information relevant for planners as well as for practitioners and patients. We shall go on to discuss *how* to evaluate mental health services, both in terms of the scales and instruments that may be useful, and the research designs the are available. In particular, we shall illustrate the range of designs with examples from one key domain of recent outstanding mental health research, namely the evidence about assertive community-based care for those with severe mental illness. In conclusion we shall discuss the key challenges of mental health service evaluation and their implications for future research and clinical practice.

> Evaluation at its best is a systematic way of learning from experience and using the lessons learned to improve both current and future action. At its worst it is an activity used to justify the selection of a scapegoat for past failures.
>
> (Sartorius 1983, pp. 59–67)

Mental health services research: definitions and conceptual framework

The development of evaluative research in psychiatry originated in the mid-nineteenth century with the tabulation of admissions, discharges and deaths in mental hospitals, this evolved through more patient-orientated statistics (both should be more appropriately referred to as monitoring than as evaluation), to the recent, increasingly sophisticated studies of community forms of care (Sartorius and Harding 1984).

Definitions and synonyms of 'evaluation' are shown in Box 9.1 (*Concise Oxford Dictionary* 1993). The etymological root of the word refers directly to 'value', although in common usage the emphasis has moved to a more technical, quantitative connotation. This reflects our view that evaluation necessarily requires both the precise measurement of aspects of treatment or service performance, and the consequent contextualisation of the measurement, so that the value of the results may be given meaning.

Box 9.1   Definitions of 'evaluate' and synonyms for 'evaluation'

evaluate *v. tr.*
1.   assess, appraise
2a. find or state the number or amount of
2b. find a numerical expression for

evaluation *n.*
1.   appraisal, valuation, assessment
2.   estimate, estimation, approximation, rating, opinion, ranking, judgement, reckoning, figuring, calculation, computation, determination

Etymology back-form. f. *evaluation* f. F *évaluation* f. *évaluer* (as e-value)

Sources: *Concise Oxford Dictionary* 1993 and *Oxford Thesaurus* 1999.

For health service research, the purpose of evaluation is often more specific. As Sartorius (1997, 239) has put it 'In its most classical form, evaluation denotes a comparison between results and goals of activity'. This moves the definition on from the description of measurements *per se* to a purposeful exercise in which measurements are tools to answer defined, specific questions. We shall show in this chapter that, in relation to the research on the wide range of 'community care arrangements'(Kluiter 1997), it is exactly the lack of

Table 9.1 Overview of the matrix model, with examples of key issues in the outcome phase

Geographical dimension	Temporal dimension		
	A input phase	B process phase	C outcome phase
1. *country/regional level*	1A	1B	1C • suicide rates • special enquiries
2. *local level* (*catchment area*)	2A	2B	2C • suicide rates • homelessness rates • imprisonment rates • outcomes aggregated at local level • physical morbidity
3. *patient level*	3A	3B	3C • symptom reduction • impact on care-givers • satisfaction with services • quality of life • disability • needs

Source: Thornicroft and Tansella 1999.

1. clear definitions on the nature of the interventions defined and
2. precise questions

that has led to such confusion in the interpretation of the research findings.

One conceptual model that may be used as a framework, not only for planning and providing, but also for evaluating mental health services is the 'matrix model' (Thornicroft and Tansella 1999). This model has two dimensions (see Table 9.1). The first dimension is geographical and has three levels (country/regional, local and patient). The second dimension is temporal and also has three levels (input, process and outcome). The 3 = 3 matrix which results from the use of the two dimensions brings into focus critical issues of mental health service evaluation, and helps to distinguish the content of this chapter (the evaluation of mental health services at the local level) from assessments made at the national/regional level, as well as from those made at the individual patient level. The second benefit of using the matrix model is that it allows the measurement of outcomes (the results obtained by treatments or services in terms of functioning, morbidity or mortality) in relation to both inputs (the resources which are put into the mental health care system) and processes (those activities which take place to deliver mental health services).

Public health context for mental health service evaluation

Methods of evaluation are constrained by the types of mental health services that exist in any particular area. The configuration of these services in turn reflects the overall conceptual approach used for their planning and implementation. One such conceptual framework is the *public health approach*, the historical origins of which, according to Eisenberg (1984), are rooted in the work of Virchow. He proposed the reform of medicine on the basis of four principles

1.   the health of the people is a matter of direct social concern
2.   social and economic conditions have an important effect on health and disease, and these relations must be the subject of scientific investigation
3.   the measures taken to promote health and to contain disease must be social as well as medical
4.   medical statistics will be our standard of measurement.

The health of populations is therefore the central concern of the public health approach. As applied to psychiatry, it means that the mental health of individuals is integrally linked with the wider social and economic health of their communities. Moreover, a consequence of adopting a public health orientation in planning mental health care is that the service components (such as a community mental health team, an in-patient unit, or an outpatient department) are viewed not only as separate elements, but also as parts of a wider *service system*. Such a system aims to provide care to all those in need within an entire local population. An alternative way to plan is to provide a range of independent service components for separate patient groups according, for example, to diagnostic or financial eligibility criteria, without reference to the population-based levels of need for such services.

Why evaluate mental health services?

The core aim of mental health services research is, in our view, to establish how far these services meet their pre-identified aims. This means that a clear statement of the service aims should be prepared well in advance of starting an evaluation. In terms of the matrix model shown in Table 9.1, service aims can be located at three levels: national, local and individual. Planners are primarily concerned with the first two, while clinicians limit their scope to the last aim. Both commit categorical errors. The local level approach alone runs the risk of disregarding the extent to which organisational

---

Box 9.2   National mental health targets for England

1. To improve significantly the health and social functioning of mentally ill people.
2. To reduce the overall suicide rate by at least 15% by the year 2000 (from 11.1 per 100,000 population in 1990 to no more than 9.4).
3. To reduce the suicide rate of severely mentally ill people by at least 33% by the year 2000 (from the estimate of 15% in 1990 to no more than 10%).

Source: Department of Health 1993.

---

arrangements do actually lead to improved outcomes for individual patients. The individual level approach alone, on the other hand, cannot address vital local level issues such as ensuring access to care for the whole population that needs it. One of the few examples of explicit service goals which have been set at the national level are the 'Health of the Nation' targets for England, which are shown in Box 9.2.

Against this background, we propose that the intended purposes of mental health services can be classified into two categories

1. the provision of effective treatments to individuals, according to the standards of evidence-based medicine
2. the fulfilment of principles which are regarded, according to both scientific evidence and clinical experience, as central to the adequate provision of mental health care.

The nine principles which we have identified for this purpose are: autonomy, continuity, effectiveness, accessibility, comprehensiveness, equity, accountability, co-ordination and efficiency. From their initials, these principles may be termed 'the three ACEs'.

The distinction and balance between inputs, processes and outcomes within mental health services are far from clear-cut for three reasons (Thornicroft and Tansella 1999). *First*, there is no consensus on the definitions of these terms and their use in the literature is widely variable. As a result the three temporal phases are often used in a confused way so that processes (such as numbers of admissions) are employed *as if* they were outcome variables. *Second*, these three categories of variables are interconnected and need to be seen as different aspects of the wider, dynamic mental health care system, and in fact patients will often want acceptable care processes *and* outcomes, so that attention to outcomes alone will miss a part of what is valued by the recipients of care. *Third*, the paradigm which best fits the tripartite sequence of input, process and outcome, is that of an acute epi-sode of illness and its consequent medical care, such as an uncomplicated infection, or a straightforward surgical intervention such as an appendectomy. This is because the acute illness paradigm assumes

1. clear start and end points for the episode
2. that outcomes are directly related to treatment inputs and to the pro-cesses of their delivery
3. that outcome is simply the difference (or health gain) between health status at time 1 and at time 2.

Many mental disorders, however, especially those treated by specialist mental health services, are chronic, relapsing and remitting conditions, which do not fit a simple acute illness paradigm.

Evaluation should be primarily used for the improvement of the service in which data were obtained, as well as in other similar services. The produc-tion of scientific publications, government reports, and training materials should only be seen as secondary aims (Sartorius 1997). A pragmatic list of reasons why evaluation of mental health services is *actually* conducted is shown in Box 9.3.

Box 9.3   Reasons why mental health service evaluation is conducted

1. To undertake studies of the outcomes of new services in experi-mental conditions (*efficacy*).
2. To investigate whether interventions which have demonstrated *efficacy* (under experimental conditions) are also *effective* (in ordin-ary, routine clinical conditions).
3. To inform future service investment decisions.
4. To stimulate planners to restructure services.
5. To sensitise politicians to service delivery gaps or problems.
6. To replicate/refute previous research, within the same region or country or international comparisons.
7. To sustain academic careers and produce publications in peer-reviewed journals.
8. To justify or to check *post hoc* the value of planning decisions already made, for example the closure of mental hospitals.

What to evaluate in mental health services?

The focus of the evaluation of mental health services remains the outcome of care. Outcomes can be measured at three levels, not only at the local

Table 9.2 Mental health service outcome measures suitable for the three levels of the geographical dimension

Outcome measure	Geographical dimension		
	Country level	Local level	Patient level
Lost occupation	<	<	<
Physical morbidity	<	<	<
Suicide and parasuicide in the general population	<	<	
Suicide and parasuicide in mental health patients	<	<	<
Homelessness	<	<	<
Special enquiries and reports	<	<	<
Standardised mortality ratios among current and former patients		<	
Symptom severity		<	<
Impact on care-givers		<	<
Satisfaction with services		<	<
Quality of life/subjective well being		<	<
Disability/social role performance		<	<
Met needs for care		<	<
Global ratings of function		<	<

Source: Thornicroft and Tansella 1999.

service level, but also upstream at the country/regional level, and downstream at the patient level. We shall therefore discuss what to evaluate in terms of these three levels, as summarised in Table 9.2.

Outcomes at the country/regional level

The classic epidemiological outcome measures at the population level are mortality and morbidity rates, but while these have also been used in epidemiological psychiatry as outcome measures, the use of such indicators taken from general medicine for psychiatry needs careful translation. This is, first, because the conditions under investigation in cardiology or oncology have a direct causal association with death, while in psychiatry the established higher mortality rates (Allebeck 1989; Harris and Barraclough 1998) are indirectly associated with mental illness, most often through suicide or risks from patients' lifestyles. Second, because morbidity indicators used as outcome measures in mental health need to be seen in a modest context: psychiatry, so far, has not been able to effect primary prevention for any form of severe mental illness.

Secondary prevention (reducing symptom relapse) and tertiary prevention (reducing the suffering consequent upon symptoms) are predominant in mental health services over primary prevention activities. In this case, the relevant outcomes in the mental health field can be subsumed within the headings of impairment (primary symptoms), disability (consequent reduced ability to perform specific skills) and handicap (limited social role performance), as formalised by the WHO *International Classification of Impairments, Disabilities and Handicaps* (World Health Organisation 1980), or outcomes may deal with other consequences of health services provision, such as service satisfaction or impact on care givers.

A frequently used outcome measure at the population level is *suicide rate*, which is shown in cell 1C in Table 9.1 (see p. 83). Rates of *homelessness* among the mentally ill (or rates of mental illness among the homeless) can also be used as an outcome indicator of the effectiveness of mental illness policies at the national level. In practice, however, we are not aware of any such studies at this level, and most such data are relevant to the local level (Bachrach 1984; Scott 1988). The same applies to the inappropriate placement in *prison* of those who would be better treated in mental health facilities (Gunn *et al.* 1991; Maden *et al.* 1995).

Outcomes at the local level

At the local level outcome indicators useful for evaluation can be made in three ways

1. by interpolating from national/country data
2. by measuring directly at the local level
3. by aggregating up to the local level information which has been collected for individuals at the patient level.

For example, rates of suicide and unemployment can be estimated using the first method, or directly measured using the second method if the appropriate information and resources exist. The second approach will provide more accurate and up-to-date information. The third approach is to aggregate up to the local level information gathered from individual patients, if institutions providing care to those local patients are willing to co-operate in data collection and collation on, for example, symptom reduction, satisfaction with services and quality of life.

Outcomes at the patient level

Since we have argued that the primary purpose of mental health services is to optimise outcomes for individual patients, then prior inputs and processes should be concentrated upon their effectiveness in terms of patient level outcomes. In this section we shall discuss the range of most commonly used domains of outcome measurement. It is noteworthy that health service evaluation in the mental health field is increasingly acknowledging the importance of other outcomes apart from symptom severity.

Traditionally *symptom severity measures* have been used most often to assess the effectiveness of the early mental health treatments. Psychiatrists and psychologists have contributed to the early development of such assessment scales to allow this research to take place (Bowling 1991, 1995, 1997; Thornicroft and Tansella 1996; Wetzler 1989; Thompson 1989; Wilkin *et al.* 1992). Recently excellent reviews of scales suitable for this purpose have been published (Wing 1996; Wittchen and Nelson 1996; Sartorius and Janca 1996). While the primary symptoms are clearly important, for most chronic mental disorders there is symptom persistence, and it is unrealistic at present to see symptom eradication as the sole aim of treatment (World Health Organisation 1980).

The importance of the *impact of caring* for those with mental illnesses upon family members and others who provide informal care has long been recognised (Creer and Wing 1974), but has only been subjected to concerted research in relatively recent years (Schene *et al.* 1994). Such research has shown that it is common for carers themselves to suffer from mental illnesses, most commonly depression and anxiety, and to worry about the future and how their relative will cope when they can no longer provide care. Moreover, many family members are most distressed by underactivity by the patient, are often poorly informed about the clinical condition, its treatment and the likely prognosis, and want to be provided with a practical action plan of what to do in future, should a crisis occur. Indeed, some services continue to convey to families the outmoded idea that carers, especially parents, are in some way to blame for the disorder or for relapses of the condition (Lehman 1994).

Patients' *satisfaction with services* is a further domain which has recently become established as a legitimate, important and feasible area of outcome assessment at the local level. This is a recognition of the contribution that patients and their carers can make to outcome assessment. Psychometrically adequate scales are those that adopt a multi-dimensional approach to assess the full range of service characteristics, which are independently administered (so that patient ratings have no consequences upon their future clinical care), and which have established validity and reliability (Ruggeri and Dall'Agnola 1993; Ruggeri 1996).

Quality of life ratings have also become prominent during the last decade, and several instruments have been constructed which reflect varying basic approaches to the topic. The first distinction is between schedules which address subjective well being only, compared with those which also measure objective elements of quality of life. The second main point of differentiation is between scales constructed for the general population, or designed for those suffering from specific disorders, including the more severe mental illnesses

(Lehman 1996). One advantage of quality of life data is that they tend to be popular with politicians who find the concept has a powerful face validity!

After symptom treatment has been optimised, usually by treatment with medication (for example for psychotic disorders) the residual *disabilities* may need quite different types of intervention (Wiersma 1996). Separate measurements of cognitive and social abilities, which are essential for an independent life, are therefore justified. Indeed, from a longitudinal perspective, social disability tends to have a less favourable course than psychopathology.

Increasing importance is being attached to the *needs* of those who suffer from mental illnesses. This new orientation marks a wider public mood that emphasises the active role of the recipients of health services as consumers, and also raises a series of important questions. How can needs be defined and by whom? Stevens and Gabbay (1991) have defined need as 'what people benefit from', demand as 'what people ask for', and supply as 'what is provided'. This applies largely to clinical data and one example is the measurement of patients' needs. In the PRiSM Psychosis Study (Thornicroft *et al.* 1998a), the assessment of individual need was made using the Camberwell Assessment of Need (CAN). The overall results of the user (patient) ratings of need from the twenty-two CAN domains (Phelan *et al.* 1995) show that epidemiologically representative psychotic individuals, half of whom are schizophrenic, have on average about seven major needs, and that about three-quarters of these are met and one-quarter are not met.

How to evaluate mental health services

This section will deal with research designs which may be applicable for mental health service evaluation. First, the measures used must be fit for the purpose, in other words, psychometrically adequate (Hall 1979, 1980; National Institute of Mental Health 1985; Steiner and Norman 1989; Salvador-Carulla 1996). Different types of evidence produced using these measures cannot necessarily be considered as equivalent. A hierarchical order has been proposed by Geddes and Harrison (1997), as shown in Box 9.4, and we shall consider each source of evidence in turn, except for evidence from expert committee reports or the clinical experience of respected authorities, which cannot be considered as types of formal evaluation.

Evidence from a meta-analysis of randomised controlled trials

Meta-analysis can be defined as 'the quantitative synthesis of the results of systematic overviews of previous studies'. Systematic overviews, in turn, are methods of collating and synthesising all the available evidence on a particular scientific question (Adams *et al.* 1996). Since RCTs are often

---

Box 9.4   A hierarchy of evidence

1a.   Evidence from a meta-analysis of randomised controlled trials.
1b.   Evidence from at least one randomised controlled trial.
2a.   Evidence from at least one controlled study without randomisation.
2b.   Evidence from at least one other type of quasi-experimental study.
3.   Evidence from non-experimental descriptive studies such as comparative studies, correlation studies and case-control studies.
4.   Evidence from expert committee reports or opinions and/or clinical experience of respected authorities.

Source: Geddes and Harrison 1997.

---

considered to produce the most sophisticated evidence on the efficacy of medical treatments, a meta-analysis conducted on well selected and relevant RCTs can be seen as the highest order of knowledge. It follows that the quality of systematic overviews is limited by the quality and quantity of the contributory trials (see Box 9.5).

Cochrane was the first to emphasise the need to bring together, within specific categories, the results of RCTs (Cochrane 1979). This approach now

---

Box 9.5   Characteristics of systematic overviews

Questions to ask about papers for potential inclusion in a systematic overview.

- Were the questions and methods clearly stated?
- Were comprehensive search methods used to locate the relevant articles?
- Were explicit methods used to determine which articles were included in the review?
- Was the methodological quality of the primary studies assessed?
- Were the selection and assessment of the primary studies reproducible and free from bias?
- Were the differences in individual study results adequately explained?
- Were the results of the primary studies combined appropriately?
- Were the reviewer's conclusions supported by the data cited?

Source: Sackett *et al.* 1991.

forms the basis of evidence-based medicine (Chalmers *et al.* 1993; L'Abbe *et al.* 1987; Sackett *et al.* 1996). Within mental health service evaluation the first meta-analyses were conducted in the late 1970s, and until recently the technique was more often applied to case-control studies than to RCTs (Adams *et al.* 1996; Lau *et al.* 1998).

The randomised controlled trial

The quintessence of the central role accorded to RCTs within medical research has been expressed by Tyrer *et al.* (1997) as well as by Korn and Baumrind (1991, p. 149): 'Randomised clinical trials are the sine qua non for evaluating treatment in man'. According to Barker and Rose (1979)

> the essence of the randomised controlled trial is that the outcome of the treatment given to one group of patients is compared with one or more other groups who are given different treatments or none at all. Allocation of individuals to the treatment and comparison groups is by random selection.
>
> (p. 96)

Pocock has further clarified the role of RCTs by saying that they can be applied to 'any form of planned experiment which involves patients and which is designed to elucidate the most appropriate treatment of future patients with a given medical condition' (Pocock 1987, p. 35). The advantages of the RCT research design have been extensively described (Kluiter and Wiersma 1996) and are shown in Box 9.6.

Box 9.6   Advantages of randomised controlled trials

- They control for many confounding variables which may exist.
- They eliminate the effects of spontaneous remission.
- They eliminate regression to mean.
- They eliminate the placebo effect.
- They are independent of rater bias if blindness is maintained.
- They are the basis for systematic reviews.

Source: Taylor and Thornicroft 1996.

At the same time, the limitations of the RCT design need to be appreciated, especially in relation to health-services research (Taylor and Thornicroft 1996; Black 1996). For the sake of brevity the main limitations and disadvantages of RCT design are shown in Box 9.7.

Box 9.7 Limitations and disadvantages in the design of randomised controlled trials

1. *Difficulties in choosing the unit or level of random allocation*
- should allocation be made at the patient level, the clinician level, the clinical team or practice level or the locality level?

2. *Difficulties in achieving random allocation*
- randomisation is not possible
- particular patient groups are excluded
- self-exclusion because of non-consent.

3. *Difficulties in obtaining consent and in maintaining motivation*
- consent may be inversely proportional to the severity of the condition
- consent may be refused because of patient treatment preferences
- retention with the trial may be affected by patient motivation.

4. *Difficulties in establishing and maintaining blindness*
- degree of blinding of subjects
- degree of blinding of staff
- degree of blinding of raters
- reactive Hawthorne effect (the effect of being studied upon those being studied).

5. *Difficulties related to the experimental conditions*
- concurrent multiple interventions in health service research trials (without a single potentially active ingredient)
- interactions between treatment components
- consistency of control ('usual treatment') conditions
- high attrition rates or loss to follow up
- large differences between conditions in which trials can take place and those of routine practice.

Source: Taylor and Thornicroft 1996.

In addition to the technical limitations of the RCT design, there are also situations in which RCTs are not applicable to specific research questions. These may be summarised as conditions in which RCTs are inadequate, impossible, inappropriate or unnecessary, as shown in Box 9.8.

In terms of assessing the quality of an RCT, Marriot and Palmer (1996) have suggested a framework of fourteen questions to be used. We shall

---

Box 9.8   Situations when randomised-controlled-trial designs are not applicable

1. *Situations in which experimentation is inadequate*
- poor generalisability – low external validity
- unrepresentative staff are included
- atypical patients are included
- treatments are not standardarised.

2. *Situations in which experimentation is impossible*
- refusal of clinicians to take part
- ethical objections to the study
- political barriers
- legal objections
- contamination between experimental and control conditions
- scale of the task – trials are required for too many treatments.

3. *Situations in which experimentation is inappropriate*
- studies conducted to reduce the occurrence of events of very low frequency
- studies to prevent unwanted outcomes in the distant future.

4. *Experimentation unnecessary*
- when the benefit–risk ratio is dramatic
- when there is a small likelihood of confounders.

Source: Black 1996.

---

illustrate the use of this grid of questions by critically applying it to a study of family-aided assertive community treatment (MacFarlane *et al.* 1996).

Quasi-experimental studies

The term 'quasi-experiment' was first used by Campbell and Stanley (1966) to refer to a situation in which the decision about whether an individual does or does not receive the intervention to be evaluated is not under the investigator's control. Random allocation of patients is not made, so selection bias may occur. In other respects quasi-experiment aims to apply the logic of RCTs to the study design, and the researcher tries to reduce this bias by making the study units, in the groups being compared, as alike as possible in terms of the most important characteristics. This approach is

Table 9.3 Criteria to evaluate the quality of a randomised controlled trial

Criteria	Criteria applied (MacFarlane et al. 1996)
1. Is the hypothesis clearly defined?	Hypothesis is stated in general terms.
2. Is the study population representative?	Not stated: patients were recruited from urban, suburban and rural mental health centers in NY State.
3. Was patient assignment randomised?	Yes.
4. Were patients, practitioners and assessors blind to the experimental intervention?	Not stated.
5. Were the groups similar at the start of the trial?	No for several variables, including 'living at home' (33% versus 59%).
6. Were the groups treated equally apart from the experimental intervention?	Yes.
7. Were all those who entered the trial accounted for at its conclusion?	Yes, 37 patients were allocated to the experimental treatment and 31 to the control condition, 3 patients in each group failed to complete treatment.
8. Was this in the groups to which they were originally allocated?	Yes.
9. Are all clinically important outcomes considered?	Yes, except costs.
10. Whose perspective do they reflect?	A range of psychosocial outcomes.
11. Is the data analysis appropriate?	Yes, mainly using analysis of variance which appears to be on an 'intention to treat' basis.
12. What is the size and precision of the treatment effect?	Not stated, no power calculation is given to justify the relatively small sample.
13. Do the likely benefits outweigh the harms and risks?	Probably, but costs of the treatments are not stated.
14. Is the conclusion supported by the results?	Largely.

known as *matching*. Characteristics chosen for matching are those expected to influence the outcomes. The over-arching aim of matching is therefore to reduce the extent of selection bias which is contributed by the variables which are matched, although this method is inferior to randomisation in that it cannot reduce the selection bias which is contributed by all other variables

There are two main approaches to matching. *Paired matching* consists of selecting individuals for the comparison group (or groups) who have closely similar characteristics to those included in the experimental group, for example in terms of age, gender and occupation. This form of pre-stratification will need to be taken into account at the data analysis stage.

A less rigorous variant is *group matching*, which only ensures that there are similar overall proportions of people, for both the experimental and comparison groups, in the various age bands, occupational groups or other pre-defined strata used for the variables chosen for matching (St Leger *et al.* 1992).

One example of the whole catchment area comparison is the home treatment study of Dean *et al.* (1993), and another is the PRiSM Psychosis Study (Thornicroft *et al.* 1998a), which compared two types of community mental health team (a single generic team against a two-team model) in closely matched geographical sectors in South London and followed up patients over a 2-year period. It showed that the outcomes on the majority of outcome variables were similar for the two models, and that both were superior to the baseline hospital-based model of care. Apart from the value of the results of such studies, they can also generate specific hypotheses to be tested in future RCTs.

In fact the RCT paradigm is most suited to short-term, single invention studies, such as psychopharmacological trials, in which blindness can be maintained more easily. It is more often the case that health-service research evaluations

1. take place in routine settings in which control over critical parameters, such as blindness, is more difficult
2. need longer term periods of follow-up
3. assess the effects of multiple, simultaneous inputs on a range of outcome measures.

This is because the specific active ingredients, and their effect size, is not yet known.

Non-experimental descriptive studies

The next type of research design included in the Geddes and Harrison (1997) typology is non-experimental descriptive studies. For the sake of clarity and brevity we shall distinguish two types of descriptive study: structured clinical practice, and everyday unstructured clinical practice. Table 9.4 shows a comparison of the key strengths and weaknesses of these two types of descriptive study, compared with the other two principal designs, as discussed above, namely RCTs and quasi-experimental studies. An example of a descriptive evaluation design is the South Verona Outcome Study (Ruggeri *et al.* 1998). The aim of this prospective study is to assess the outcome of mental health care using a multi-dimensional perspective, and graphical chain models, a new multi-variate method which analyses the relationship between variables conditionally, i.e. taking into account the effect of antecedent or intervening variables.

Table 9.4 Comparison of the characteristics of four types of clinical research design

Study characteristic	Randomised clinical trials	Non-randomised clinical trials (quasi-experimental studies)	Structured clinical practice (routine outcome studies)	Unstructured clinical practice
Defined acceptance/exclusion criteria	√	?	√	√
Inclusion of whole patient populations			√√	√√
Adequate sample size	√	√	√	
Clear controlled conditions	√	√		
Bias reduction by double blindness	√			
Bias reduction by randomisation	√			
Standardised measures	√	√	√√√	
Regularly repeated outcome measurements	?	?	√	
Long-term follow up		?	?	?
Power of statistical analysis	?√	? ?	?√	
Hypothesis generation	√	√	?√	√
Generalisation	?	?	?√	
Lack of constraint by ethical committee			√√√	√√√
Explicit patient consent unnecessary			√√	√√
Low cost for data collection			√	√√

Source: Thornicroft and Tansella 1999.

Table 9.5 Key challenges to rigorous and relevant evaluation of mental health services

- clarifying who is asking the research question and why
- asking clear research questions
- evaluating already established as well as newly proposed services
- providing sufficient funding for long-term health service research
- ensuring quality assurance for research proposals
- balancing internal and external validity
- specifying the type of intervention to be evaluated
- specifying the precise nature of the control condition
- identifying the active ingredients of treatment
- specifying the key characteristics of the patient groups to be treated
- using representative patient samples
- only using standardised instruments relevant to each type of evaluation
- overcoming resistance from clinical staff
- implementing the results of evaluation when the evidence is strong enough

Conclusions

What are the central challenges that mental health service evaluation will face in the future? (see Table 9.5).

We consider that the first issues to address are the need to *clarify who is asking the research question and why.* On occasions a call for funding is initiated by a central governmental or research body acting for the wider health service, and commissioning targeted research which has been identified as a national priority. On the other hand it is also common for research workers to take the initiative and to bid for grants to fund studies which test hypotheses which the researchers themselves have formulated or selected. These two different approaches have important implications. Externally commissioned research for defined programmatic areas are often linked to political or policy initiatives which have shorter time constraints. By comparison, investigator initiated studies may have a far more limited impact since they may reflect concerns of the research staff more than those of service planners or clinicians.

Studies of mental health service evaluation *which ask clear research questions* are still relatively few. This is in part because the tradition of research in this field is primarily that of unfocussed descriptive studies, and because only recently have the methodological tools necessary for analytical studies (which address specific and refutable hypotheses) been used at the service level.

In addition, there remains an imbalance between the evaluation of new service models compared with *research upon established clinical practice.* In most service systems the majority of expenditure is for traditional inpatient and outpatient provision, about which there is remarkably little research-based evidence. It will therefore be important in future to evaluate *post hoc* current but unproven service configurations, especially those which are widespread and expensive, as well as innovative interventions. In future such studies will need *longer-term funding*, commensurate with the frequently long-term course of the mental disorders treated by the services which they evaluate. At the same time an increasing investment in health services research in many economically developed countries needs to be accompanied by a commitment to systems of *quality assurance* for research proposals, so that only studies which can answer their stated hypotheses are funded.

A fine balance is also needed between *internal and external validity*. Internal validity is most often satisfied by RCTs which examine questions of the efficacy of specific interventions. On the other hand, external validity (generalisability) is usually better addressed by larger scale clinical studies in routine settings, under which conditions the RCT design may not be feasible. It will often be appropriate to see these two designs as sequential: first establish if an intervention is efficacious, and then test whether it is effective.

Commonly mental health service evaluations *fail to specify the interventions to be tested, and to give a detailed description of the control condition.* While it is common to find a description of the overall service organisation, what is often missing is detail about the treatment capacity of the services being studied, and the precise nature of the interventions provided to patients. This issue has bedevilled research reviews and systematic overviews, for example, on the range of services which have been described variously as assertive community treatment, intensive case management and community care arrangements (Burns and Santos 1995; Scott and Dixon 1995; Marshall 1996; Kluiter 1997; Mueser *et al.* 1998).

A further necessary future step is to identify the *active ingredients* of such services, a major research agenda. It will be necessary to distinguish and assess the separate effects of

1. size of case load
2. clarity of local operational policies and programme fidelity
3. qualification of the care workers
4. degree of continuity of care
5. the specific illnesses/disorders of the patients treated
6. the extent of the hours of operation for the service
7. patient compliance with the treatments offered, especially medication
8. the flexibility of the programme to provide individualised treatment packages.

Furthermore, future research will need to *specify the key characteristics of the patient groups to be treated*. This has most often been done in the past in terms of diagnostic group. Rather than proceed to further dissection of diagnostic categories, it may be more useful to have valid descriptors for typical clinical populations which may in future include biological and genetic markers. For the present it is necessary for research purposes to be much more specific about ill-defined terms such as, for example, 'severe mental illness'. Related to this is the challenge to include in studies *patients who are clinically or epidemiologically representative.* The former are patient samples which are essentially similar to larger groups of patients under treatment in a similar type of service elsewhere, while the latter are population-based samples.

An important requirement within mental health service evaluation is that only *standardised measures* are used. While this is now common, it is not yet established that translations of original instruments need to be re-standardised in their secondary languages, or that application of measures used for one particular patient group to another distinct group should not proceed until the scale has been restandardised and recalibrated to the second population, also using focus groups (Becker *et al.* 2000). This issue becomes increasingly important in times of high rates of international migration.

In many types of health service research, a barrier to effective studies is *resistance from clinical staff.* There are several reasons that contribute to these negative attitudes. As Sartorius (1997) has pointed out, they include the following

- evaluation has often been used for cost cutting instead of advancing a treatment programme
- research may precede a reform of services which is not welcome to staff
- the results of evaluation are sometimes used to justify a decision which has already been made
- studies absorb resources which could be dedicated for clinical purposes
- the analysis of results often takes a long time so that they cannot be used for any practical purpose.

For research to proceed, such staff concerns may need to be adequately addressed. Ultimately, one of the most severe challenges is to ensure that the results of mental health service evaluation are disseminated and that, when the evidence is strong enough, research findings are translated into *policy and clinical implications* which are then implemented.

Chapter 10

Conceptual limitations of randomised controlled trials

Mike Slade and Stefan Priebe

Introduction

The previous three chapters have presented a strong case for the gradual aggregation of high-quality evidence, where 'evidence' ideally comprises findings from randomised controlled trials (RCTs). This chapter is intended to make the case for other sources of evidence. The intention is not to argue for the merits of other approaches to garnering knowledge – that will be left to the remaining authors in this section. Rather, the intent of this chapter (at the risk of appearing overly negative) is to indicate the shortcomings of an over-reliance on RCTs as the sole source of credible evidence.

Using evidence as the basis for deciding on and prioritising between health interventions is more important than ever before. The long-term goal is to ensure that every decision, from what help to offer a mildly depressed patient who has consulted their family doctor, to how to reduce the stigma of mental illness, will be underpinned by research evidence. So are RCTs likely to provide the evidence necessary for the planning, development and evaluation of health services? It will be argued that there is a need to embrace a broader understanding of what constitutes evidence for at least three reasons. First, RCTs identify groups using diagnoses, which obscures the variation within groups. Second, there are conceptual problems with the notion of generalisation. Third, the evidence base itself is biased.

Diagnostic samples

Randomised controlled trials of interventions group subjects by diagnosis, with the goal of producing recommendations regarding treatment strategies. This implies that diagnosis is a sufficient description on which to make treatment decisions. It should be noted that this view is not often stated by practising clinicians, probably for a number of reasons. First, it may not be a view that is held. Second, professional protectionism may preclude stating this view, since if treatment can be manualised then the arguments for increased salary and status for mental health practitioners are weakened. Third, it may be seen as an academic and hence non-clinical question, leading to the 'category error' of statements such as 'but people have a right to know what's wrong with them' (Johnstone 1997, p. 33). The centrality of diagnosis in understanding mental disorder leads to deterministic algorithms for treatment, such as the comprehensive flow chart of appropriate pharmacological treatment strategies for schizophrenia (Taylor 1996).

However, people who are grouped on the basis of diagnosis may be heterogeneous, with RCTs which focus on diagnosis producing inconsistent findings because of variation attributable to individual differences. This is typically addressed by controlling for sociodemographic and other variables seen as relevant (e.g. psychiatric history, symptom severity, treatment setting), but there is no consensus as to which variables should be controlled for. Moreover, the methods of controlling for the influence of potentially confounding variables are purely quantitative, so qualitative differences are missed. For instance, in the case of an age difference between two groups, years of age of patients may be controlled for as an influential factor in a statistical analysis. Yet, similar age differences in years might have a very different impact depending on how old the patients are and how age interacts with other factors. Even small differences in age may make two groups qualitatively different, a difference which is not controlled for by quantitative statistical procedures.

Conceptually, the use of diagnosis to define a group is predicated on the assumption that all people with diagnosis of mental disorder X (e.g. paranoid schizophrenia) are fundamentally similar to each other, with a few differences explained by moderating variables. It cannot control for unrecognised influences, such as the service itself, and ignores the dynamic nature of mental disorders that current diagnostic classifications fail to capture.

Furthermore, the use of treatment protocols derived from diagnosis-based RCT evidence has the potential to focus clinicians on diagnosis-based interventions, rather than developing individualised formulations and intervention strategies. A practical result is that, in general, people who meet diagnostic criteria for schizophrenia are always prescribed anti-psychotic medication, even though the evidence indicates it will be ineffective (and, due to side-effects, on balance harmful) for some patients.

An alternative view is that people are fundamentally unique, with a few similarities described by some of them all matching operational criteria for a particular disorder. This alternative view has produced the development of treatments which are symptom focused (rather than diagnosis based), such as cognitive-behavioural therapy. At the conceptual level psychiatry has attempted to defend itself from this critique, but these defences are argued from within a positivist framework, rather than making a 'paradigm shift' (Kuhn 1962). For example, Reznek (1991) proposes that 'Something is a (mental) illness if and only if it is an abnormal and involuntary process that does (mental) harm and should best be treated by medical means' (p. 163), with the implication that the word 'best' has some objective (universally shared) meaning. Mojtabai and Rieder (1998) use empirical evidence to challenge a symptom-based approach to psychiatric research, without considering the difference between reliability and external validity. They argue that if syndromes can be more reliably assessed than symptoms, then this elevates syndromes as the appropriate focus for psychiatric research. However, being able to reliably describe a concept (e.g. Father Christmas) does not make it real, and runs the risk of treating as a real thing something which is no more than a label.

In the currently dominant diagnostic classifications of DSM-IV and ICD-10, the conventional distinction between syndrome and diagnosis has been blurred. Most diagnoses in these manuals are based on lists of defined symptoms, a certain number of which have to be present for justifying a given diagnostic category. Simple algorithms are used leading to a high reliability and questionable validity of diagnoses (Priebe 1989). The underlying nosological concept of diagnoses remains unclear so that diagnosis is a particularly problematic – and possibly often meaningless – criterion for grouping patients in clinical studies.

Generalisation

Inferential statistics are central to current approaches to mental health research, involving the assumption that a result can be generalised, and is representative of something. The P value indicates the probability of a finding occurring by chance given the presumed variance of the outcome criterion in the 'total group', and hence the extent to which the finding is representative of the population from which the sample was taken. However, this use of inferential statistics only makes sense if one can identify to which other samples, settings and times the result can be generalised. This may not be possible. For example, recent studies investigated the effectiveness of two patterns of clinical services in London (Thornicroft et al. 1998b) and of deinstitutionalisation in Berlin (Hoffman et al. 2000). To which patients do the findings of these studies generalise? For patients in other districts of London or Berlin, for patients in all inner-city districts in western Europe, for patients across the world, or just for other patients with the same characteristics at the same place and the same point of time (in which case representation would lose its meaning)? No criteria have been proposed for establishing what the results are representative for. The criteria for characterising samples and settings are, in general, so weak and dependent on historical and social interpretations, that the principle of representation may not apply. Without the principle of representation and inferential statistics, however, RCTs and meta-analyses would lose their conceptual and methodological basis. By extension, the unit of analysis in future research investigating mental health services and systems may have to be the service, and not a patient in the service. This means using number of services in a power analysis, and not number of patients, which will in practice be impossible for many research questions.

In summary, it is difficult to specify the extent to which RCTs based on diagnostic clusters can be generalised. If inclusion criteria are tightly specified, then the results relate to a very specific sample and hence cannot be generalised to other clinical settings. If the inclusion criteria are loosely specified, then the sample is inadequately characterised, so the degree of individual variation will mean that results are influenced by both the intervention and individual characteristics (and hence cannot be generalised). This balance will always be an imperfect negotiation.

The evidence base

If care is to be provided on the basis of evidence, then it follows that equal opportunity should be available for all types of relevant research evidence to be gathered and considered. This requirement is not met for at least four reasons.

First, the methods of natural science may be not applicable to the study of mental health. For example, the assessment of height or electrolyte levels is straightforward since they can be directly measured. The assessment of psychological characteristics such as severity of depression, or conviction in delusions, necessarily requires proxy measures. For these characteristics, there cannot be a 'true' measure because they are not observable. It is tempting, therefore, to ignore them. However, as Robert McNamara (US Secretary of State during the Vietnam war) is reported to have said 'The challenge is to make the important measurable, not the measurable important'. The compelling reason to include consideration of characteristics such as 'quality of life', 'beliefs', 'motivation' and 'self-esteem' is that these may be precisely what go wrong in mental disorder.

Whilst symptoms and psychological constructs cannot be directly observed, interactions can. Indeed, all symptoms need to be presented in some type of interaction to be noticed by mental health professionals. Mental disorders are expressed and treated in social interactions, so that those interactions are inevitably at the centre of mental health research. The explanatory methods of social science, as opposed to the descriptive methods of natural science, will be needed to understand these interactions and processes.

Second, RCTs are particularly appropriate for interventions for which treatment integrity can be shown – the patient receives an intervention which is no more and no less than what is intended. However, mental health care is a complex phenomenon, comprising at least three different types. It is a circumscribed diagnostic or therapeutic intervention, it is a more complex programme or service, and it is a comprehensive mental-health-care system (Burns and Priebe 1996). At the therapeutic level psychopharmacological drugs, for instance, are well defined by their chemical structure, but the way psychological and social interventions are provided may vary appropriately between patients and between therapists. For service programmes and systems, the situation is even more complex. Service descriptions are often used as technical terms, which assumes that they can be clearly defined and that the definition can be applied and makes sense elsewhere. It is, however, impossible to define language – terms have no copyright, language changes, translations vary, jargon varies across professions and regions, the use of terms is influenced by various interests, and a complete definition would require so many rules as to be impossible to use. Treatment integrity is relatively easy to ensure for pharmacotherapy, relatively difficult to ensure for individual psychotherapeutic and psychosocial treatments, and practically impossible where the intervention is a complex package of care or a care system.

This is illustrated by the findings from the Schizophrenia Patient Outcomes Research Team (PORT) review of outcome studies in schizophrenia (Lehman and Steinwachs 1998a), which made thirty treatment recommendations, of which twenty-five were positive. These comprise seventeen concerning pharmacotherapy, two concerning ECT, one concerning family therapy, one concerning individual and group therapies, and four concerning services (vocational rehabilitation and assertive treatment). The use of RCTs as the means by which evidence is gathered leads to a lot of evidence regarding pharmacotherapy, less concerning other types of intervention, and little if any undebated, positive evidence about service organisation. To illustrate the point, the only PORT recommendation regarding service configuration is assertive community treatment, which is a subject of active disagreement amongst researchers in the UK (Burns *et al.* 1999a; Thornicroft *et al.* 1999). The use of RCTs has therefore not produced widely accepted evidence for mental health services.

A third reason for the disparity in available evidence is bias. Researchers who undertake any research will have particular values and beliefs, which in mental health research may (for example) lead them to investigate one intervention rather than another, or to present findings confirming rather than refuting their beliefs. This appraisal bias is recognised within social science research, and attempts are made to separate the roles of participant and observer, but is much less recognised in mental health research. There may also be availability bias – a skew in the number of studies of sufficient quality for inclusion in a review. For example, the PORT review (whose first author is a psychiatrist) produced nineteen positive recommendations related to physical treatments and only four to psychological, social and vocational approaches, thus underlining the role of pharmacotherapy in schizophrenia. Another review, carried out by psychologists, was much more optimistic regarding the role of psychological and social interventions (Roth and Fonagy 1996). Bias in the research process is unavoidable, but can be minimised using the methods of other social sciences.

A fourth reason for the disparity is economic considerations. The funding of research is not a level playing field, with the budget from pharmaceutical companies for research into psychotropic medication dwarfing the tax-funded budget allocated to other types of intervention. Pharmacotherapy and related research is aggressively marketed by pharmaceutical companies, including the use of promotional material citing data which may not have been peer reviewed (e.g. 'data on file') (Gilbody and Song 2000). Furthermore, the available data may be selectively presented, such as one trial of olanzapine which has been published in various forms in eighty-three separate publications (Duggan *et al.* 1999). This compares with very little active marketing for psychological or social interventions. Furthermore, high-quality recent studies suggest that the effectiveness of antidepressants (Khan *et al.* 2000) and novel antipsychotics (Geddes *et al.* 2000) has been exaggerated. Although only suggesting, not demonstrating, that scientific principles have been compromised by commercial imperatives, it is clear that economic factors influence the provision and availability of evidence.

Overall, RCTs in medicine have been used for evaluating well-defined and standardised treatments. The importing of this approach into mental-health-service research strengthens the position of pharmacotherapy (which tends to be a standardised and well-defined intervention) compared with psychological and social interventions, and underlines the link between psychiatry and other specialities in medicine. Regarding RCTs as the gold standard in mental-health-care research results in 'evidence-based' recommendations which are skewed, both in the available evidence and the weight assigned to evidence.

Conclusion

The equating of evidence with RCTs has been challenged in other branches of medicine (Feinstein and Horwitz 1997). However, specific issues arise in mental health. We have argued that samples based on diagnosis are inevitably heterogeneous, and even if they could be made more homogenous it is not clear to what the RCT results based on such samples could be generalised. RCT evidence does not meet the requirement to provide equally weighted and fairly evaluated evidence for all aspects of mental health services.

At a more fundamental level, it is worth noting that some questions cannot even be addressed using RCTs. As noted by Goldberg (1991), RCTs only allow existing interventions to be compared, and cannot create new approaches or policies, they cannot indicate gaps in knowledge, and so cannot be the only source of information. Similarly, RCTs cannot be used to investigate issues where the number of cases is very small, such as the effects of a national mental health policy. Overall, the use of RCTs as the highest form of evidence means that the ability to have feedback between theory and observation is reduced. If RCTs are the only form of valid high-quality evidence, then where will the conceptual advances come from? Where will the loop exist between what is thought to work (based on RCT evidence) and what actually happens in practice? How will the understanding be developed to inform decisions as to *which* model of mental disorder will be most helpful for an individual patient?

These questions highlight the special situation that mental health research occupies, by spanning both the natural and social sciences. Evidence based on RCTs has an important place, but to adopt concepts from only one body of knowledge is to neglect the contribution that other, well-established methodologies can make. Randomised clinical trials cannot be used to answer all questions, and it is an illusion that the development of increasingly rigorous and sophisticated RCTs will ultimately provide a complete evidence base. In one sense this is not a new observation – informed commentators note that RCTs are not suitable for questions of (for example) aetiology, diagnosis and prognosis (Sackett and Wennberg 1997). However, a hierarchy of evidence with meta-analyses of RCTs uncritically placed at the top continues to be widely propagated in both the academic literature (e.g. Guyatt *et al.* 1995; Geddes and Harrison 1997; Greenhalgh 1997; Roth and Fonagy 1996) and mental health policy (e.g. Department of Health 1999). There is no universally applicable hierarchy of methods of gathering evidence.

If mental health researchers are to ask all possible questions, to evaluate the evidence in a disinterested fashion, and to present the results in a balanced and non-partisan way, then there needs to be more use of established methodologies from other approaches, some of which will be considered in Chapters 11 to 13. The long-term challenge is not just to apply currently dominant methodologies more rigorously, but to develop new approaches for providing adequate evidence, which can account for the complexity of mental health care. A first step may be to bring together methodologies that exist in natural and social sciences, rather than to work in distinct fields with little collaboration among researchers from different methodological backgrounds (Chapter 21, this volume).

To end, we advocate the development of a multi-method approach to enquiry in mental-health-services research. It is therefore appropriate to highlight a lesson which has been learnt in another field. The seminal review by Martinson (1974) of offender rehabilitation programmes considered all published reports in English between 1945 and 1967, and the full version ran to 1,400 pages. He concluded

> I am bound to say that these data, involving over two hundred studies and hundreds of thousands of individuals as they do, are the best available and give us very little reason for hope that we have in fact found a sure way of reducing recidivism through rehabilitation. This is not to say that we have found no instances of success or partial success; it is

only to say that these instances have been isolated, producing no clear pattern to indicate the efficacy of any particular method of treatment.

(Martinson 1974, p. 49)

As noted by Pawson and Tilley (1997), the problem at one level is the impossible criteria for success, in which an intervention 'works' only if it produces positive outcomes in all trials in all contexts. However, the relevance to mental health services is that the pattern of developments in research approaches is depressingly similar, with an increased emphasis on methodologies which cost more and more to implement (larger samples, mega-trials, increased programme fidelity, etc.), in the (mistaken) belief that interventions will ultimately be categorised into 'effective' and 'ineffective'. If mental-health-service researchers are to move beyond the limits of randomised controlled trials, then new methodologies and innovative ways of synthesising evidence will be needed. This theme will be returned to in Chapter 21.

Acknowledgements

We are grateful to Derek Bolton, Gene Feder, Elizabeth Kuipers and James Tighe for their comments.

Chapter 11

The role of qualitative research methods in evidence-based mental health care

Brian Williams

Introduction

The rise in evidence-based medicine over the past decade has led to an ever-increasing emphasis on research centring on hypothesis testing. Such testing has generally taken the form of either randomised controlled trials (RCTs) or, more recently, meta-analyses and some systematic reviews. Given the context of increasing financial costs, and expectations of longevity and quality of life, it is not surprising that the most emphasis, effort and funding has been centred on these hypothetico-deductive-based designs. Such designs are clearly the most rigorous in identifying the relative effectiveness of interventions and forms of service provision. This is likely to continue indefinitely, and so it should.

The alternative to hypothetico-deductive-based designs is generally regarded as one that stems from a more inductive-based reasoning.[1] The human mind has a natural capacity for inductive thought; we explore the empirical world, seek patterns in what we see and attempt to make sense of it (Hume 1978). Where patterns appear to emerge, we may internalise laws as explanatory devices and adopt them in our day-to-day activities. However, this does not mean that they are true, even if they appear to have a predictive capacity.

The history of inductively derived knowledge reveals a host of false theories, which suggests that it may not represent the most effective or efficient approach to informing an evidence-based health-care system. In July 1886 members of the Medico-Psychological Association met at the Bethlem Hospital. At this meeting Dr Geo Savage presented a paper entitled 'A Case of Insanity Cured by the Removal of a Beard in a Woman'. There followed

---

1 'With *deductive* reasoning, the investigator starts with general ideas and develops a theory and testable hypotheses from it. The hypotheses are then tested by gathering and analysing data. In contrast, *inductive* reasoning begins with the observations and builds up ideas and general statements and testable hypotheses from them for further testing on the basis of further observations.' (Bowling 1997, p. 104).

a general discussion on the relationship between facial hair and insanity in which Dr Savage clarified that

> they were not discussing the whole subject of beards in relation to insanity, although that merited a paper apart. All connected with chronic lunatics must have seen very fine beards. He had got at least a dozen photographs. Undoubtedly there was a greater tendency with chronically insane women to develop beards than with others.
>
> (Savage 1886, p. 301)

Simply observing events and associations without subjecting theories to rigorous testing (where possible) frequently proves problematic. The reliance on inductively generated knowledge alone has probably been the greatest hindrance to the development of truly evidence-based health-care. Given such a comment, where does this leave the essentially, inductively based qualitative research methods?

The recommendations contained within the proliferating clinical guidelines are based on a ranking of research designs originating from the US Agency for Health Care Research and Quality. Each design is associated with a graded level of evidence, with the highest being a meta-analysis or systematic review of RCTs (see Box 11.1).

Box 11.1   (see also Box 9.4) Classification of evidence levels (Sign 1999)

Ia   Evidence obtained from meta-analysis of randomised controlled trials

Ib   Evidence obtained from at least one randomised controlled trial

IIa   Evidence obtained from at least one well-designed controlled study without randomisation

IIb   Evidence obtained from at least one other type of well-designed quasi-experimental study*

III   Evidence obtained from well-designed non-experimental descriptive studies, such as comparative studies, correlation studies and case studies

IV   Evidence obtained from expert committee reports or opinions and/or clinical experiences of respected authorities

* refers to a situation in which implementation of an intervention is outwith the control of the investigators, but an opportunity exists to evaluate its effect.

Evidence ranking usually places well-conducted systematic reviews and meta-analyses at the top, RCTs close second and observational studies lower down. However, it is essential to recognise that this ordering is not only determined by issues such as the vulnerability of specific designs to issues such as confounding or bias, but also to the question being asked. Rankings for clinical guidelines are those which are appropriate for answering questions of cause and effect (generally, what outcome does a specific intervention produce?). An RCT would not provide a high level of evidence for answering other questions such as the prevalence of particular conditions, or the time course of a disease. Such questions would best be answered by a cross-sectional observational study and cohort study respectively. Consequently, level of evidence is not an inherent attribute of a design or methodological approach alone, but is also dependent on the question for which evidence is being sought.

Qualitative methods seek to answer different questions to those of RCTs, and for those types of questions they potentially provide a high level of evidence, higher than that of the RCT. 'Potentially' remains an important qualification since (as with any research) the level of evidence produced is also dependent on the rigour of the study itself. Just as a poorly designed or conducted RCT provides weak evidence so too with a qualitative project.

In assessing the role of qualitative research in relation to evidence-based mental health care three questions therefore become important.

1. What questions can be answered (with a high level of evidence) by qualitative methods?
2. What are the qualities of a rigorous, well-conducted qualitative study?
3. Are the questions that qualitative studies can answer useful in designing and implementing an evidence-based mental health service?

The remainder of this chapter addresses these questions in turn. Key issues of data collection, sampling and analysis, which are common to the various types of qualitative research (i.e. in-depth interviewing, focus groups and participant observation),[2] are explained along with their advantages and disadvantages.

What questions can qualitative studies answer?

The subject matter of qualitative research is not the physical world itself but rather how it is interpreted and understood by individuals, societies and cultures. Consequently, it is concerned with exploring people's perceptions

---

2 The remaining designs, including consensus methods, case studies and action research are more seldomly used. Details on their design and use can be found elsewhere, see Bowling 1997; Hart and Bond 1996; etc.

of the world, their beliefs, attitudes and experiences, and conceptualising these in ways that are both meaningful and useful. It attempts to achieve understanding rather than explanations. Within contemporary health care such perspectives are important for two reasons. First, the move towards more patient-centred care suggests that the meaning which an individual attaches to a clinical problem should be regarded as important and addressed where possible (Stewart *et al.* 1995; Williams 1995; Williams and Grant 1998). Second, the ongoing concern with health and illness behaviour (risk taking, adherence to prescribed regimen, appointment keeping, etc.) largely depends on a knowledge of people's attitudes and beliefs, as the content of most social cognition models in health psychology demonstrates (Conner and Norman 1998).

The contribution that qualitative methods can make to the design and implementation of evidence-based mental health care may become clearer by initially considering how well they can answer three types of questions.

1. What exists? A qualitative approach provides a high level of evidence when answering this type of question.
2. Questions of process. A qualitative approach provides a moderate level of evidence when answering these types of question.
3. How many or how often? The level of evidence provided by a qualitative approach to this type of question is theoretically high but practically very low.

What exists?

Qualitative research can provide a rich and rigorous descriptive base of people's experiences, beliefs and attitudes upon which subsequent explanatory research can be based. In many circumstances it is difficult for a researcher, who is an outsider to an experience or a social or cultural group, to have an informed insight into the world in which these people inhabit. For example, Barham and Hayward's study of the experience of people with schizophrenia living in the community identified a variety of issues that were of immense importance to the individuals themselves. These included issues of exclusion (housing, employment and social life), burden (the consequences of disclosure of psychiatric status) and reorientation (the development of new ways of coping) (Barham and Hayward 1991). Similar studies have successfully described the meaning and experience of people with depression (Lewis 1995) and general affective disorders (Karp 1992).

While questionnaires may be of some use in identifying such issues they have two disadvantages. Since the generation of questions largely depends on the views of the researcher, key issues may be omitted and irrelevant ones included. Perhaps more importantly, there can be threats to various types of validity. Many of the assumptions upon which a data collection tool may be based may not hold. Questionnaires assume a fixed meaning in the use of language; however, particular words or phrases may hold different meanings (or none at all) for the people being studied. In an examination of the use of satisfaction questionnaires among people referred to a community mental health team, Williams discovered that ticking a box indicating 'satisfaction' with the service did not always mean that the patient had evaluated the service or even had a positive experience (Williams *et al.* 1998). While some patients were really expressing confidence in the staff (Owens and Batchelor 1996), others meant that though they had had bad experiences they were not holding the staff to blame for these.

Qualitative data and analysis can generate new concepts with precise definitions. Where these are grounded in the data and generated in the light of the research questions being asked or the wider issues of concern, they can have enormous relevance for subsequent quantitative research, whether that be in terms of questions of prevalence, explaining behaviour or in designing effective interventions. Qualitative research is therefore a powerful way of identifying what exists, conceptualising findings and providing precise definitions of key issues.

Questions of process

In addition to the descriptive questions addressed above, qualitative research can also play an important role in illuminating processes of change, both at an individual and an organisational level. This may involve shedding light on decision-making processes, or exploring health or illness behaviour, or identifying how organisations respond to change. Quantitative research can infer cause and effect either directly through experimental studies, or indirectly through correlations in cross-sectional studies. However, the actual processes by which these causes are *mediated* are often less open to quantitative analysis. Qualitative research can examine the specific processes that an intervention sets in motion, and examine how these lead to a particular outcome. In this case the qualitative data is attempting to throw light on a statistical occurrence. For example, quantitative research has indicated that a substantial proportion of people with mental health problems deviate from prescribed drug regimens. A qualitative study by Rogers has identified a variety of reasons for such behaviour. In particular medication was often managed in a way that allowed individuals to continue drinking alcohol, and visiting the pub with their friends, thereby maintaining social networks (Rogers *et al.* 1998).

Qualitative studies are not, however, unproblematic in providing explanations of process. Since qualitative sample sizes are generally small they cannot provide an answer as to the overall importance of any particular issue which is identified. For example, Rogers' study cannot provide any indication of what proportion of non-adherence can be explained by the desire to drink alcohol. Such an answer would require a further quantitative study.

While interviews and/or observations may shed light on human behaviour it is important that data relying on individuals' own reports of the reasons for their behaviour are regarded tentatively. The context of an interview often means that individuals reflect on their experience and behaviour, and provide explanations which may make sense of what occurred but which may not necessarily have been instrumental at that time. Where possible, further quantitative research might prove helpful. This is particularly common in informing new psychological models of behaviour or operationalising concepts in current models.

For the reasons highlighted above, and the fact that behaviour and general decision-making may include biological elements, the contribution of qualitative methods in this area should best be regarded as important but incomplete. They cannot provide a stand-alone answer. Consequently, questions of how something comes to occur may best be answered through a combination of both qualitative and quantitative approaches. The contribution of qualitative research in this context may best be described as generating hypotheses, and the level of evidence provided might therefore be described as 'moderate'.

How many or how often?

Useful and meaningful quantification is entirely dependent on a precise definition of the thing to be counted. Since qualitative methods are a powerful tool for identifying what exists and for generating useful concepts with precise definitions, it would appear theoretically possible and advantageous to use qualitative methods for ensuring validity while assessing issues of prevalence and incidence. One thousand people could be interviewed in depth and the number of people with particular views could be categorised. One could even use several coders and assess inter-rater reliability (Mays and Pope 1995). This might be methodologically desirable in that each interview would permit the respondents' views to be thoroughly explored and the meanings clarified so that any misinterpretation of questions or answers was minimised (i.e. to ensure validity). In practice this is rarely if ever done. In-depth interviews are time consuming to arrange, conduct and analyse. Interviews with twenty people may take a minimum of 2 months to collect and prepare for analysis. Data analysis is a slow and laborious process as transcripts need to be carefully scrutinised and every few phrases considered for coding. Six months for this process is not excessive. Qualitative studies do not represent good value for money when answering quantitative questions.

What are the qualities of a rigorous, well-conducted qualitative study?

Typical quantitative research involves a linear progression from a specific research question, through to data collection and then, once completed to

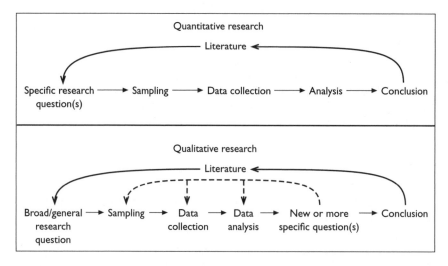

Figure 11.1 Research processes for qualitative and quantitative research

analysis (see Figure 11.1). Such a sequence assumes that the researcher has sufficient information about the research subject to generate a specific question. Since qualitative research is concerned with identifying what exists and in particular how *other people* see and experience the world it would be inappropriate to design a study around what appears important to an uninformed outsider.

A more effective and efficient way of progressing is by designing a study with a broad and general question, which makes few assumptions about the topic under study. A qualitative research question frequently indicates that the aim is to 'explore', 'identify' or 'describe'. The reaction of many to such questions is that if one asks a vague question then one will get a vague answer, and is that really useful to anyone? Probably it isn't. For this reason, the research process simply commences with a broad, overarching question. As data are collected and analysed, new, more specific questions arise. This then feeds back into the selection of a new and more specific sample, which is more relevant to the new question. In addition, analysis can feed back into new questions of the existing sample, or into the analysis of interviews already conducted. This presents a dynamic cycle of data collection and analysis, which is carried out until no new issues arise from the data.

This dynamic process indicates that while qualitative research is essentially an inductive exercise, the most specific findings stem from those which involved an inductive–deductive cycle. Where newly generated questions are allowed to feed back into the research process at either the sampling, data collection or analysis stages there is the possibility to engage in theory or hypothesis testing.

In practice qualitative studies vary from those which involve a simple linear progression mirroring quantitative research in the sequential timing of each stage to those which include numerous 'feedback' loops to the sampling, collection and analysis stages. For those that employ a simple linear progression data are collected, transcribed, analysed, then conclusions are drawn and written up. While such studies may be of some use, the issues identified and new concepts presented are generally vague, leaving a multitude of questions unanswered.

Sampling

For practical reasons qualitative research is not generally concerned with questions of frequency. As a result, large random samples are not employed. Since questions are of the exploratory 'what exists?' type, samples are selected in order to identify as wide a range of issues, experiences, beliefs and practices as possible. The size and statistical representativeness of the sample is therefore of less concern than the quality of the information elicited from it. Four types of sampling strategy for qualitative research exist.

Convenience sampling

This is a quick and easy form of sampling that involves selecting individuals who are easily accessible to the researcher and are able and willing to participate. However, those who are 'inconvenient' to sample may represent an important study group with specific experiences, beliefs or concerns which are relevant to the overall research question.

Snowball samples

'Snowballing' refers to the process by which a sample is drawn sequentially by asking participants to suggest, and frequently approach, other people to be involved in the study (usually friends, work colleagues or relatives). This represents a well-proven method of overcoming access problems where the topic of study is particularly sensitive (e.g. drug misuse, sexual behaviour). As with convenience sampling there is a possibility of significant omission as the sample is recruited from within a network of individuals.

Theoretical sampling

Theoretical sampling arguably facilitates the most rigorous qualitative studies. An initial series of individuals or groups representing a wide range of likely views and experiences are studied. Subsequent data analysis raises new questions that may feed back into the creation of a new sample by informing the selection of individuals who would best be able to throw light on the issues raised. This feedback may consist of one of two types. First, individuals might be selected in order to identify how the issues already raised vary in new contexts. Second, selection can be used to facilitate hypothesis testing through processes of falsification. Individuals can be interviewed who may prove to contradict the initial findings and developing theory. In these circumstances, the developing theory is either abandoned or modified to incorporate the new finding.

Purposive sampling

This technique involves the identification and subsequent selection of individuals who are likely to have as wide a range of views, experiences and behaviours as possible. The strategy is therefore employed to inform highly exploratory questions where the research is simply attempting to establish 'what is out there'. A practical problem is in knowing what variables are likely to cause variation in views or experiences. In these cases it is not unusual or unacceptable to employ a random sampling strategy. The initial sampling selection of a theoretical sampling strategy is often purposive.

Data collection

The two most common forms of data collection are in-depth interviews and focus groups. Each has its advantages and disadvantages and may be appropriate or inappropriate depending on both the research question and the characteristics of the study participants. However, it should be stressed that the choice of data collection is not either one form or the other; both collection methods may be used in a single study.

In-depth interviews

In-depth interviews attempt to provide an environment and method by which the content, meaning and significance of an individual's experiences and beliefs can be identified and made explicit. In-depth interviews are frequently described as 'unstructured' to set them apart from semi-structured and structured interviews used in much survey research. In-depth interviews are particularly useful in situations where the subject matter is sensitive or where individuals may have beliefs which they would be unwilling to express in a group context. The format also permits the interviewer to discuss their interpretation and understanding of what the participant has reported. This preliminary step of 'respondent validation' makes a useful contribution towards the rigour of the study.

In-depth interviews are time consuming to arrange, conduct, transcribe and analyse. Consequently, they do not represent a cheap option even though sample sizes tend to be relatively small (generally between twenty and sixty individuals). Furthermore the success or failure of the study is not entirely dependent on the appropriateness of the research design. The key research tool is the interviewer. An experienced, reflective and skilled interviewer can produce a rich data set while a poor interviewer can generate data which is biased and of poor quality.

Focus groups

Focus groups consist of between six and twelve generally similar or like-minded individuals being guided through a series of topics by a facilitator. Members of the group are encouraged to talk among themselves rather than addressing themselves to the facilitator or researcher (this may or may not be the same person). This slight detachment from the discussion enables the researcher to examine not only individuals' beliefs but also the interaction between members of the group. Analysis of such interaction can reveal the arguments that are employed in justifying particular beliefs or stances. By creating and observing the interactions within a social group it may also prove possible to identify social norms and values in a way in which a one-to-one interview could not possibly do (Barbour and Kitzinger 1998). By employing both individual interviews *and* focus groups it can also be possible to identify discrepancies between an individual's 'private' and 'public' accounts thereby revealing some of the effects of group pressure and/or interaction.

While focus groups make it possible to involve a larger number of participants in the overall study sample, there are a number of common problems. Depending on the study population it may prove difficult to identify times and dates that are suitable to all group members. Some individuals find group discussions intimidating and may refuse to attend or may contribute little to the discussion, particularly if there are one or two dominant personalities.

Data analysis

In the vast majority of cases in-depth interviews and focus groups are tape recorded and transcribed, thereby providing a written document to analyse. In some cases recording may prove impossible or unacceptable, and in these circumstances extensive field notes are taken and submitted to analysis. Data analysis exists at both the data collection and formal analysis stages of the research process. Given the relatively unstructured nature of in-depth interviews and the broad-ranging nature of discussion within groups, the choice of what question to ask is dependent on the interviewer constantly listening and analysing what has gone before. In order to access relevant and important issues the interviewer must be able to separate the important from the unimportant and choose which avenue to pursue in further questioning.

Historically, relatively little has been written about the analysis of qualitative data. Consequently, the process has remained somewhat enigmatic. Data are collected and then somehow miraculously transformed into an array of key findings. Faced with a set of transcripts the researcher is attempting to identify what issues exist (experiences, beliefs, etc.) and then how they change or vary across contexts or relate to one another. Sections of text that appear important and are broadly similar in meaning are grouped together and given a conceptual label or code. Once a large number of these codes have been developed it is possible to compare them with each other. At this stage a number of things may occur. First, two codes may appear so similar that they are joined. Second, it may be apparent that one code contains quotes of different kinds and can then be subdivided. Third, one code may be identified as a property of another. As this process continues concepts and their definitions are constantly refined and the relationships between issues become explicit.

Through the analysis the researcher generates concepts which accurately embody and represent the data. However, there are various ways in which the same phenomenon can be legitimately grouped together and coded. For example, if the objects in an office were to be listed they could be grouped in a variety of different ways: by material, by function, by colour. However, while different researchers may generate conceptualisations, both of which are valid, one may be more useful than the other or 'fit' the data better. Returning to the items in an office, if I was moving office then grouping objects by size or weight may be more helpful than by colour. It is important, therefore, to carry out coding with the research question, or range of possible applications of the research findings, in one's mind. Given the role of choice in both the questioning at interview stage and the generation and codes from transcripts, there is an aspect of qualitative research which has been described as an 'art'.

Attempts have been made to deconstruct the analytic procedure and reproduce a systematic 'how-to' guide. The most influential of these has been the detailed 'constant-comparative' technique outlined by Anselm Strauss and Juliet Corbin (Strauss and Corbin 1990). However, others exist in the form of analytic induction (Robinson 1951) and logical analysis (Williams 1981). The key point is that the analysis involves a continual attempt to falsify what has been generated. Where contradictions arise the concepts and theory are either abandoned, modified or added to. In this way it is possible to generate a theory or model which describes and suggests an explanation of how experiences, beliefs and behaviours vary over a wide variety of contexts.

Documenting rigour: validity and reliability

As with quantitative research, issues of rigour must be addressed at every stage of the research process, i.e. sampling, data collection and analysis. In order to facilitate an assessment of rigour the researcher must document the relevant steps in each of these stages and make them available so that the reader can arrive at an informed opinion of the trustworthiness of the findings. The key features to document have become more explicit in recent years with the development of explicit evaluative criteria for systematic reviews and meta-analyses. Many of these are based on new research evidence, which suggests possible sources of bias. For example, it is now increasingly common for RCTs to report concealment (i.e. how the process of randomisation was kept separate from those involved in the delivery of an intervention). The need to document the research process remains of equal importance for qualitative research. Achieving this is somewhat more problematic, particularly with regard to analysis. Quantitative research can merely report the use of a statistical test since what that test does is fixed by a set of precise and unambiguous rules.

Describing the process of analysis of a specific qualitative study is desirable and should contain a detailed description of what was coded, and how and why new cases were sought, how falsification was sought and in what ways new concepts were identified and theory was modified. The aim is that by providing this 'audit trail' it should be possible *'to create an account of method and data which can stand independently so that another trained researcher could analyse the data in the same way and come to essentially the same conclusions'*. (Mays and Pope 1995, p. 110). In practice, the creation of this audit trail has proved difficult, although the increasing use of computer software to facilitate data coding means that a systematic log of codes, their history and inter-relationships is becoming possible. The second problem is in making such a lengthy description of the research process available to the reader. The increasing willingness of journals to allow qualitative papers a higher word limit is helpful, as is the potential for longer documents to be made available online.

Within the detailed description of the research process a variety of procedures have been included which help ensure validity and reliability.

Sampling

Sampling bias is increasingly likely with the use of convenience and snowballing strategies. Purposive and theoretical sampling strategies both attempt to recruit with the aim of identifying as wide a variety of issues as possible. These are the preferred strategies and must be described in detail by the researcher. Random samples may be problematic as they are likely to omit individuals with more uncommon views and are therefore an inefficient device for identifying variety. This could be addressed by adopting a highly stratified random sample. However, with a small sample size this becomes almost identical to a purposive sample.

Data collection

Interviewer bias remains a constant possibility. Questioning within interviews can be informed by many of the same rules that apply to questionnaire design, in particular avoiding leading questions (Patton 1990). More open-ended questions are appropriate since closed questions make assumptions about the interviewee's views (they may not fit into a simple 'yes/no' dichotomy). Quotations contained in the final report should include the preceding question for the reader to assess the context in which the response was provided. Other issues of context should also be reported which may have influenced the respondent. Was anonymity guaranteed? Where was the interview conducted, in private or public, in a doctor's surgery or the interviewee's home?

Data analysis

An explicit description of the research process is essential in enabling an assessment of the reliability and validity of the findings. While different analytic strategies may have been employed it is important that the researcher has looked for disconfirming cases, and where this has occurred, explained the consequences. The search for falsification ensures against much selective coding and interpretation. Other, additional techniques include involving more than one researcher in both the coding and interview processes. This is becoming increasingly common and enables an assessment of rater agreement.

A process of 'respondent validation' is commonly used to improve confidence in the interpretation of meanings and processes. This entails feeding back findings to research participants to see if they regard them as an accurate and reasonable account of their views or experience. This can be carried out at various stages, within an individual interview, midway through analysis and as a final check on validity at the conclusion of the study.

A helpful list of evaluative criteria has been produced by Mays and Pope and is reproduced in Box 11.2. As with all critical appraisal, it is important not to disregard a study in its entirety for particular methodological weaknesses. It is important to identify what the study can still tell us despite those weaknesses or failings. There are few perfect studies.

Are the answers that qualitative studies can provide useful in designing and implementing an evidence-based mental health service?

Studies mentioned earlier in this chapter have indicated that results produced from qualitative studies may be useful in a number of areas. An

Box 11.2   Questions to ask of a qualitative study (Mays and Pope 1996)

- Overall, did the researcher make explicit in the account the theoretical framework and methods used at every stage of the research?
- Was the context clearly described?
- Was the sampling strategy clearly described and justified?
- Was the sampling strategy theoretically comprehensive to ensure the generalisability of the conceptual analyses (diverse range of individuals and settings, for example)?
- How was the fieldwork undertaken? Was it described in detail?
- Could the evidence (fieldwork notes, interview transcripts, recordings, documentary analysis, etc.) be inspected independently by others; if relevant, could the process of transcription be independently inspected?
- Were the procedures for data analysis clearly described and theoretically justified? Did they relate to the original research questions? How were themes and concepts identified from the data?
- Was the analysis repeated by more than one researcher to ensure reliability?
- Did the investigator make use of quantitative evidence to test qualitative conclusions where appropriate?
- Did the investigator give evidence of seeking out observations that might have contradicted or modified the analysis?
- Was sufficient of the original evidence presented systematically in the written account to satisfy the sceptical reader of the relation between the interpretation and the evidence (for example, were quotations numbered and sources given)?

evidence-based mental-health-care system relies on research addressing a range of questions through an ongoing process. Figure 11.2 shows the various stages that a service must go through if it is to arrive at a point at which it can claim to be delivering an evidence-based service that is meaningful to the patient and others.

Earlier reference to studies of patients' experience of mental health problems (Barham and Hayward 1991; Karp 1992; Lewis 1995) demonstrates that it is possible to identify issues of importance and concern from the patient's perspective. Once these have been identified and described in detail it may be possible to assess the practical and financial feasibility of a service addressing them alongside traditional clinical goals. This may become increasingly important as services seek to follow policy calls for more patient-centred care (Department of Health 1984; 1998).

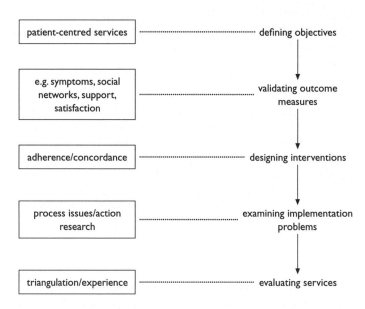

Figure 11.2 The role of qualitative studies in the design and implementation of evidence-based mental health care

   Once objectives have been identified a natural step is to objectify these into reliable and valid outcome measures. The increasing development of patient-centred outcomes (often generic or disease-specific health-related quality of life measures (Bowling 1995)) has resulted in a large number of measures with variable quality. While issues of reliability are addressed relatively easily, validity continues to be more problematic. Early stage qualitative research can help establish content validity (Oppenheim 1997) and be used subsequently to ensure correct interpretation of established measures (Williams 1994).
   In-depth interviewing may also identify the underlying rationale for sets of concerns or behaviour. These may therefore inform the design of interventions to address those concerns, or, more commonly, to change problematic aspects of health or illness behaviour. For example, a study that involved interviewing women with post-natal depression revealed that many women were concerned that if diagnosed as 'depressed' their baby might be taken away, as it demonstrated their inability to cope. The interview data not only highlighted the existence of this concern but also pointed to sets of underlying health beliefs about the cause and nature of depression which fuelled this concern (Williams 1995). The data therefore pointed to both the problem and a possible solution. Behavioural issues may also extend to health professionals. Increasing emphasis is being placed on the appropriate implementation of clinical guidelines in an attempt to provide an increasingly

evidence-based health-care system. For example, qualitative studies are currently ongoing under the 'Implementation of Research Findings' theme of the NHS research and development programme.

Finally, qualitative research has been used extensively in the evaluation of health services. Since the NHS Management Inquiry in 1984 called for collation of the evaluations and experience of patients and the community there has been a growing number of both qualitative, quantitative and triangulated (combination of both) studies of patients' views (Department of Health 1984; Sitzia and Wood 1997). The purpose of this research has laid a premium on using methods that can produce findings in a form that accurately embodies patients' views, and yet still has sufficient quantitative dimension to inform decision making about the desirability of making appropriate service delivery changes (Lebow 1983; Williams et al. 1998).

Conclusions

When conducted rigorously qualitative research can provide a high level of evidence in answering particular questions. Such questions may also be useful in contributing towards the design and implementation of evidence-based mental health care. Having made this point two further issues are worth considering. First, as with any research method or design qualitative research makes a contribution, nothing more. The delivery of evidence-based health care relies on answering and addressing a sequence of questions as outlined in Figure 11.2. Such a sequence mirrors the existence of a chain – it is only as strong as its weakest link. An RCT is useless if it is using the wrong outcome measures. Similarly, identifying patients' concerns or goals through a qualitative study is unlikely to lead to substantial changes in services unless an intervention can be tested to see if they can be addressed.

A final consideration concerns the nature of knowledge and evidence itself. Qualitative research generally starts from the philosophical premise that the acquisition of knowledge is problematic. While the world may be seen and experienced we can never know it fully or be certain that what knowledge we have is actually true. What we can ascertain is whether the constructions or models of the world that we have developed appear to make sense of, explain it and/or have some predictive capacity. This philosophical stance is common to many qualitative and quantitative researchers, in particular Karl Popper (Popper 1959; 1963). Whatever the research design or method that is employed there is a sense in which the results remain at theory level. They may be useful and have predictive capacity, but they may not be true. Such theories should be used until they are disproved; at which point they may be abandoned or modified. The recent Health Technology Assessment (HTA) review on qualitative methods summarised the situation well.

The goal of all research in HTA should be to establish knowledge about which we can be reasonably confident, and to provide findings that are relevant to policy makers and practitioners. Therefore, decisions about whether qualitative or quantitative methods (or a combination of both) are most appropriate to a particular research problem should be made on the basis of which approach is likely to answer the question most effectively and efficiently.

(Murphy *et al.* 1998a, p. iii)

Chapter 12

Studying psychiatric practice without *P* values: what is the place of anthropological inquiry?

Annie Bartlett

Introduction

Anthropology is an academic discipline that is both independent of psychiatry and at times closely linked. For anyone who thought that anthropology consisted of films on Channel 4 about exotic islands in the South Pacific, this chapter may come as something of a revelation. Its title is deliberately both positive and questioning. Positive, in the sense that it argues that there continues to be a place for anthropological inquiry in our research repertoire as mental health professionals. Questioning, in that it remains to be seen how acceptable anthropological inquiry is in the current research climate. Hence the reference to *P* values in the title.

This chapter will describe anthropology, its historical and contemporary approach, compare its approach in general terms with that of psychiatry and specifically with other research strategies, and outline the ways in which anthropology has already been used in mental health research and how it might be used in the future.

What is anthropology?

Conventionally anthropology is thought of as the study of mankind, as the Greek origins of the term imply. It is usual to think of the subject in two parts, physical and social. Physical anthropology studies the evolution of human kind. This chapter is solely concerned with social anthropology which focuses on people as social animals, specifically their beliefs, behaviours and belongings as part of a social group. It characteristically considers religious and moral beliefs, how people work and play, and aspects of their material world. It looks for similarities between people to establish cultural norms. It is immediately apparent that it is distinct from psychology and psychiatry whose primary focus is the individual psyche, and in the case of psychiatry the abnormal psyche.

Historical approaches

The origins of modern social anthropology are in a period of Western colonialism. This shaped the approach, possibilities and preoccupations of early anthropologists. Although this may at first sight seem a long way from contemporary psychiatric practice, the reflections on the methodological approach of the time are pertinent to psychiatric research today.

Early anthropologists were almost always white men. They studied the exotic other. For the most part they left northern Europe for colonies of their own country. They brought back copious notes, and many, often valuable, artefacts of the small-scale societies they studied. This was not a two-way traffic. No one from Ghana was studying village life in Gloucestershire and removing seventeenth century portraits from the local manor house to take home. They recorded the aspects of society that were probably fundamental but certainly different from that with which they were familiar. British anthropology in the first half of the twentieth century comprised pioneering documentation of kinship systems, political structures, economic and legal systems, the structure of settlements and the material of everyday life (Evans-Pritchard 1940; Fortes 1945; Leach 1954; Malinowski 1919). At the time their approach was ground breaking and involved rejection of the eighteenth and nineteenth century idea of evolutionary progress.

> the approach was naturalistic and empirical in intention, if not in practice; generalizing and above all genetic. Their thought was dominated by the notion of progress, of improvement of manners and customs from rudeness to civility, from savagery to civilization; and the method of investigation they elaborated, the comparative method, was chiefly employed by them for the purpose of reconstructing the hypothetical course of this development. It is in this respect that the anthropology of today is most at variance with that of yesterday.
>
> (Evans Pritchard 1951, p. 42)

With the confidence that came from being part of twentieth-century patriarchy these men thought that if they wrote down what they found, then they would understand the society in question, as it was at that time. They mistook being systematic for being objective; they believed that they were creating a scientific record. Their reputations have not stood the test of time without qualification. It transpired that Malinowski's scientific record was compromised by a revealing diary (Malinowski 1967). The Nuer had run away from Evans-Pritchard though he seemed immune to the meaning of this. Leach had lost his research notes but wrote a highly influential book on the political systems of Burma without them. They published in Europe for a highly select audience. The people who had told them about their lives seldom if ever found out what had been said about them.

Anthropology has moved on since then, but the early days of anthropology contained disturbing parallels to current research practice in psychiatry. Most professors of psychiatry are white men, who use a positivist paradigm to study the individual in society. Most of what is published is not shared with the people, or subjects of inquiry.

Crisis of confidence

Anthropology had a crisis of methodological confidence, as did other social sciences. First, it realised that almost without exception anthropologists had failed to establish the views of women from the societies they studied (Ardener 1975). The records of society were in fact records derived from contact with men, purporting to be the general view. Second, as a new generation of anthropologists emerged in the now independent ex-colonies the western world view was challenged. Western preoccupations in research began to be seen as just that, and as only sometimes relevant to the indigenous people. The white men had missed the point. They had not identified what mattered, just what mattered to them. It became clear that their *a priori* knowledge had contaminated the direction and implementation of their research. Third, the claims of anthropologists about the generalisability of their findings were undermined by an inability to replicate studies and by others who said it was different in the next village.

Current approaches

Anthropology in particular and social sciences in general have avoided the empirical paralysis that might have followed from these important critiques. They now use a more reflexive approach. It is now crucial to consider the context in which the research is undertaken, the reasons why the research topic has been singled out, and the relations of the anthropologist and informants (Okely and Calloway 1992). This has lent a transparency to accounts that was absent from early work. Anthropology has become, perforce, more sophisticated in its understanding of the impact of the researcher on the research process, particularly on data collection.

Anthropological work is now undertaken all over the world and is conducted by individuals trained in anthropological method in many different countries. Work is done both on small communities and in parts of complex urban societies. In the UK the subtleties of social identity and practice have been explored by a generation of anthropologists undertaking 'anthropology at home' (Jackson 1987; Okely 1996).

However the claims to ethnographic authority characteristic of earlier writing have been tempered by the crisis of positivism (Crapanzano 1986; Geertz 1983), paradoxically accompanied by a robust body of writing on anthropological method.

Methodological comparisons

This section deals specifically with a comparison of empirical anthropology, as practised today, with the quantitative approach usually adopted by those studying disease and illness, including psychiatric disorder. This is to subsume a number of different quantitative approaches, for example epidemiological, intervention studies together. Equally, in practice anthropologists do not just use participant observation, which was their hallmark technique.

Perhaps the single most important distinction between anthropological inquiry and quantitative techniques applied to mental health problems is the difference in importance attached to indigenous categories of meaning. For an anthropologist, understanding how people describe and frame their world is the place to start. The single most important task is to find out what people say, do and think, both in their own words and through their own actions. So, for an anthropologist considering drug use in south London, it will be more important to know the meanings attached to drug-taking behaviours, the social context in which certain drug vocabulary is used, and how the drug culture operates, not only in clinics but outside. From this raw material, conceptual analyses are derived with discernible fidelity to the original data set. These analyses privilege indigenous categories of societal analysis. In contrast the medical world uses largely pre-existing categories of analysis. Psychiatry has traditionally left itself open to criticism by researching from a framework clinically imposed on a rebellious patient group who contradict the value attached by psychiatry to such terms as schizophrenia. The pre-existing frameworks used often unthinkingly by researchers may be either offensive or unintelligible to the patient group. The personal investment in them by the researchers may lead to their relevance to the population in question being neglected. A possibly apocryphal tale from outside mental health was of research into a new analgesic which established much physiological data on the drug, including serum levels at different doses, but failed to clarify from the patients its analgesic efficacy, or as it might be better put, whether the pain went away.

Anthropologists start each study from a position of ignorance. The inductive method of research favoured in anthropology allows indigenous categories of meaning to emerge during the course of data collection. Neither their significance nor their definition is clear at the start. One consequence can be that they may remain poorly or ambiguously defined. Quantitative work prefers operational definitions. As in life, anthropology is about the social world in which words and phrases can have multiple meanings and context-dependent usage. This is not a problem if the intention is to obtain a complex real-life understanding as opposed to a reductionist one. The attempt at reductionism in psychiatry, in its desire to be seen as experimental and scientific, has been confounded by the plasticity of many crucial terms, for example anxiety and depression, whose everyday use undermines any ascribed professional meanings. An anthropologist would address this dilemma by exploring the multiple meanings. The result is that anthropological categories have high validity.

It must be obvious that the application of statistical manipulation to such unstable anthropological real-life categories is a non-starter. As a result, the anthropological product is less opaque than many quantitative papers, which require the reader either to take things on trust or to become statistically literate. The widespread application of statistical tests to variables or categories with limited meaning allows them to be numerically transformed, and has given the P value its remarkable status. But for certain kinds of data, anthropology encourages the counting and comparison of kinds of things (events, people, cassava, turnips). Economic anthropologists may be particularly concerned with what can sensibly be numerical data, but their work is the exception within anthropology as a whole.

The desire to discover meaningful analytic categories through the work also flags up the great strength of anthropological inquiry. You can find out the unexpected. More than that, you can incorporate the unforeseen and unexpected into the process of inquiry. This can result in a major shift in focus away from the original aims of the study. This is a very different experience from those of us who find there is nowhere on the structured questionnaire to write down the illuminating aside that the last patient produced. The rigidity of much quantitative research is both its strength and its weakness. The fluidity of anthropology, likewise, is both its strength and its weakness. But anthropology explicitly allows for the possibility of radical analysis. All too often quantitative work refines existing ideas to death without breaking new ground. This could result in a poverty of ideas within psychiatric research dominated by this outlook.

Like other qualitative methods, anthropology provides 'thick description' (Geertz 1993) of the social phenomena being described. The analysis should be embedded in a social context brought alive by the local detail and accessibility of the writing. The specific nature of the study is of course at the expense of breadth. But anthropology is not epidemiological in its intention. A reflexive approach applied to all stages of the research is evident in modern anthropology. The relationship of the identity of the anthropologist to the 'other' is an important element in the research and the final publication.

To some extent the dichotomy established here between styles of inquiry is false. This is because some researchers are flexible and have training in a range of research techniques. However the dichotomy is helpful in emphasising the need to choose horses for courses. Some research techniques will be appropriate to some research agendas and contexts but not to others.

The process of anthropological inquiry

For anyone embarking on psychiatric research which is informed by anthropology, or more ambitiously is contemplating the possible value of a full blown ethnography, or simply reading anthropology with a critical eye, this section will explain the likely broad brush approach. It is not a substitute for handbooks on ethnography, nor does it dwell at length on the methodological issues facing modern-day researchers. It is inappropriate that anthropology is judged by the standards and preoccupations of other research approaches. However, it is important, both theoretically and practically, that there are criteria against which anthropology can be judged. Within anthropology there are two schools of thought. The first is exemplified by writers such as Miles and Huberman (1984) who describe their position as 'soft-nosed logical positivism'. They want to document the process of data analysis in particular. They are opposed to what they see as the 'magical' and 'artistic' approach of writers like Clifford (1988) who see anthropology as just another kind of writing. What follows panders to the first school of thought, but pays lip-service to the second. It suggests ways in which the value of any given piece of work can be judged from within the discipline's own paradigms.

Questions

A combination of globalisation and information overload places contemporary anthropology in a very different situation from that of 100 years ago. In the past the adventure of anthropology was, in part, documenting what was completely unknown. Now more is known, even if less is certain. Setting the agenda from existing information is necessary. It is rather like knowing the point of departure. You can identify the aims you started with, even if they fall by the wayside, you can also document the journey you subsequently undertake.

But establishing aims is different from defining hypotheses. Aims will be broad, and honest in their implicit message that the focus may alter and narrow. Early hypotheses do not fit with the spirit or the reality of anthropological inquiry. They are useful where the research focus is precise and built on a large body of well-established data. They imply evidence-based foreclosure on lines of inquiry that is inappropriate when venturing into the unknown.

Access

Anthropologists are nosy. When they venture into your world they are both inquisitive and sceptical about what you say you are doing. They see your explanation of your way of life and, in the case of psychiatric practice, work as just one of a number of ways of seeing the world. They probably do not share your belief in the way the world is, but they may hide this well and/or cheerfully admit complete ignorance. Hammersley (1983) reports a number of anthropological attempts to gain access to the world of medical staff. Without recognisable prestige, acquired through personal friendship or the status of a partner, hospitals have been unwelcoming places.

Reflections on the process of access are not just the personal knowledge of the researcher, rather they are integral to many projects as they shed light on the value system of the institution. My own access to a highly secure hospital took several years to achieve, in contrast to other projects in the same place, and was a revealing exercise. Anthropologists are refreshingly upfront about why they undertake particular projects. More transparency of this kind would be welcome in much mental health research.

Ethics

Anthropologists have been less than explicit about their ethics. They have nothing that approaches the rigour of a medical ethics committee, though perhaps therefore nothing so inconsistent either (Cohen *et al.* 1996). Their position is historically understandable. It was assumed at first that studies were either morally neutral, or helpful, in bringing to the west an understanding of non-western society that would otherwise be absent. In cultures with significant illiteracy, and to whom such a procedure would be entirely alien, an individual consent form would be bizarre.

But with anthropological projects in literate, complex societies at a time when the best intentioned research is not seen as morally neutral, this position requires revision. For anthropologists working with patient populations ethical scrutiny is likely to be essential. Where the patients are that much more vulnerable by virtue of mental health problems and perhaps involuntary hospitalisation, failure to address ethical concerns is unacceptable. The difficulty raised is that of the spirit of anthropology projects. It is difficult to obtain meaningful consent for very open-ended projects. The danger is that in allowing for the unexpected, any consent obtained is potentially meaningless. Individual consent in a group situation will badly affect the attempt at naturalism and does not allow for the real-life entry of other participants to the research field. My own view is that for participant observation studies, individual consent should not be attempted. But in such studies there is a need both for explanation of the project and for considerable sensitivity on the part of the researcher not to hound unwilling participants.

Medical ethical committees dealing with projects like this are likely to be concerned and inexpert. There is a case for external scrutiny by those with relevant methodological expertise. There may also be a role for ethical minimum standards to reduce the chance of prejudiced arbitrary decision making.

Resources

Social-science funding bodies in the UK have far less money than the large medical grant bodies. The latter may rarely fund pure social-science projects but may fund projects with social-science elements. Anthropology is often done on behalf of voluntary-sector organisations and governments in non-western countries. Research in western societies will be done by people employed by or studying in higher education, often working alone. Medical anthropologists who work as clinicians will find the opportunity for fieldwork frequently constrained by clinical schedules.

Data collection

The characteristic form of anthropological data collection is through participant observation, recorded in the form of field notes. Anthropologists go to the field, in many cases a literal as well as a metaphorical statement. Participant observation is a term that disguises different degrees of participation and observation. The variability may be in terms of the general approach, will correspond to the possibilities in the research setting (I learnt to play snooker in the high security hospital), and will vary within a given day and from day to day. The process will give access to both ordinary and extraordinary events, both of which will be revealing about custom and belief. The technique will usually involve much informal conversation with participants as well as offering the opportunity for more systematic interviewing or observation in relation to areas of interest. So, for instance, studying decision making in multi-disciplinary teams might involve shadowing a member of the team, sitting in on ward rounds, and then asking questions of all team members about the decisions made.

Recording of field notes is often difficult. Many, like mine, are written in the lavatory rather than in front of people. Field notes are both systematic and idiosyncratic. In themselves they represent only part of what the anthropologist uses in analysing and writing. Their function is in part to trigger memory. They can include recordings, drawings, personal reflections, chunks of dialogue, lists of vocabulary and schema for social interactions, and the placing of material objects. They may well be supplemented by documentary material, for example case notes, newspaper articles, colonial agricultural records.

Field notes are huge, and a common sensation of anthropologists looking at their own is to feel inadequate to the task of analysis, and that they are drowning in data.

Data analysis

Anthropological studies are usually published without detail on data analysis. Qualitative work has historically been vulnerable to the criticism that the process of analysis has not been demonstrated and some authors have devoted considerable energy to tidying up anthropology's act (Miles and Huberman 1984; Hammersley 1992). Other writers relish the subjective, creative elements of the process and ignore these rather anxious attempts to make anthropology acceptable to those immersed in other styles of inquiry (Clifford 1986).

There is an inherent difficulty in describing the analysis of field notes. At a crude level there is agreement that it involves immersion, descriptive and analytic coding, interrogating the data (checking for negative cases, qualitative correlation, triangulation of data sources) and moving between levels of data as a conceptual framework develops. But, when the process is undertaken rigorously it is hard to describe. Even if it is rigorously described it is hard to verify. Equally it is true that much of the quantitative paradigm cannot be checked from the write-up itself. As with field notes you would have to go back to the raw data. Describing the analysis of field notes would also make unexciting reading. In a discipline that prides itself on accessibility this would be unfortunate. For large databases there are computer programmes that assist with coding and retrieval. Not everyone likes them and people may still prefer the cut-and-paste technique of old which can be more efficient. Whatever the technique of computer programming, nothing is a substitute for thinking about the meaning of the data.

Data analysis will result in some ideas testable in the data and some that cannot be examined within the data but which require further work. Some people conceptualise research as a continuum, where you start with vagueness and uncertainty and progress from qualitative to quantitative studies, arriving in medicine at the randomised control trial! Anthropology invites further research on the ideas that are generated by the data analysis. In reality many of these areas of research are limited by the methods that can be sensibly applied; this is particularly true of human subjects living in social groups. Powerful and convincing theory may be developed but there may be practical limits to narrow empiricism.

Writing and publication

We live in an era of 'impact factors' and 'bottom lines'. Anthropology and its insights do not sit easily with either. Unless prestigious psychiatric journals and their editors change their outlook, anthropology applied to mental health issues will only rarely find a home in either the *British Journal of Psychiatry* or the *British Medical Journal*. This is a disincentive to researchers. Equally importantly, it is doubtful whether those brave enough to submit to such journals are reviewed by those competent in the relevant methodology.

The best anthropology, and that which will stand the test of time, is both scholarly and literary. It is likely to be lengthy and often appears in book form. The best of anthropology is a good read, in fact in the same way that some psychiatric authors, for example Aubrey Lewis (whose son is an anthropologist), Peter Scott and Anthony Clare are a good read. So the consolation prize for the ambitious researcher is that when the neuro-imaging papers have been consigned to the dustbin, someone may still read your monograph. It will remain readable because it will give a complex, illuminating and satisfyingly complete picture of the social group you have described, and because certain individuals will still leap out of the pages.

Assessing the value of studies

Most people reading this chapter will be reading anthropology, not doing it. The terms scholarly and literary used in the previous paragraph are useful because people can research well but write badly, and vice versa. The evaluation of scholarly and literary merit tells you whether what you are reading is any good, i.e. that in describing and analysing the beliefs, behaviours and belongings of a given social group, the author has produced a valid representation. Although your opinion as a reader is, like the work, subjective, it can and should be based on criteria that are explicit.

The previous sections have attempted to describe briefly how anthropological work is done. In terms of the scholarly merit of a piece of work, these stages and reference to them in any publication are helpful. But the fact that something is not mentioned does not mean it has not happened, merely that it is hard to tell. In general terms, it is wise to consider how the development of the project is explained, including limitations on access and the extent and volume of systematic inquiry. Where field note material *per se* is used its purpose and representativeness should be clear, for example it is legitimate to use the most memorable quote to illustrate a point supported by other data, it is not legitimate to use it to suggest that all informants agreed when they did not. Detailed analysis contributes to the plausibility of unexpected results, and descriptions of context, referencing and evaluation of work in the same field are all important. In a study of drug addicts that made no reference to types of drug used, circumstances or financing of drug taking, it would be implausible if you were told that the informants funded their habit exclusively from the sale of their families' antique jewellry. The development of theory from empirical data should show evidence of reasoning, and consideration and exclusion of competing explanations. Ultimately of course the reader may decide that, however rigorous the work, it is unimportant.

They are probably less likely to reject it if the work is convincingly written. Part of that judgement is down to the factors given above. But the reader is wise to be wary; narrative flow, imagery and rhetorical devices will all make a favourable impression (Crapanzano 1986). Wilful obscurity and the use of unnecessary social-science jargon will alienate many readers and can disguise woolly thinking.

Anthropology and mental health

This section will discuss the ways in which anthropology has already impacted on the field of mental health. This is a highly selected review in order to be able to discuss each piece of work in some detail. As the approaches have been affected by changes in thinking in anthropology generally, a chronological approach is adopted. Having said that the contribution of anthropology is primarily

1. the concepts of disorder and their relationship to cultural norms
2. the approaches to care by psychiatric services and the cultures established within institutions.

Historical studies

In the early days of anthropology, the interest in the exotic led to the collection of manifestations of distress in different parts of the world. There were detailed descriptions of phenomena that were apparently unique to non-western societies, but which at the same time were considered to be variants of western disorder, for example amok, latah, koro (Yap 1965; Littlewood and Lipsedge 1985). These were incidental observations for the most part, not an attempt to develop illness ethnography in particular settings. Another strand of this early approach was, put simply, to see if the shaman had schizophrenia. Valued members of small-scale societies who had authority over the use of certain rituals, not infrequently involving trance states, were scrutinised to see if their observed experiences could be attributed to disease. There was a corresponding lack of enthusiasm for detecting culture-bound syndromes among white populations living in western Europe and North America (Littlewood and Lipsedge 1985).

Meanwhile the consequences of attributing disease labels indiscriminately to large numbers of the population were becoming clearer. Western Europe and North America had incarcerated ever increasing numbers of individuals in asylums (Jones 1993). The extent to which the illness labels were ever justified has been eloquently debated (Hare 1983; Scull 1979). Scull (1989) argues that it was a useful way of mopping up the unwanted – the poor, the black, the Irish, the unmarried mothers, etc. Certainly my own interest in institutions was informed by meeting, as a medical student, an unmarried mother in her fifties, she had spent her late teenage years, as well as the rest of her life, living in a mental handicap institution in Epsom.

The impetus for deinstitutionalisation came in part from the work of Goffman (1961). *Asylums* is a book that everyone should read. It is both deeply flawed as a work of anthropology and enormously important. It illustrates how truth can, and sometimes should, transcend method. Goffman worked as a fitness instructor in a large asylum. Asylums in the US were often very much larger than those in England. Goffman used the cover of his work to observe life in the asylum. He documented social practices of remarkable rigidity which allowed patients little room for personal expression. Using the established language of anthropology he described initiation rituals, or 'how you become a patient'. Such a process involved 'a series of abasements, degradations, humiliations and abasements of the self' (Goffman 1961, p. 24). This last sentence reflects the tone of the four essays and explains in part why the work was controversial. The other shocking strategy was to see similarities between psychiatric hospitals, concentration camps and prisons, and to stress similarities at the expense of difference. This was not an accident. He was discussing the theory of institutions and, as an anthropologist, he was refusing to take at face value what the psychiatrists and nurses said they were doing.

From the point of view of an anthropologist the work is infuriating. There is no exegesis of method other than glancing reference to field notes used as a source of verbatim quotation. As an empirical piece it fails to explain how it arrived at its conclusion or indeed how Goffman got access. As a theoretical piece it is powerful and convincing.

It could be juxtaposed with the work of Rosenhan (1981) who neatly combines the two foci of anthropology in psychiatry indicated above. He describes the concepts of illness played out in different psychiatric hospitals. Rosenhan (1981, p. 308) argues that the diagnoses of mental illness may be 'less substantive than many believe them to be'. The timing of his work meant he was addressing a central anxiety in Anglo-American psychiatry. Using covert techniques, participant observation researchers gained admission to psychiatric hospitals as patients. They complained of voices saying thud, empty and hollow and otherwise gave factual accounts of their life histories (apart from name and occupation). They denied symptoms from the point of admission and behaved normally on the wards apart from writing notes. The length of stay was 7 to 52 days, averaging 19 days. The eight patients were prescribed 2,100 pills during these admissions. Although staff were unable to detect sanity, patients did rather better and accused the researchers of being journalists. Examination of notes on the pseudo-patients also indicated that life histories were distorted to fit the diagnosis. The paper also includes interesting reflections on staff–patient contact and the powerlessness and depersonalisation of individuals when they became patients.

Both Rosenhan and Goffman share anthropological scepticism about the value psychiatry attaches to its ideas, terminology and procedures. It is interesting that both were originally published in mainstream journals: Goffman in *Psychiatry* and Rosenhan in *Science*.

Although both these pieces of work have stood the test of time and contain insight of relevance to contemporary psychiatry, it is wise to point out that other work has fallen by the wayside. Bateson's work (1956) on the 'double bind' children of schizophrenogenic mothers was prominent in multiple choice questions as an example of discredited ideas about schizophrenia. Possibly its dubious longevity owed something to its catchy phrases which were certainly all that most training psychiatrists knew about the study. This is an example of rhetoric outweighing scholarly considerations.

Recent work

The majority of recent work has focused on categories of illness. This has involved critiques of earlier research practices and understanding of illnesses, and concern about the way in which contemporary psychiatry has exported its own ideas of pathology, reliant on an explicitly western mind–body dualism. It has measured abnormality in a range of non-western settings with varying degrees of scientific and anthropological rigour (see Leff 1988 for summary, Carstairs and Kapur 1976, Kleinman 1986 for anthropologically informed examples).

Although a range of disorders have been studied the test case for much of this thinking has been the International Pilot Study of Schizophrenia (IPSS) and its successor projects (World Health Organisation 1973, Sartorius *et al.* 1986). These studies are epidemiologically based with considerable attention given to the translation of terms used in standardised diagnostic instruments developed in Europe and the United States. They were international in that they involved psychiatric centres worldwide. Their outcome has been characterised as 'universalist' in that they stressed the similarities in incidence and presentation of disorder in the centres and only mentioned in passing differences in presentation and outcome.

Kleinman (1977, 1987) has argued that western diagnostic formulations are inappropriate to non-western societies. He terms this 'category fallacy'. He argues that without an understanding of indigenous concepts of illness in a given society, the measurement of western diseases may be a wasted effort, and invalid. Not only will disease that does not correspond to suffering be identified, but suffering that does not correspond to disease will be missed. In the same vein, post-diagnosis, therapeutic effort will be misplaced and there may be a failure to recognise elements of caring which contribute to good outcome because they do not match western response to psychiatric disorder. Prognosis in schizophrenia may well be better with support offered by extended rather than nuclear families. This was a finding Kleinman felt had been underplayed in the IPSS study. This position has been described as 'cultural relativism'.

This debate between epidemiological universalists, concerned with comparison and similarity, and anthropological cultural relativists, concerned with individual cultural circumstance and local detail, is Evans-Pritchard brought up to date. Neither position is always likely to be right.

In his own empirical studies of illness and help-seeking behaviours in non-western societies, Kleinman (1986) described existing patterns of presentation and care. The lines of argument developed by Kleinman and Leff are now rehearsed in relation to post-traumatic stress disorder. Summerfield (1995) has vehemently opposed the internationalisation of this new diagnosis because it is both irrelevant and misleading. The occurrence of post-traumatic features after what are often societal, rather than isolated individual traumas, may be best dealt with by economic and social regeneration rather than individual counselling.

The impact of globalisation on many societies means that the purity of belief systems that might have pertained in earlier years is unlikely to continue to do so. The exposure of many communities to western systems of thought, for example via satellite television, means that ideas will mix and change. This is not a new phenomenon, but one with a contemporary spin. The Indian system of rural health care established after independence is an interesting example of absorption and culturally specific regurgitation of allopathic medicine, first brought as part of the colonial regime, alongside the older traditions of Ayurvedic medicine. The challenge for those providing health care may be in keeping up with the patients. A good example of this from multicultural Britain is the study of Punjabis in Bedford (Krause 1989), where the presentation of illness owed something to the beliefs that the original migrant group brought with them, something to the mutation of belief brought about by living in the west, and something to the next generation of the community born in Britain.

The anthropological critique of illness categories has also found expression in this country in the work of Rack (1982), who bizarrely writes as though all psychiatrists were from the majority white community, and Littlewood (1990) who does not. This is best illustrated with regard to the understanding of schizophrenia in the Afro-Caribbean population. The alarming statistics of admission, and in particular compulsory admission, were reported as simple statistical findings. Explanations were offered which questioned the ethnocentricity of diagnosis or speculated crudely on the cultural situation of first and second-generation Afro-Caribbeans (Littlewood and Lipsedge 1988). Even so, it is striking that there has been little large scale anthropologically informed work on this topic despite both the moral importance of the work and the cost to the health service.

As psychiatric institutions have affected a smaller proportion of the population it is understandable that they have ceased to be a focus of anthropological activity. An exception to this has been the work of Barratt (1988a; 1988b). He used participant observation in an acute psychiatric unit dealing with schizophrenia. Once again he drew attention to the fact that psychiatric units do not do what they say they do, and his study indicated the continuing importance of informal categorisation of patients even with modern, and more rigorous diagnostic systems. The relationship between linguistic representation of patients and quality of care is a further avenue of research.

Although anthropology and psychiatry have a long-standing relationship, anthropology has been unsettling to psychiatry. This is a function of its stance in relation to belief systems of any kind, and its agnostic method of inquiry. There are signs that psychiatry can withstand cultural critique and better work may emerge. Examples of this include the incorporation of an anthropologist into the MacArthur study of risk and the multimethod approach of the World Mental Health Report (Desjarlais *et al.* 1995). The World Mental Health Report uses epidemiological studies alongside anthropological studies to make the best use of both. Its wide-ranging and authoritative analysis of mental health problems is rooted in an understanding of the cultural context in which they are manifest. This piece of comparative work is interesting not least because it suggests that many of the problems they identify are not solved by wealth, and they resist the obvious temptation to provide an overarching simple analysis.

The way forward

Future areas of inquiry

Anthropology within the field of mental health is a flexible approach. It can be used to critique studies where a cultural perspective can add to the value of the work. It can also be used as an empirical approach in its own right. It may be more useful than other approaches in accessing certain groups who may be suspicious of research linked to clinical work, and in obtaining specific kinds of information about psychiatric practice.

In Britain it may be better than other approaches because of its emphasis on the informant's world-view where the following cultural frameworks can be used

1. the disenchanted, for example homeless people, drug users, ethnic minorities, gays and lesbians
2. service users (where professional paradigms are not as valuable as indigenous categories of meaning)
3. mental health practitioners
4. health service management.

As a method, the establishment of an ethnographic record can be useful for

1. obtaining private rather than public opinions on sensitive subjects
2. detailed examination of process (decision making, attribution of events) *in vivo*

3. documentation and analysis of implicit and explicit symbolism in psychiatric practice (including the meaning of microspace, for example offices, and macrospace, for example hospital architecture)
4. understanding the political and kinship systems of mental health practitioners and how they change
5. capturing meaningful quality standards and outcome measures as they develop and change.

Working in mixed-method teams

Multicentre studies are in fashion. It is early days to assess their value. But they may offer a way forward in mental health work where the poverty of previous methodology is acknowledged. Mixed skills in a team can make for more robust work. Anthropologists skilled in self-reflexion in research, and good at looking sceptically at accepted conceptual frameworks, can be 'added value'. There is no shortage of up-and-coming researchers with talent and experience in qualitative and quantitative research. The future of research in mental health must lie in the rejection of the rigidity of traditional research paradigms which privilege professionally generated psychiatric explanation, and which owe much to the easily criticised medical model. To satisfy the demand for evidence-based medicine, a broader approach, which can include where appropriate both an anthropological perspective and, at times, ethnographic work, is necessary.

Chapter 13

Individual case studies

Nick Alderman

Introduction

Studies of the individual recipients of mental health services have much to offer. For the rehabilitation practitioner the goal of such studies has been described succinctly by Wilson (1991, p. 247): *'is my treatment the cause of this person's change?'*

In this chapter the contribution made by study of the individual to the evidence-based mental health services will be reviewed. Utility of individual case study methods will be illustrated through their application to the fields of neurology, neuropsychology and neuro-rehabilitation. Reasons for this are twofold

1. people with acquired neurological disorders clearly illustrate some of the problems of attempting to apply group methodologies to clinical populations
2. the advantages of using these methods are particularly relevant in meeting the needs of neurological patients whilst most clearly demonstrating benefits regarding evidence-based outcome measurement.

Their nature, types of information generated, and issues regarding generalisation will be illustrated using examples from clinical work.

Limitations in utilising group experimental methodologies in evaluating clinical outcome

Application of group comparison methodologies in determining treatment efficacy became the norm during the 1950s: this tradition was attributed to the growth of inferential statistics which began two decades previously with the work of Fisher. Before then, individual case studies had provided the dominant focus for inquiry (Hersen and Barlow 1984).

Group methodologies continue to enjoy longevity in the evaluation of mental health outcomes (Blackburn *et al.* 1981). However, they are not flawless. Hersen and Barlow (1984) drew attention to several potentially limiting factors. First, there are ethical concerns about withholding treatment from a control group, whilst withdrawing treatment from an experimental group who may continue to benefit raises similar problems. Second, group studies may be expensive, difficult to sustain and constrain other clinical activities. Finally, there may be difficulties in recruiting sufficient numbers of homogenous participants, that is, people who not only present with the same problem, but are also matched regarding demographic and other characteristics.

In addition Wilson (1991) argued that group designs lack flexibility in meeting individual patient needs (for example, the option to adjust treatment to progress). This further highlights ethical and practical concerns about these methods.

Special difficulties in using group experimental methodologies with neurological patients

Neurological patients encompass a wide variety of clinical conditions including traumatic brain injury, stroke, degenerative disease, cerebral tumour, infection, anoxia and other conditions such as Korsakoff's Syndrome (Wilson 1991). Their characteristics highlight the difficulties associated with group methodologies and other procedures.

Problems arising through lack of participant homogeneity are especially heightened with regard to traumatic brain injury (Wood 1987). Difficulties other than those created by the need to match participants within and between groups on demographic factors are clearly evident. For example, traumatic brain injury rarely leaves a person with one identifiable problem. Instead, people routinely acquire a range of cognitive, emotional, behavioural, physical and functional impairments which interact to produce unique symptom-led profiles of bewildering complexity. This issue was ably summarised by Mateer and Ruff (1990, p. 278) when they stated that *'no two head injuries are alike'*. Wilson (1991) commented that such people are almost certain to present with a combination of problems, and that these are rarely identical. Further difficulties in creating homogenous groups arise through the need to match participants regarding a range of additional variables including the severity of injury, and location and size of brain lesions (Mateer and Ruff 1990). The problem of grouping people together on the basis of cognitive impairment was highlighted by Colthart (1991) who said the probability of a cognitive system being damaged in exactly the same way is negligible. He illustrated this in respect to the naming system which was hypothesised to be potentially impaired in up to 16,383 distinct ways.

Further difficulties arise when data are pooled. For example, group averages obscure individual outcome. This problem of the 'averaging artefact' is well known (Chassan 1967; Sidman 1960). However, because lack of homogeneity within groups of people with acquired neurological disorders is greater than in most other clinical populations, this artefact is exaggerated further (Wood 1987; Wilson 1991). Deciding whether a particular intervention may benefit a patient on the basis of change in group averages may be tenuous (see Alderman *et al.* 1999a for an example of how abnormal variance masked individual change in the rehabilitation of challenging behaviour).

Another problem is the rarity of some conditions (Wilson 1991). Accounts of phenomena such as visual object agnosia, persistent reduplicative misidentification syndromes and the Cotard delusion make fascinating reading. However, gathering sufficient numbers of people who present with such conditions is rarely practical.

Finally, whilst there is evidence that neurorehabilitation may be beneficial (Cope 1994) it remains the case within the UK that services are underdeveloped and poorly resourced. A good example of this concerns people with acquired brain injury and challenging behaviour (Greenwood and McMillan 1993; Medical Disability Society 1988) and scarcity of resources will certainly prejudice group methodologies.

It is evident that the contribution made by group study to evidence-based practice is not without its criticisms. Issues regarding homogeneity, ethical and economic considerations may limit the ability to implement these methods and draw meaningful conclusions regarding treatment efficacy. Problems with homogeneity are further exaggerated amongst neurological patients, rendering use of group methods even more questionable. Whilst some areas of investigation positively endorse this approach, for example the study of the executive system (Burgess 1997), single case methods have been advocated as providing the principal tool of enquiry with this group (Alderman *et al.* 1999a; Alderman and Knight 1997; Colthart 1991; Mateer and Ruff 1990; Wilson 1991; Wood 1987).

Approaches to the study of the individual

Two principle approaches have evolved

1.   the uncontrolled/descriptive approach
2.   single-case experimental designs.

Uncontrolled/descriptive case study approach

The study of individuals was prominent in the early histories of physiology and experimental psychology: until adaptation of group methods in the middle of the twentieth century it was the dominant means of informing and developing practice within psychiatry (Hersen and Barlow 1984).

Some of the earliest descriptive case studies concerned neurological conditions. Probably the first was the account given by Broca in 1861 regarding one of his patients who could not speak intelligibly; at autopsy Broca identified the brain area responsible and thus began the tradition that continues today of mapping brain–behaviour relationships (Hersen and Barlow 1984). Other neurological conditions were first identified and studied through descriptions of individuals. For example, Pick (1903) identified a variant of reduplicative paramnesia through his observations of a 67-year-old woman with degenerative brain disease. Subsequent accounts of environmental reduplication, for example by Head (1926) and Paterson and Zangwill (1944), lent further validity to the nature of this disorder. Other types of reduplicative paramnesia were also identified using this method, for example, the Capgras Syndrome (Capgras and Reboul-Lachaux 1923).

Descriptive case studies continue to fulfil an important role in the study of acquired neurological disorders. A good example of this is evident from the recent publication of an entire volume concerning cognitive neuropsychiatry in which the descriptive case study provides the vehicle for the investigation of a wide variety of neurological and psychiatric conditions (Halligan and Marshall 1996). The editors testify to the versatility of this approach, in which interviews, cognitive tests and neurological findings are incorporated alongside behavioural observations.

Descriptive cases continue to provide a means of investigation within applied neuroscience. It is especially relevant in aiding understanding of potential causes and mechanisms of particular conditions. For example, study of individual cases is fundamental to the process of evolving models of domain-specific cognitive functions. Colthart (1991) argued that cognitive-neuropsychological analyses of individual cases to understand what has gone wrong must precede treatment. Without models to aid understanding of why a patient behaves as they do, treatment may amount to no more than educated guesswork.

However, uncontrolled/descriptive case studies are inadequate methods of determining treatment outcome. For example, one patient within a series described by Alderman *et al.* (1999a) was physically aggressive 451 times during the first 8 weeks that he participated in a neurobehavioural programme; in the 8 weeks prior to discharge the number of aggressive incidents was 33. These data suggest that the programme was effective in reducing aggression. However, although this is a tempting conclusion, there is no more than weak correlational evidence to substantiate this: it could be that the patient's aggression was reduced for another reason, or that the second 8-week period was unrepresentative of the patient's behaviour. The case study was 'uncontrolled' in that there is no indication that either conditions were maintained consistently, or that variables were systematically manipulated and effects on behaviour measured. Consequently, it is erroneous to state that what appears to be a good outcome was attributable to treatment.

Other omissions within this patient's account help to illustrate why the uncontrolled/descriptive case study approach cannot be used to reach valid conclusions concerning treatment efficacy. First, there was no definition of the target behaviour: interpretations of what constitutes physical aggression may vary widely between people making recordings. Second, data lacked serial dependency: there was no way of determining any trend in behaviour that may be attributed to treatment. Third, there was no indication regarding the conditions under which behaviour was recorded: was it logged within therapy sessions or throughout the day? What were the expectations levied on the patient? It may be that during the first 8 weeks many efforts were made to initiate therapy: this may have elicited much of the aggressive behaviour. A consequence could be that by the second recording period staff expectations had become reduced in order to avoid assault, thus provoking little of this behaviour.

Purely descriptive accounts of treatment in the absence of any attempt to collect data are inherently even weaker (Horton and Howe 1981). In the absence of attempts to define relevant variables, consistently measure the behaviour that is the object of change, and systematically manipulate treatment, the uncontrolled case study method cannot demonstrate outcome. When this is the goal, single-case experimental design methodologies should be employed.

Single-case experimental designs

These methodologies address the above issues by minimising variance in data from all sources other than that attributable to treatment.

There is insufficient space to relate a detailed history regarding the development of the scientific method to the study of the individual: instead, the reader is referred to the definitive work on this subject by Hersen and Barlow (1984). In brief, disenchantment with limitations of group comparison approaches, growth in the popularity of behaviour therapy, and the desire to retain the credibility of measuring treatment efficacy using scientific methods, all contributed to what became known as 'applied behaviour analysis'. Shapiro is accredited as one of the first practitioners to report the application of scientific methodology to clinical work in an attempt to isolate treatment effects (Shapiro and Ravenette 1959; Shapiro 1961, 1966), thus demonstrating that independent variables could be defined and systematically manipulated within a single case, thereby enabling the experimental approach to be utilised in the evaluation of therapeutic techniques.

Methodologies developed that embraced the scientific approach whilst retaining the ability to enable treatment to be designed to meet individual patient needs (Campbell and Stanley 1963; Chassan 1967). These utilise the patient as their own control. Consequently, many disadvantages of group comparison methods are circumvented. Homogeneity is not an issue (but remains important when a series of cases are compared). Economic constraints are reduced. Patients receive treatment free from the lottery of assignment to a control group, and without the need to wait until sufficient subject numbers have been recruited. Ethical concerns are reduced, as these designs have the flexibility to meet individual needs whilst retaining the ability to demonstrate 'cause-and-effect' relationships.

Types of methodology

Single-case experimental designs utilise scientific principles in order to

- precisely define treatment methods (independent variables) and the target behaviour or skill (dependent variable)
- quantify and measure the dependent variable
- minimise variability to isolate the effect of each independent (treatment) variable
- systematically manipulate independent variables
- measure the effects this has on the dependent variable
- establish reliable 'cause-and-effect' relationships that demonstrate treatment efficacy.

Flexibility of approach means that unique methodologies tailored to individual needs are designed. Most are based on two types of design: the 'reversal' or 'withdrawal' design, and the 'multiple baseline' approach. Each have qualities that lend themselves to different clinical situations in which reliable knowledge concerning cause-and-effect relationships is sought.

Common features and assumptions

All single-case experimental designs require the dependent variable to be defined using objective, replicable criteria. For example, it is insufficient that observers record 'aggression': some may define swearing and assaults as aggression, whilst others record only physical assaults. Without objective criteria, unwanted variance will hinder data interpretation.

After defining the dependent variable, recordings of its frequency and/or duration are required. Different methods are available, including continuous observation, interval recording and time sampling (Wood 1987). Recordings are made under standardised conditions. When more than one observer is employed, reliability checks should be undertaken.

Designs incorporate at least one observation period in which the natural occurrence of the dependent variable is measured. This 'baseline', or no-treatment, condition provides a standard against which treatment efficacy is determined. Thus the patient is their own control. Ideally, repeated measurement of the dependent variable is undertaken until it is clear that there is a stable trend. If, for example, there was a decreasing trend in the frequency of aggressive behaviour prior to the introduction of treatment, conclusions regarding efficacy will be confounded.

Only one treatment method should be manipulated if its therapeutic effects are to be determined. However, clinical and ethical demands may not always allow this.

Finally, a lettering convention is used to refer to different phases within a design. The baseline is labelled A, the B phase represents what happens to the dependent variable when treatment is introduced, and other letters (C, D and so on) are used to reflect the effect of other interventions.

The two most reported methodologies will now be examined. Examples will be given regarding neurological patients, references will be cited for the inquiring reader to study, and more complete examples will be presented from the author's own clinical work.

Reversal or withdrawal designs

Hersen and Barlow (1984) remind us that measurement of the impact of treatment on a dependent variable in the absence of baseline information represents no more than an uncontrolled case study. To identify reliable cause-and-effect relationships, contrasts must be made between conditions in which treatment is available and those where it is not. At its simplest this represents an A–B design, where repeated measures taken of the dependent variable are continued following the introduction of treatment. Examples within neuro-rehabilitation include the use of aids to improve executive functioning (Burke *et al.* 1991) and reduction in challenging behaviour using a holistic multiple-component neurobehavioural programme (Alderman *et al.* 1999b).

An A–B design is presented in Figure 13.1. This demonstrates the effect of a behaviour modification intervention, response cost (Alderman and Burgess 1990, 1994; Alderman and Ward 1991) on ritualistic behaviour demonstrated by FO, a 27-year-old male who sustained brain damage through viral infection. Figure 13.1 shows a reduction in these behaviours (compulsive hip thrusting and rocking) following the introduction of treatment.

However, design limitations only allow weak conclusions to be made regarding treatment efficacy, because it remains unknown whether the change measured following the introduction of treatment occurred by chance.

These data also reflect some other clinical and ethical concerns regarding single-case experimental designs. In order to resolve the above, the treatment should be withdrawn and evidence of its effectiveness is apparent if the frequency of ritualistic behaviour subsequently increases. However, for the therapist, being asked to retract a strategy that allows them to purposefully engage a patient, for no other reason than satisfying the curiosity of the programme designer, may be unacceptable. Also, it may be hard to justify withdrawing treatment to demonstrate efficacy (for example in the management of self-injurious behaviour) or prove impossible to do so (for example patients admitted into a specialised rehabilitation service).

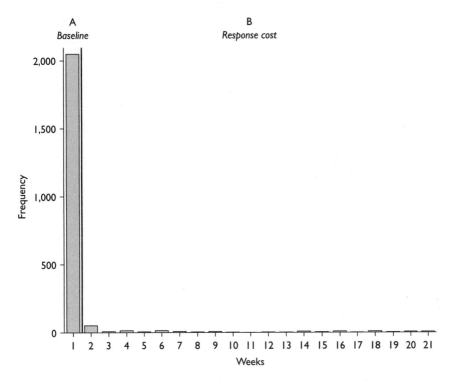

Figure 13.1 Investigation of the effect of response cost on the weekly frequency of FO's hip thrusting and rocking using an 'A-B' single case experimental design. (NB. During the 'A' or baseline phase attention was withdrawn from FO, during the 'B' or treatment stage response cost was implemented.)

Conflicts between clinical needs, ethical considerations, and a desire to inform evidence-based practice can sometimes be resolved. If treatment is to be no more than educated guesswork it is necessary to assess the patient in order to determine what methods would be most beneficial. Indeed, a number of practitioners have advocated that the area of behavioural assessment is of special relevance given the difficulties imposed by neurological damage on other forms of appraisal (Wood 1987; Davis *et al.* 1994; Treadwell and Page 1996; von Cramon and Matthes-von Cramon 1994). Within this domain single-case experimental design has much to offer.

For example, consider again FO. Neuropsychological examination reflected memory and executive difficulties: problems with the ability to monitor both his own behaviour and cues within the environment were especially highlighted. Monitoring difficulties are thought to drive some behaviour disorders (Alderman 1996; Alderman *et al.* 1995; Alderman and Knight 1997). A range of neurobehavioural interventions have been found to be

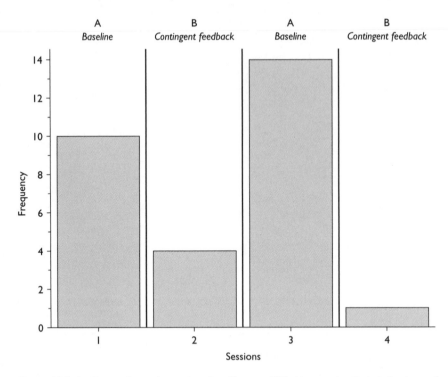

Figure 13.2 A pilot study to determine the effect on FO's bizarre ritualistic behaviour of immediate feedback and contingent reinforcement using an 'A-B-A-B' single case experimental design. (NB. Each bar represents the total number of target behaviours observed in a 14 minute session: during 'A' no attention was given to this, in 'B' FO received immediate feedback he had engaged in these behaviours.)

effective in such cases which provide consistent, immediate feedback to patients immediately contingent upon the behaviour of interest. To test the appropriateness of a self-monitoring deficit hypothesis regarding FO, an A–B–A–B reversal design was implemented as part of a behavioural assessment. The patient was observed during a 14-minute period within a morning break over 4 consecutive days in which the frequency of hip thrusting and rocking was recorded. The two A phases comprised the baseline conditions in which no attention was paid to these behaviours by staff. In the B, or treatment phases, feedback was provided to FO each time he engaged in these behaviours. A tangible reinforcer was available at the end of 14 minutes if these had reduced below a specified number.

Results are shown in Figure 13.2. This suggests a cause-and-effect relationship in that the target behaviour was low when feedback was available and high when it was not. It was on this basis that the intervention reflected in Figure 13.1 was implemented. Whilst the A–B design used in isolation provided weak evidence regarding treatment efficacy, use of reversal methodology in the behavioural assessment that preceded this, confirmed its efficacy without compromising clinical or ethical concerns.

The minimum design necessary to demonstrate efficacy is the A–B–A methodology: introduction of treatment in the B phase is predicted to influence the frequency and/or duration of that behaviour being measured, which would return to baseline levels in the second A phase (McLean et al. 1987). However, withdrawing beneficial treatment heightens clinical and ethical concerns: introduction of a second B phase primarily addresses these rather than adding any significant credibility (Hersen and Barlow 1984). A good example of A–B–A–B methodology regarding aggressive behaviour in an adult with traumatic brain injury has been described by Persel et al. (1997). Murdoch et al. (1999) demonstrated effectiveness of visual feedback in the treatment of speech breathing disorders following childhood traumatic brain injury. However, A–B–A designs may be used within behavioural assessment prior to the introduction of a more ambitious course of treatment using an A–B methodology.

An advantage of these designs is the flexibility they offer the clinician who wishes to contribute to evidence-based practice whilst meeting individual patient needs. For example, when treatment should begin immediately, efficacy may still be determined using a B–A–B approach (Yuen 1993). These designs are not limited to alternation of A and B conditions. Having determined the impact of one treatment, efficacy of others may also be assessed. What interventions are used, and when, may be driven by change in the patient. In this way, designs evolve in a manner that is not always predictable: however, these methodologies continue to facilitate objective assessment of treatment.

Figure 13.3 illustrates this, showing spitting frequency during 30-minute sessions exhibited by a 25-year-old male with acquired brain damage. An A–B–A–B–C design was used to assess the efficacy of two reinforcement methods. Following a baseline phase, an intervention based on the principle of differential reinforcement of low rates of behaviour (DRL) (Alderman and Knight 1997) was introduced. A reduction in spitting occurred. As spitting frequency increased in the second A phase, the likelihood that the reduction was attributable to treatment was confirmed. Following the reintroduction of DRL (as the benefits of this approach had been confirmed) in the second B phase, the frequency of spitting remained low. It was therefore clinically desirable to use a more demanding variant of differential reinforcement, that of incompatible behaviour (DRI: see Alderman and Knight 1997). A C phase was added in which no spitting occurred. The point is that whilst the design began in A–B–A format to establish treatment efficacy, clinical progress led to this being extended to meet individual needs as they evolved.

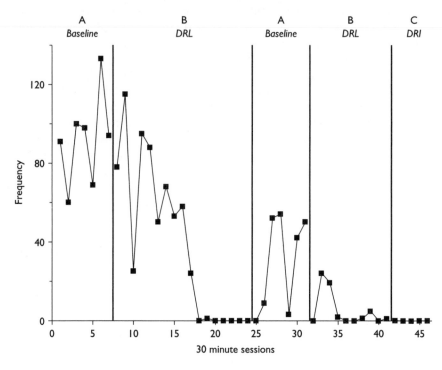

Figure 13.3 Illustration of a variant of a reversal design employing an 'A-B-A-B-C' methodology to investigate the effects of two differential reinforcement approaches on the frequency of spitting exhibited by an adult male following stroke. (NB. Attention was withdrawn contingent on spitting in 'A', DRL was implemented in 'B', and DRI in 'C'.)

More complex examples of these designs within neurorehabiltation are in the literature. For example, Kearney and Fussey (1991) used an A–BC–B–BC–A methodology to demonstrate the influence of contingent music on head positioning.

Multiple baseline designs

Whilst reversal and withdrawal designs are flexible, they are not always appropriate. First, treatment cannot always be withdrawn. Second, learning may occur so when treatment is discontinued the dependent measure may not return to baseline levels (Youngson and Alderman 1994): whilst this is desirable in rehabilitation, it creates difficulties in establishing cause-and-effect relationships. Similarly, effects of medication may persist. Under such circumstances, multiple baseline designs are appropriate. Again, the reader is referred to Hersen and Barlow (1984) for an extensive discussion regarding these points.

One feature is that two or more dependent variables are measured concurrently. Treatment is extended initially to one variable and, following evidence of change, it is successively extended to the others. If change only occurs when treatment is introduced, it can be reasonably argued that chance is not responsible for this. These designs are weaker than reversal and withdrawal methodologies as the controlling effects of treatment on each variable are not directly demonstrated. Instead, its effects are inferred from a lack of change in untreated dependent variables. Nevertheless, they can provide a valid alternative.

Three principal types of multiple baseline design are available. The first is across behaviours: several behaviours exhibited by one individual are selected for treatment. The second is across subjects: there is one dependent variable and treatment effects are demonstrated when it is successively introduced to three or more people exhibiting the same behaviour. The final variant is across settings: again, one dependent variable shown by one person is targeted. Efficacy is evaluated by measuring the target behaviour separately in three or more situations and successively introducing treatment to each of these.

Use of multiple baseline designs with neurological patients appear to be numerous and to extend to many areas of rehabilitation including reduction of aggression (Hegel and Ferguson 2000; Burke and Lewis 1986; Alderman and Knight 1997), improving continence (Garcia and Lam 1990), motor learning (Shiller *et al.* 1999), memory training (Gray and Robertson 1989), visual neglect (Robertson *et al.* 1988) and hand function (Barry and Riley 1987).

An example applied to rehabilitation of executive impairment is shown in Figure 13.4. YB, a 22-year-old male, had sustained a traumatic brain injury. The design was a multiple baseline across behaviours (where each 'behaviour' was a skill to be acquired). YB was preparing to live in his own flat and a rehabilitation goal was to increase kitchen hygiene maintenance by teaching him efficient ways of cleaning the work surface, floor and windows. Four age-matched, neurologically healthy male peers were observed completing these tasks: performance records were used to construct a sequenced check-list of separate task-parts for each chore. During the baseline (A) stage, YB was observed completing each task. A sequence score was obtained for each (expressed as a percentage) which quantified the efficiency with which he completed these tasks in relation to his peers. During the B phase, the intervention was introduced which consisted of a graduated system of giving instructions to counter executive functioning difficulties. When observed to deviate from the correct sequence, YB was given a general prompt that he needed to rethink what he was doing; if necessary a second prompt was given to specifically inform him of what task he needed to do.

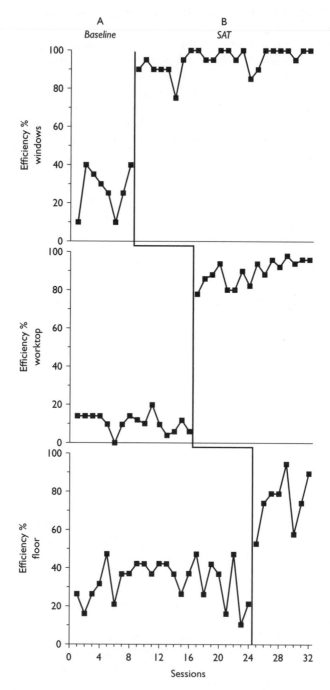

Figure 13.4 Example of a multiple baseline across behaviour single case experimental design. This demonstrates the impact on YB of Strategy Application Training on learning kitchen hygiene skills.

Figure 13.4 shows that YB's efficiency in completing each task increased following the introduction of this 'strategy application training' approach; because efficiency only increased contingent on implementation of this approach for each chore, it can reasonably be inferred that this brought about improvement.

Like reversal and withdrawal designs, multiple baseline methodologies are flexible. When it suits the needs of the individual patient, elements from both categories of design may be incorporated (for example a second A phase to determine the longevity of treatment).

Summary and concluding remarks

Single-case methods have been discussed and illustrated regarding neurological patients. These patients' characteristics highlight limitations of group methodologies, whilst emphasising benefits of single-case methods. The principal thrust of this book is to determine the contribution of various methods in informing evidence-based practice. How useful are single-case methods in this respect?

First, what are the benefits? A principal advantage is that they provide means by which answers to clinical questions are sought together with information concerning treatment efficacy, whilst circumventing problems inherent in group methodologies. The latter have been highlighted: poor homogeneity, ethical concerns, economic limitations and practical difficulties can be avoided using single-case methods. These empower clinicians to meet two different, sometimes antagonistic needs: individual patient requirements in treatment, and enablement of the process of scientific scrutiny of efficacy necessary to inform evidence-based practice.

A further consideration also supports study of the individual within neurorehabilitation. This concerns homogeneity. As was stated earlier, the range of problems acquired through neurological damage is diverse and complex. Three points need to be made concerning this issue in relation to single-case studies. First, it is rare to find two individuals with exactly the same difficulties. Second, assessment using traditional interview methods should be avoided: it is recognised that lack of awareness and reduced insight are associated with acquired brain injury (Sazbon and Groswasser 1991; Wilson et al. 1996; Burgess et al. 1998). Finally, problems exhibited by neurological patients are attributable to complex interactions between variables. Consequently, the best means of assessing brain–behaviour relationships is through environmental manipulation as this can be carefully controlled. Hypotheses concerning aetiology may then be tested through further manipulations (Beaumont 1983; Wood 1987). When supplemented with information concerning cognitive status, this approach enables brain–behaviour relationships to be determined by controlling antecedents and contingencies, whose effects may be determined by measuring behaviour. This is particularly helpful when attempting to determine reasons underlying behaviour in people who have severe cognitive impairment and/or communication problems. Single-case experimental designs provide ideal methodologies to enable this.

Second, what kind of information do they provide? Descriptive uncontrolled case studies generate qualitative and quantitative information but do not facilitate objective assessment of cause-and-effect relationships. Consequently, they cannot reliably inform practice. This purpose is best served by single-case experimental designs which facilitate clinical intervention, and produce data which inform both practice and academic theory: these ultimately contribute towards evidence-based treatment.

Quantitative information generated through single-case experimental designs cannot be subjected to the usual range of parametric statistical procedures because serial dependency violates assumptions concerning independence: a range of alternative tests has been proposed (Kazdin 1984). Procedures that determine the presence of trends in data sets have a particularly useful role to play: the simplified form of time-series analyses proposed by Tyron (1982) lends itself well to this task.

Finally, how generalisable are findings from single-case methods? This question highlights limitations of the approach. Whilst their flexibility renders them ideal in meeting individual needs, the down side is that data are unique to that person. Suppose a number of neurological patients are recipients of the same treatment. Pooling data to determine treatment generalisation would be erroneous for the reasons espoused earlier. Whilst all have brain damage, the nature and extent of this will vary from person to person. Poor treatment homogeneity will also mitigate against pooling data: whilst the same method may be used, differences in application will be evident when modified to meet individual needs. This was illustrated by Alderman and Knight (1997) who reported the efficacy of differential reinforcement. Whilst treatment took the same general form, it was operationalised differently for each of three patients to meet their unique needs: a multiple baseline was used in one case and reversal designs in the others, the baseline durations were different and interventions varied in detail according to individual needs.

Hersen and Barlow (1984) argued that generalisation is best determined through systematic replication. Cases are not directly comparable. Instead, potential influences on treatment from a range of variables, including those of different settings and therapists, are examined. For example, each of the patients described by Alderman and Knight (1997) successfully demonstrated that differential reinforcement led to a reduction in challenging behaviour within a specialised environment. Generality amongst people was demonstrated as the technique was found to work with three individuals. Further steps in replication to investigate generality would include study of efficacy in different environments and with different therapists. Systematic replication enables general conclusions to be drawn regarding efficacy with a specific population as opposed to one or two individuals.

In a review of the literature regarding treatment of aggression following traumatic brain injury, Alderman *et al.* (1997) highlighted a further point regarding replication. Whilst single-case methods provided the chief means of assessing efficacy of a number of treatment methods, replication was hindered by failure to report wider information. For example, severity and type of brain injury were not described in most studies, information regarding cognitive status was generally absent, and what constituted a 'baseline' was invariably missing. This is especially relevant. The whole purpose of single-case experimental designs is to isolate and control variability so that the influence of treatment may be determined. Contingencies to behaviour are always present and will influence this. It is imperative that these are identified to fully understand what is happening within the 'no-treatment' phase which precedes treatment (Davis *et al.* 1994).

In summary, problems with homogeneity are exacerbated amongst neurological patients. This, and other difficulties reviewed here support the use of single-case methods in providing the means of first choice to inform evidence-based practice. These methods provide clinicians with tools that enable individual needs to be met whilst satisfying methodological criteria so that enquiries about treatment efficacy may be reliably conducted.

Section 3

Applying the evidence

Chapter 14

Applying the evidence: pharmacotherapies

John Cookson

The history of drug treatments in psychiatry

The modern era of effective drug treatments in psychiatry began over 50 years ago with the discovery in 1948 by John Cade in Australia of the use of lithium salts in mania, and by French scientists in 1952 of the use of the synthetic phenothiazine, chlorpromazine, as an antipsychotic; older 'pragmatic' treatments such as bromides could then be discarded (Shorter 1997). Plants with medicinal uses affecting the mind include St Johns Wort (Hypericum alkaloids), which has only recently been confirmed in randomised controlled trials (RCTs) to have antidepressant activity.

(Maidment 2000)

The synthesis by chemists, particularly in Germany, of sedative drugs in the nineteenth century, was the start of the modern pharmaceutical industry. Chloral was synthesised in 1832 and found to be a sedative in 1869; it became widely used in psychiatry although was prone to abuse and addiction. There were also cases of sudden death among patients on chloral.

Sakel (1930) thought that insulin-induced hypoglycaemic coma could relieve opiate withdrawal problems, and suggested its use in schizophrenia, claiming success in 1934. Insulin units were set up in many hospitals; in some centres insulin coma was repeatedly induced using increasing doses of the drug until convulsions occurred. By 1944 insulin-coma therapy was the main physical treatment recommended for acute schizophrenia for instance by Sargant and Slater (1946, 1948, 1963) in London. However in 1953 Bourne, a junior psychiatrist, challenged its efficacy calling its use 'a therapeutic myth' (Bourne, 1953). Several academic psychiatrists wrote in its defence but the controlled trial which followed, comparing insulin coma and barbiturate-induced sleep, failed to demonstrate any advantage of insulin-coma therapy (Ackner 1957). The use of this dangerous and ineffective treatment gradually ended and the antipsychotic drugs took its place.

Controlled trials

To prove efficacy in psychiatric conditions, it is necessary to design studies that take account of spontaneous improvement, and of bias in the observer or patient, as well as non-specific factors such as the special attention received by the patient. This is achieved by having a treatment and a control group, and assigning patients at random to receive either the new treatment or a comparator. The trial is conducted double blind (neither the doctor nor the patient knows which treatment is received until all the data from the whole trial are gathered and complete). This powerful design (the randomised double-blind controlled trial) was conceived by Bradford Hill during World War II and strongly advocated by him from 1946. Randomisation is particularly important because it can remove bias arising from any demographic or other unpredictable factors in the patient that may affect their response to the treatments.

Placebo

If the new treatment is much better than the standard treatment, then only a treatment and a control group are needed. If, however, the new drug is thought to be about as effective as standard treatment and if the change in condition could be liable to spontaneous improvement, then the efficacy of the treatment can only be proved by comparing the drug with a placebo. Regulatory authorities in many countries require two 'pivotal studies' in separate and independent centres to demonstrate a drug's superiority to a placebo, before the drug can be licensed for use in a psychiatric condition. It is best (ideally) to include both placebo and standard treatments as comparators since this will show whether the standard treatment is effective under the circumstances of the trial. Otherwise the trial fails as a test of efficacy and is a 'failed trial'.

The inclusion of a placebo in a study means that patients cannot be included if they require immediate active treatment, if, for example, they are severely disturbed.

The placebo effect

Patients may get better when treated with tablets that do not contain any active drug. This is called the 'placebo' effect (from Latin meaning 'I shall please'). This effect was exploited in former times when inert substances (placebos) were given by apparently successful physicians to 'treat' patients. Today placebos are used in orthodox medicine only as research tools in clinical trials. However the 'placebo effect' may add on to the pharmacological effect where an active drug is used and can therefore be an important part of clinical practice.

On the other hand patients may complain of side effects when given placebo treatments. This has been called the 'nocebo' effect (from Latin meaning 'I shall harm'); this effect has its most extreme form in 'voodoo death'.

On the positive side, factors contributing to the placebo effect include the patient's confidence in the treatment, their suggestibility, their belief in the potency of a remedy, which may depend in part on its striking colour or bitter taste, their acceptance of the doctor's 'gift' of tablets as symbolic or magical, involving concern or care, and the prestige of medical knowledge. These factors may therefore be as important as an individual drug's pharmacological action in determining the benefits and acceptability of treatment. On the other hand, distrust, together with preconceived notions about side effects, toxicity or dependence, may detract from the beneficial actions of the drug.

In psychiatry a medication is seldom prescribed without a dialogue between the doctor and patient. The patient's decision to seek help can herald some improvement. Often the first contact will have entailed the doctor taking a detailed account of the patient's symptoms and background, and providing some explanation in terms of medical diagnosis or formulation of the psychological problem. Reassurance and encouragement may have been given, as well as the offer of further help. These in themselves are powerful interventions in some cases, and affect the trust and expectation of the patient.

Placebo responses in clinical trials

In order to prove the efficacy of a new treatment it is necessary to control for the coincidental action of non-specific factors. This is achieved using a placebo-controlled design. In such a design, the improvement that is seen to occur in the group of patients receiving placebo may arise from any of the above factors. Table 14.1 lists these factors, together with other processes

Table 14.1 Factors contributing to an improvement in the condition of a patient on a placebo

Patient	Illness	Doctor	Previous drugs
Trust	Spontaneous recovery	First interview	Side effects
Expectation	Fluctuating severity	Explanation	Withdrawal/rebound
Suggestibility	Engagement with doctor	Reassurance	Delayed effects, e.g. of depot injection
Decision to seek treatment	Psychotherapy	Physical examination, investigations	'Rescue' medication
Change of environment, e.g. hospital admission		Bias	

that are controlled for by the inclusion of a placebo group. The latter processes include spontaneous improvement as part of the natural history of the illness, the decline in side effects resulting from previous medication that was stopped, and the course of any symptoms arising from discontinuation such as rebound exacerbation of the treated condition. During the early stages of the trial it may be permitted to administer limited amounts of additional medication to calm the patient or to help them sleep; this 'rescue' medication is often a benzodiazepine, and is assumed not to have profound enduring beneficial effects. With both depression and the negative symptoms of schizophrenia, improvement arises from the social stimulation of repeated contacts with the investigator. The continuing contacts between the doctor and patient may amount to psychotherapeutic interventions, unless this is deliberately and perhaps unethically avoided within the design of the trial. The beneficial effect of simply giving attention to people is known as the Hawthorne effect, after an electricity plant where it was found to improve productivity. Finally, the assessment of improvement may be biased by the enthusiasm or other feelings of the doctor for the treatment under investigation.

Placebo response rates

The proportion of patients improving on placebo varies even among groups of patients with the same diagnosis. For instance in depressive illness the rate varies from 25 per cent to 60 per cent. In schizophrenia it may vary from 20 per cent to 50 per cent depending upon the criterion of improvement that is used, and other factors. Patients who are chronically ill show lower placebo response rates. The placebo response in mania is commonly thought to be small, but in clinical trials placebo response rates as high as 25 per cent are found.

Time course of drug–placebo differences

In studies of depression the difference in improvement in the group of patients on active treatment compared with the group on placebo increases gradually, with little difference until about 2 weeks of treatment and the full difference developing by 6 weeks. In schizophrenia too the advantage of the active treatment develops slowly, with much of the difference becoming apparent between 2 and 6 weeks, but it increases progressively for several months. The use of placebo in studies of mania is especially difficult because of the need for 'rescue' medication in more severe cases.

Analysis of the data

Patients who drop out or are withdrawn because of side effects, non-response or recovery, pose difficulties for the analysis of the data. When studying the results of a trial it is important to know whether the scores from these drop outs have been included in the graphs and subsequent analyses. For studies testing efficacy, it is preferable to include the data from all patients who entered the trial and received at least one dose of medication. This is called the 'intent to treat' population. To analyse the results, the scores of patients who drop out early may be carried forward to later time points. This is known as the 'intent to treat analysis with last observation carried forward'. Sometimes graphs are presented with data only to the time of drop out, and this has the effect of exaggerating the improvement shown in the rest of the graph. Alternatively, only those patients who complete the full duration of the study are considered (completer analysis). Analysis of the intent to treat population helps to avoid bias that could arise from allowing individuals to be excluded for special reasons.

If the active comparator (the established drug with proven efficacy in the condition) leads to more early drop outs through side effects, the new drug with fewer side effects may appear spuriously to have greater therapeutic efficacy on intent to treat analysis with last observation carried forward. Likewise, if there are many early drop outs through lack of improvement in the placebo group, then the advantage of the new and effective drug may appear somewhat exaggerated on intent to treat analysis with last observation carried forward, because patients will have remained on it longer and have greater time for improvement. However this method of analysis is clearly fairer than completer analysis, because it will include all the placebo responders.

Standards of evidence

Apart from the parallel-group randomly assigned double-blind placebo-controlled trial, other lesser standards of evidence may provide the earliest indications that a treatment is effective. Box 14.1 lists the types of evidence that may support the use of a treatment, in decreasing order of their conclusiveness.

Box 14.1   Hierarchy of the quality of evidence for the efficacy of a treatment (see also Boxes 9.4 and 11.1)

1. Clear advantage over placebo in at least one randomised controlled trial, preferably replicated at a different centre.
2. Series of cases compared to a non-randomised control series.
3. Consecutive series of cases described by a respected authority.
4. Dramatic results in an uncontrolled series of cases.
5. Single case report.

Systematic reviews and meta-analysis

When several RCTs have been reported with similar designs, these can be ana-lysed together using the method of meta-analysis. This allows the consistency of the findings to be examined, and an overall conclusion to be drawn about the effect size, using the pooled data. The technique of a 'funnel plot' can identify whether there is a gap in the data, suggesting that there are missing data, this may arise from the researcher's desire to publish positive findings.

The methods of systematic review are intended to identify all available data relevant to the subject being studied. As well as searching a variety of computerised databases, it is important to try and include unpublished findings; these may be more negative than those that have been published. They may be obtained by personal communication with investigators, or by approaching pharmaceutical companies and seeking internal reports on studies that were not published.

Size of treatment effect and number-needed-to-treat

Beyond establishing that a treatment is more efficacious than placebo in a condition, it is important to know the magnitude of the benefit, or the size of the 'treatment effect'. This enables the doctor to tell the patient how likely it is that the treatment will help them; it also enables comparisons to be made with other treatments for the same condition, or indeed for different conditions. One of the simplest measures of size of treatment effect is the difference in the percentage of people improving on the treatment, from the percentage who improve on the placebo (also known as the absolute risk reduction). To make this comparison, improvement must be defined at the start of the trial using a criterion that can be readily recognised. As an example, the change in the overall clinical state might be used, and the percentage of patients counted who are 'much improved' or 'very much improved' according to the Clinical Global Impression Scale. Alternatively, if a well-known and validated rating scale is used, then a patient might be defined as improved if their score falls below a defined threshold, or if their score decreases by the average amount (for example, 20 per cent or 50 per cent) by the end of the trial.

This measure of treatment effect size can be converted to the number-needed-to-treat (NNT), by dividing the difference into 100. For example, in the treatment of depression there is commonly a difference of about 33 per cent between the proportion of patients who improved on the antide-pressant drug and the proportion who improved on placebo. The number-needed-to-treat is then 100/33 or about 3. This means that in order for the drug to bring about improvement in one patient, three patients must be treated, one of whom would have improved on placebo and the third patient will remain unwell. For a drug that is always effective in an otherwise untreatable chronic condition the number-needed-to-treat is 1. A treatment with a large number-needed-to-treat might be considered useful if no other treatments are available, or if it is used as an adjunct to other treatments that are only partially effective and it has few side effects. At present many research reports do not provide sufficient information about effect size. Later in the chapter, Table 14.4 summarises the results of influential clinical trials in different conditions, showing the drop out rates, effect size and number-needed-to-treat. Similarly the frequency of adverse effects can be described in terms of a number-needed-to-harm.

Other measures of effect size

The difference in effect between two treatments can also be described using the scores on rating scales, as the difference between the mean scores on drug and placebo divided by the standard deviation of the scores, this is also called the effect size.

Efficacy versus effectiveness

We have seen that the efficacy of a treatment is established by means of double-blind randomised trials with placebo control groups, carried out in carefully selected patients under relatively ideal circumstances. Both the patients and the clinicians taking part in these specialised trials are atypical and the results may not be generalisable to other patients (see Boxes 14.2 and 14.3).

In clinical practice it is important to know what advantage accrues for everyday patients who are started on a treatment compared with those who are not, and when other interventions are allowed as their doctor judges necessary. This is called the 'effectiveness' of a treatment. In general,

---

Box 14.2   Patients entering efficacy trials

Mildly or moderately ill
Treatment-resistant
Informed consent
Physically fit

Age 18–65
No drug or alcohol dependence
Not at risk of pregnancy

Receiving limited other therapy

Box 14.3 Limitations of trials of efficacy

Atypical patients are entered
Atypical clinicians take part
Strict entry criteria reduce the generalisability
Early drop outs bias the interpretation
Outcome measures are subtle
Adherence is high
Numbers are small and rare side effects are not detected

---

treatments that are inconvenient or are associated with unwanted side effects are less effective because patients discontinue them before deriving the full benefit. Effectiveness is also measured in RCTs, but the conditions of entry are relaxed so that larger numbers may be included in treatment (the 'pragmatic trial') as shown in Table 14.2. By continuing to monitor the condition of patients who stop treatment, rather than carrying forward the last value before they discontinued, a further indication may be gained of the effectiveness of the treatment that was started. The outcomes are then compared after a set interval, for example 1 year. In this way some treatments of proven efficacy may appear much less effective in the routine clinic. A third method of assessing outcome is the 'naturalistic' study, but this does not include randomised assignment and is therefore open to many sources of bias.

Consensus statements and clinical guidelines

The complexities and costs of modern medicine have forced a sea change in therapeutic decision making. Today, clinicians are more often expected to be influenced by published guidelines and consensus statements. Indeed, in some countries 'managed care' arrangements effectively remove from clinicians any individualised choice of therapy by stipulating exactly the sequence of treatment options in a given illness. However, in an age of litigation, guidelines can become a constraint on clinicians and consensus statements may simply repeat what the guidelines have enshrined as 'correct'.

Ideally, both consensus statements and clinical guidelines should be predominantly evidence based. The guidance they provide should essentially be a summary of a systematic review of published data, which may include meta-analyses. There is some room to accommodate individual views of clinicians, for example where there are gaps in the evidence base. Where individual views are allowed to dominate, guidelines merely represent the ideas of the most forceful contributors and may be wildly at odds with published data.

Table 14.2 Characteristics of follow-up studies

	Efficacy studies	Naturalistic studies	Pragmatic trials
Purpose	To prove efficacy	To assess effectiveness	To compare effectiveness
Drug	Unproven treatment	Established treatment	Proven treatment
Comparator	Placebo	Observe practice	Standard treatment
Size	Small numbers	Large numbers	Enrol large numbers
Consent	Informed consent	No consent	'Uncertainty principle'
Recruitment	Highly selected	All patients	Few excluded
Staff	Research staff	Usual clinician	Interested clinicians
Allocation	Randomise	Clinician's choice	Randomise
Observation	Double-blind	Open follow-up	Open follow-up
Other therapy	Limit other treatment	Any other treatment	Other treatment as needed
Adherence	Avoid drop outs	Lower compliance	Allow change
Measures	Subtle rating scales	Observe outcome	Clear end-point
Analysis	Intent to treat with last observation carried forward	Descriptive analysis	Follow up after drop out

Guidelines should also closely match what is already done in clinical practice. Clinicians are, by nature, only inclined to change habits gradually and tend to reject wholesale change. Sadly, many published guidelines are rather too dependent on individual views and recommend practice that is quite different to current practice. Even when they are well constructed, guidelines and consensus statements are, for one reason or another, widely ignored.

Nevertheless, prescribing in psychiatry is likely to be increasingly influenced by guidelines and consensus statements. In the UK, the National Institute of Clinical Excellence publishes guidance on a number of treatments. The role of the individual clinician may evolve into that of assessing the cogency of any guidelines and then learn to be guided but not governed by them.

Lessons from lithium

The case of lithium illustrates the importance of RCTs and of placebo controls and double blindness, and also the influence of new treatments on practice.

The pivotal studies, which were the basis for the use of lithium, were carried out more than 25 years ago. Some psychiatrists came to regard lithium as a specific treatment for bipolar illness. In the US, FDA approval for lithium was granted in 1970, and by then, lithium therapy was widely regarded as the treatment of choice for bipolar mood disorder. It was also used extensively in Europe.

This development had a major impact on the treatment of bipolar disorder in the US. When Baldessarini (1970) compared the frequency of affective illness to schizophrenia in patients discharged from hospital before and after the introduction of lithium, a reciprocal pattern was noted, with an increasingly frequent diagnosis of bipolar illness and a decreasing frequency of schizophrenia.

Subsequently the definition of bipolar mood disorder was broadened to include patients with mood-incongruent psychotic features, who would previously have been regarded as having schizoaffective disorder or schizophrenia. Thus the availability of lithium and the wider use of standard diagnostic systems have led to the diagnosis of bipolar disorder in patients who might previously have been diagnosed as schizophrenic, at least in the US.

Many of the RCTs of lithium were carried out before this shift in the diagnosis of bipolar disorder. This may help to reconcile the often quoted expectation that lithium is 'effective for all but 20 to 40 per cent of bipolar patients' with recent studies which suggest that lithium is far less effective.

Earlier trials may need to be reconsidered in the light of new evidence. Over the past 25 years there have been two further discoveries which necessitate a reappraisal of the place of lithium in treatment (Cookson 1997)

1. the occurrence of permanent neurological sequelae as a result of acute lithium toxicity (Schou 1984)
2. the recognition that mania may occur as a result of abrupt discontinuation of lithium (Mander and Loudon 1988).

Following Cade's (1949) description of the anti-manic effects of lithium, based on an open study, there were four placebo-controlled studies of lithium in mania that used a crossover design. These were conducted in Denmark by Schou *et al.* (1954) and later in double-blind designs in England by Maggs (1963) and in the US by Goodwin *et al.* (1969) and Stokes *et al.* (1971). In a total of 116 patients on lithium, there was an overall response rate of 78 per cent, much greater than the placebo response rate (40 per cent in one study). Mogens Schou working in Aarhus, Denmark remained a robust advocate of lithium treatment, developing with Amdisen methods for monitoring blood lithium levels to avoid serious toxicity, and conducting further studies to carefully document its effects and side effects.

An early challenge from the Institute of Psychiatry described lithium as 'another therapeutic myth?' (Blackwell and Shepherd, 1966). Nevertheless lithium gradually assumed an important role in the management of mania and the prophylaxis of bipolar manic-depressive illness. It was not until 1994 however that the first parallel-group double-blind placebo-controlled study of lithium in mania was performed by Bowden *et al.*, in the course of investigating a new treatment with valproic acid (see pp. 172–3). Even in 1997 Moncrieff argued that lithium was 'a myth'. Admittedly the size of the benefits claimed for lithium by the early enthusiasts has had to be revised downwards.

Lithium's effect takes a few days to begin and 2 to 3 weeks to reach its peak (sometimes even longer). This limits lithium as a treatment for acute mania and makes monotherapy risky for all but the mildest cases. Usually clinicians must initiate other types of treatment for acute mania. Commonly, when a rapid response is required, treatment is initiated with anti-psychotic medication. Interpretation of the ten large, double-blind comparative trials of lithium versus placebo in the prophylaxis of bipolar patients requires attention to the details of study design. In some cases, this tends to produce results that over-estimate the benefit of lithium for routine clinical practice.

Two studies used double-blind discontinuation, with patients already on lithium being assigned randomly either to continue on lithium or to switch to placebo. In the study by Baastrup *et al.* (1970), 55 per cent of patients who switched to placebo and none of those who continued on lithium relapsed within 5 months. However this design is severely undermined by the occurrence of lithium withdrawal mania.

The required prospective design was used by Coppen *et al.* (1971) in the UK, by Prien *et al.* (1973) in the US, and in five other smaller studies. Overall of 204 patients on lithium prospectively, about 35 per cent relapsed in the study period (which varied from 4 months to 3 years), compared to about 80 per cent of 221 patients on placebo (Goodwin and Jamison 1990).

Applying the evidence for lithium

Table 14.3 shows the evidence from placebo-controlled trials for the efficacy of lithium. First as treatment for acute mania, Bowden *et al.* (1994) compared valproate (as Divalproex) to lithium or placebo in a 3-week parallel-group double-blind study of 179 patients, half of whom had previously been unresponsive to lithium. The proportion of patients showing 50 per cent improvement was greater for valproate (48 per cent) and lithium (49 per cent) than for placebo (25 per cent). The striking result here is that neither lithium nor valproate given alone as monotherapy is effective in a majority of patients, even using the modest criterion of outcome of this study. This points to the need for combination treatments in most patients.

Second, the use of lithium as prophylaxis for bipolar disorder was impressively effective (Prien *et al.* 1973), but the drop-out rate for side effects was extraordinarily low, and quite untypical of the use of lithium in routine practice. Even the most enthusiastic centres find that about half of the patients who start on lithium discontinue it within 1 year (McCreadie and Morrison 1985), however a quarter of patients do remain on it for over 10 years.

A 5-year follow up conducted in Naples (Maj *et al.* 1998) of all patients commenced on lithium, showed only 23 per cent continuing on it without recurrence for 5 years. Another 29 per cent had continued lithium and suffered a recurrence, but had a reduction in the amount of hospitalization by more than 50 per cent compared to the pre-treatment period. Only 39 per cent of patients were managed for 5 years on lithium alone. Most of those who stopped lithium did so on their own initiative; the most common reasons given were

- perceived ineffectiveness (37 per cent)
- side effects (28 per cent)
- no need for the medication (18 per cent)
- found it inconvenient (12 per cent)
- felt a loss of drive (5 per cent).

The poor concordance of bipolar patients with treatment plans involving lithium indicates the importance of 'psycho-education'. A group of bipolar patients, who had relapsed in the previous year, received nine sessions of psycho-education aimed at recognising the early features of relapse and preparing the patient and clinician with an action plan. The treated group showed a 12-month relapse rates for mania of 18 per cent, compared with 46 per cent in the control group (effect size 28 per cent, with 95 per cent CI, 6–49 per cent) (Perry *et al.* 1999).

Table 14.3 Lithium trials: drop out rates, response rates and number-needed-to-treat

Diagnosis	Treatments (number of patients)	Duration	Criterion of improvement	Drop outs due to inefficacy %	Drop outs due to adverse events %	Response %	Effect size %	Number-needed-to-treat (95% CI)
Mania (Bowden et al. 1994)	valproate (n = 68)	3 weeks	50% less Scale for Affective Disorders-mania (SADS-M)	30	6	48	23	5 (3–14)
	placebo (n = 73)			51	3	25		
	lithium (n = 35)			33	11	49	24	5 (3–22)
Bipolar maintenance (Prien et al. 1973)	lithium (n = 101)	2 years	no relapse	11	1	57	38	3 (3–4)
	placebo (n = 104)			40	0	19		

Official guidelines on lithium and mania

The Guidelines of the American Psychiatric Association (1996) advise the use of antipsychotics in mania only as 'adjuncts' to mood stabilisers (particularly lithium or valproate) or to ECT, when mania is associated with agitation, dangerous behaviour or psychosis. The guidelines recognise also that antipsychotics or benzodiazepines may be useful to 'enhance compliance' with mood stabilisers, or while those drugs are developing their effect. The Guidelines do not define what is meant by agitation in the context of mania, and this is ambiguous.

More recently, practice guidelines from the Department of Veterans Affairs recommend first-line treatment with lithium for 3 weeks, followed by a change to 'a different mood stabiliser' if there is no response, or a combination with an anticonvulsant if there is a partial response (Bauer et al. 1999). If the manic patient has psychotic features (delusions or hallucinations), antipsychotic drugs should be given if they are judged to be needed. It is acknowledged that mood stabilisers may take several weeks for a maximal response, and that during this time the patient with mania may require 'adjunctive' antipsychotic medication for 'severe agitation'. It is stated that antipsychotics may exacerbate post-manic-depressive episodes or induce rapid cycling; but this is a matter requiring further study.

Current practice

In Europe, where antipsychotics are widely regarded as a first-line treatment for acute mania (Licht 1998), psychiatrists view the American guidelines with scepticism. Lithium is often combined with an antipsychotic drug added for patients who are known to have responded to it in the past or as an adjunct for those who remain manic after about 2 weeks of adequate doses of an antipsychotic drug.

In view of the American Psychiatric Association Guidelines (1996), it might be expected that American psychiatrists would use antipsychotic drugs sparingly, and less often than their counterparts in other countries. However, the difference in approach may be more theoretical than real (Cookson and Sachs 2000). In centres in both the US and Europe, surveys show that the majority of manic patients discharged from hospital are still taking antipsychotic medication and remain on it after 6 months (Licht et al. 1994; Cookson, this volume). This may signify that the Guidelines are more conservative about the use of antipsychotics than the clinical situation is judged to warrant.

Applying the evidence for antipsychotics

Table 14.4 shows the results of two efficacy trials in schizophrenia. First, in acute schizophrenia there is a substantial improvement with a robust

Table 14.4 Schizophrenia trials: drop out rates, response rates and number-needed-to-treat

Diagnosis	Treatments (number of patients)	Duration	Criterion of improvement	Drop outs due to inefficacy %	Drop outs due to adverse events %	Response %	Effect size %	Number-needed-to-treat (95% CI)
Acute schizophrenia (Cole et al. 1964)	phenothiazine (n = 338)	6 weeks	Much or very much improved on the clinical global impression scale	2	3	75	52	2 (2–3)
	placebo (n = 125)			29	0	23		
Schizophrenia maintenance (Hirsch et al. 1973)	depot injection fluphenazine (n = 40)	9 months	no relapse	9		92	58	2 (2–3)
	placebo (n = 41)					34		

Table 14.5 Adherence to depot medication and associated relapse rates in 1 year. Data from an East London clinic (total number = 298) (Cookson and Duffelt 1994)

Depot medication received %	Proportion of patients %	Relapse rate %
More than 90%	60	13
70–90%	21	29
Less than 70%	15	42
Not known	4	–
Total	100	19

number-needed-to-treat. Nevertheless a number of patients do not improve and these patients will need special therapy because of their resistance to treatment. Second, antipsychotics are capable of preventing relapses of schizophrenia, again with a robust number-needed-to-treat.

In practice, however, non-compliance is a common problem both with medication given as depot injections by a community psychiatric nurse (see Table 14.5), and with oral medication using modern atypical antipsychotics that have fewer side effects. This non-compliance has direct consequences that are reflected in relapse rates.

More systematic efforts may be made to overcome this reluctance to accept treatment. In one research study, treatment with six sessions of 'compliance therapy' (psycho-education and cognitive therapy, lasting from 3 to 4 hours) was compared to non-specific counselling, in seventy-four psychotic patients following admission to hospital. The relapse rate of 63 per cent at 12 months in the control group was reduced to 41 per cent in the treated group (effect size 22 per cent); however the relapse rates were high in both groups (Kemp *et al.* 1998).

Conclusion

The discovery of methods for proving efficacy and detecting side effects of drugs has enabled us to treat severe mental illnesses such as bipolar disorder and schizophrenia with more confidence. It has also revealed the short-comings of current treatments in terms of both efficacy and tolerability. These methods, combined with pharmaceutical innovations, offer hope for the development of better treatments.

Chapter 15

The outcome of psychoanalysis: the hope for the future

Peter Fonagy

At first we hope too much, later on, not enough.
(Joseph Roux, *Meditations of a Parish Priest*, 1886)

Background

In 1903, in his contribution to Loewenfeld's book on obsessional phenomena, Freud wrote 'the number of persons suitable for psycho-analytic treatment is extraordinarily large and the extension which has come to our therapeutic powers from this method is . . . very considerable' (Freud 1904, p. 254). Earlier, in a series of three lectures on hysteria given by Freud in October 1905, he asserted 'And I may say that the analytic method of psychotherapy is one that penetrates most deeply and carries farthest, the one by means of which the most effective transformations can be effected in patients' (Freud 1905, p. 260). His therapeutic optimism persisted for at least two decades. In 1917 he writes 'Through the overcoming of these resistances the patient's mental life is permanently changed, is raised to a higher level of development and remains protected against a fresh possibility of falling ill' (Freud 1916–17, p. 451). Fifteen years later, however, his optimism apparently wilted and he claimed 'never [to have] been a therapeutic enthusiast' (Freud 1933, p. 151). In one of his last strictly psychoanalytic writings, Freud (1937) decisively repudiated earlier statements on the prophylactic aspects of analysis. By this time perhaps he was 'hoping for too little' and he devastatingly added

> One has the impression that one ought not to be surprised if it should turn out in the end that the difference between a person who has not been analysed and the behaviour of a person after he has been analysed is not so thoroughgoing as we aim at making it and as we expect and maintain it to be.
>
> (p. 228)

Recognising the limited benefit that analysts are likely to observe following years of treatment, he added 'It almost looks as if analysis were the third of those "impossible" professions in which one can be sure beforehand of achieving unsatisfying results' (p. 248). The other two endeavours deserving of similar empathy are, of course, education and government.

This was the state of affairs half a century ago. What hope is there in the era of empirically validated treatments (Lonigan *et al.* 1998), which prizes brief structured interventions, for a therapeutic approach which defines itself by freedom from constraint and preconception (Bion 1967), and counts treatment length not in terms of number of sessions but in terms of years in the same numerical range? Can psychoanalysis ever demonstrate its effectiveness, let alone cost-effectiveness? After all, is psychoanalysis not a qualitatively different form of therapy which must surely require a qualitatively different kind of metric to reflect variations in its outcome? Symptom change as a sole indicator of therapeutic benefit must indeed be considered crude in relation to the complex interpersonal processes that evolve over the many hundreds of sessions of the average three to five times weekly psychoanalytic treatment. Little wonder that most psychoanalysts are sceptical about outcome investigations.

What surprises one, given this unpropitious backdrop, is that there is, in fact, some suggestive evidence for the effectiveness of psychoanalysis as a treatment for psychological disorder. Before reviewing this evidence, let us briefly outline the generally agreed hierarchy of research designs which tends to be applied to outcome studies in psychotherapy (Roth and Fonagy 1996). Broadly, at the bottom of the hierarchy are case reports and case series studies, which at best establish an expectable time frame for change. Slightly above sit prospective pre–post studies, which can document the nature and extent of change. To be preferred are comparison studies where the effects of an intervention are contrasted with no treatment or treatment as usual (sadly the latter two conditions are often not very different). The gold standard is a randomised controlled trial (RCT) comparing the index treatment with another treatment of known effectiveness or a good placebo control. Most evidence for psychoanalysis is at the case study level. There are, however, exceptions.

The evidence base of psychoanalytic treatment

Psychoanalysts have been encouraged by the body of research which supports brief dynamic psychotherapy. A meta-analysis of twenty-six such studies has yielded effect sizes comparable to other approaches (Anderson and Lambert 1995). It may even be slightly superior to some other therapies if long-term follow up is included in the design. One of the best designed RCTs, the Sheffield Psychotherapy Project (Shapiro *et al.* 1995), found evidence for the effectiveness of a sixteen-session psychodynamic treatment based on

Hobson's (1985) model, in the treatment of major depression. There is evidence for the effectiveness of psychodynamic therapy as an adjunct to drug dependence programs (Woody *et al.* 1995). There is ongoing work on a brief psychodynamic treatment for panic disorder (Milrod *et al.* 1997), and there is evidence for the use of brief psychodynamic approaches in work with older people (Thompson *et al.* 1987).

There are also psychotherapy process studies that offer qualified support for the psychoanalytic case. For example, psychoanalytic interpretations given to clients, and which have been judged to be accurate interpretations are reported to be associated with relatively good outcome (Crits-Christoph *et al.* 1988; Joyce and Piper 1993). There is even tentative evidence from the re-analysis of therapy tapes from the National Institute of Mental Health Treatment of Depression Collaborative Research Program that the more the process of a brief therapy (cognitive-behavioural therapy and interpersonal therapy) resembles that of a psychodynamic approach, the more likely it is to be effective (Ablon and Jones 1999).

Evidence is available to support therapeutic interventions that are clear derivatives of psychoanalysis. However, there is a certain degree of disingenuity in psychoanalysis embracing these investigations. Most analysts would consider that the aims and methods of short-term once-a-week psychotherapy are not comparable to 'full analysis'. What do we know about the value of intensive and long-term psychodynamic treatment? Here the evidence base becomes somewhat patchy.

The Boston Psychotherapy Study (Stanton *et al.* 1984) compared long-term psychoanalytic therapy (two or more times a week) with supportive therapy for clients with schizophrenia in a randomised controlled design. There were some treatment specific outcomes, but on the whole clients who received psychoanalytic therapy fared no better than those who received supportive treatment. In contrast, in an effectiveness study of psychoanalytic treatments conducted with ninety-nine outpatients at the Institute for Psychoanalytic Training and Research Clinical Center (Freedman *et al.* 1999), investigators concluded that there were incremental gains in patient-perceived outcomes when session frequency was increased from one to either two or three weekly sessions. Effectiveness ratings also showed incremental gains when 24 months of therapy was compared to 6 months of therapy.

In another recent RCT (Bateman and Fonagy 1999), individuals with a diagnosis of borderline personality disorder were assigned to a psychoanalytically oriented day-hospital treatment or treatment as usual, which in the vast majority of cases included a psychiatric day hospital. The psychoanalytic arm of the treatment included therapy groups three times a week as well as individual therapy once or twice a week over an 18-month period. There were considerable gains in this group relative to the controls in terms of suicidal and self-mutilating behaviour, depressive and anxiety symptoms, and social and interpersonal functioning. These differences were not only maintained in the 18 months following discharge but increased, even though the day-hospital group received less treatment than the control group (Bateman and Fonagy submitted). A further controlled trial of intensive psychoanalytic treatment for children with chronically poorly controlled diabetes reported significant gains in diabetic control in the treated group, which was maintained at 1 year follow up (Moran *et al.* 1991). Experimental single-case studies carried out with the same population supported the causal relationship between interpretive work and improvement in diabetic control and physical growth (Fonagy and Moran 1991). The work of Chris Heinicke also suggests that four or five times weekly sessions may generate more marked improvements in children with specific learning difficulties than a less intensive psychoanalytic intervention (Heinicke and Ramsey-Klee 1986).

One of the most interesting studies to emerge recently was the Stockholm Outcome of Psychotherapy and Psychoanalysis Project (Sandell 1999). The study followed 756 persons who received national-insurance-funded treatment for up to 3 years in psychoanalysis or in psychoanalytic psychotherapy. The groups were matched on many clinical variables. Four or five times weekly analysis had similar outcomes at termination when compared with one to two psychotherapy sessions per week. However, in measurements of symptomatic outcome using the SCL-90 (a symptom check list), improvement on 3-year follow up was substantially greater for individuals who received psychoanalysis than those in psychoanalytic psychotherapy. In fact, during the follow-up period, psychotherapy patients did not change but those who had had psychoanalysis continued to improve, almost to a point where their scores were indistinguishable from those obtained from a non-clinical Swedish sample. While the results of the study are positive for psychoanalysis, certain of the findings are quite challenging. For example, those therapists whose attitude to clinical process most closely resembled that of a 'classical analyst' (neutrality, exclusive orientation to insight) had psychotherapy clients with the worst, commonly negative, outcomes.

Another large pre–post study of psychoanalytic treatments has examined the clinical records of 763 children who were evaluated and treated at the Anna Freud Centre, under the close supervision of Freud's daughter (Fonagy and Target 1996). Children with certain disorders (for example depression, autism and conduct disorder) appeared to benefit only marginally from psychoanalysis or psychoanalytic psychotherapy. Interestingly, children with severe emotional disorders (three or more Axis I diagnoses) did surprisingly well in psychoanalysis, although they did poorly in once or twice a week psychoanalytic psychotherapy. Younger children derived the greatest benefit from intensive treatment. Adolescents appeared not to benefit from the increased frequency of sessions. The importance of the study is perhaps less in demonstrating that psychoanalysis is effective, although some of the effects on very severely disturbed children were quite remarkable, but more in identifying groups for whom the additional effort involved in intensive treatment appeared not to be warranted.

Several prospective follow-along studies using a pre–post design have suggested substantial improvements in patients given psychoanalytic therapies for personality disorders (Høglend 1993; Monsen *et al.* 1995a, 1995b; Stevenson and Meares 1992). However, these were all uncontrolled studies, with populations whose symptomatology is recognised to fluctuate substantially, and so the evidence can give us few reliable indications as to which particular subgroups may benefit from a psychoanalytic approach.

The Research Committee of the International Psychoanalytic Association has recently prepared a comprehensive review of North American and European outcome studies of psychoanalytic treatment (Fonagy *et al.* 1999).[1] The committee concluded that existing studies failed to unequivocally demonstrate that psychoanalysis is efficacious relative to either an alternative treatment or an active placebo, and identified a range of methodological and design problems in the studies described in the report, including the absence of intent to treat controls, heterogeneous patient groups, lack of random assignments, the failure to use independently administered standardized measures of outcome, and so on. Nevertheless, the report, which covers over fifty studies, is encouraging to psychoanalysts. Despite the limitations of the completed studies, evidence across a significant number of pre–post investigations suggests that psychoanalysis appears to be consistently helpful to patients with milder (neurotic) disorders and somewhat less consistently so for other, more severe groups. Across a range of uncontrolled or poorly controlled cohort studies, mostly carried out in Europe, longer intensive treatments tended to have better outcomes than shorter, non-intensive treatments. The impact of psychoanalysis was apparent beyond symptomatology, in measures of work functioning and reductions in health-care costs. Moreover, a number of studies testing psychoanalysis with 'state-of-the-art' methodology are ongoing and are likely to produce more compelling evidence over the next years. These include the Munich Psychotherapy of Depression Study, the Cornell Comparison of Transference Focused Psychotherapy (TFP) and Dialectical Behaviour Therapy (DBT), the Munich–New York Collaborative Study of the Psychodynamic Treatment of Borderline Personality Organization, the Helsinki Psychotherapy Study, and the Anna Freud Centre Prospective Study of Child Psychoanalysis, Psychoanalytic Psychotherapy and Cognitive-Behavioural Therapy for the Treatment of Severe Emotional Disorder.

---

1 The report is available at cost of reproduction from the IPA, Broomhills, Woodside Lane, London N12 8UD and can be downloaded free from www.ipa.org.uk.

The need for a methodology

The development of research instruments is an essential part of this increasing methodological rigour. A significant gap in the field until now, which has hindered the cumulative construction of a psychoanalytic knowledge base, is the absence of even a rudimentary classification system to describe clinical cases. There is an urgent need to develop a nosology acceptable to psychoanalytic clinicians. A group of German psychoanalysts has already evolved operationalised psychodynamic diagnoses that could function in conjunction with or independently of DSM-IV (Arbeitkreis 1996; Cierpka *et al.* 1995). Other similarly operationalised nosologies are under development in Geneva, Barcelona and Stockholm. A comprehensive approach to the classification of predominant mechanisms of defence has also been undertaken in the US (Crits-Christoph *et al.* 1988).

Measures are also required to verify that psychoanalytic treatment has indeed taken place. This involves two challenges: first, the description of psychoanalytic treatment in a form that permits assessment, and second, a method of demonstrating therapist adherence and competence in the delivery of a specific treatment. To measure adherence we must use a manual. Yet with two preliminary exceptions (Clarkin *et al.* 1998; Fonagy *et al.* unpublished manuscript), no one has yet attempted to manualise psychoanalysis. The difficulties in manualising psychoanalytic treatments are obvious. Manuals usually describe brief treatments in a session-by-session sequence. They are most successful when treatments do not depend on the productivity of the patient, when the theoretical base provides a relatively unambiguous formulation of the disorder, and when treatment techniques may be directly linked to these formulations. In contrast, psychoanalysis is a long treatment that relies completely on the material brought by the patient, with techniques easy to prescribe but which depend on the creativity and intuition of the analyst for their competent application. Moreover, it is impossible to achieve any kind of one-to-one mapping between psychoanalytic technique and any major theoretical framework; psychoanalytic theory is largely not about clinical practice. Even when psychoanalysts are working within the same theoretical framework, they find great difficulty in arriving at a consensus as to the presence or absence of a psychoanalytic process.

The absence of an operationalised definition of what psychoanalysis is should not deter us; rather, this uncertainty necessitates a systematic examination of the psychoanalytic process. This research might ultimately identify the most generic critical components of the treatment, which could then be tested for effectiveness and ultimately cost-effectiveness. Several current research programmes have the potential to systematise the psychoanalytic process in this manner. Krause (Anstadt *et al.* 1997; Krause 1997) has studied reciprocal facial affect expression in the therapeutic dyad. Bucci (1997) has developed a coding system of referential activity, which involves the tracking of connections between non-verbal systems and the communicative verbal code (Bucci and Miller 1993). Perhaps the most promising approach makes use of a relatively simple instrument called the Psychotherapy Process Q-set (Jones et al. 1993). This 100-item instrument provides a basic language for the description and classification of treatment processes in a form suitable for quantitative analysis. Entire therapeutic hours are rated by sorting the Q items, and statistical analysis is used to identify potential underlying structures of interaction. Time-series analysis is then used to assess changes by exploring the unfolding over time of different variables.

A final empirical approach with potential is based on the assumption that a psychoanalytic process is effective, at least with certain groups of patients, because it engages modes of mental functioning that were defensively inhibited by the patient in the process of early adaptation to conflict-ridden environments (Fonagy et al. 1993). The capacity to represent mental states of self and other in the context of attachment relationships has been the focus of the work of this group (Fonagy 1995; Fonagy et al. 1991). A superior level of reflective (mentalising) ability may be the long-term outcome of effective psychoanalytic treatment in childhood. The freeing of reflective capacity is argued to be a key component of therapeutic change in psychoanalysis (Bleiberg et al. 1997) and could be routinely monitored as an index of the psychoanalytic process. This approach is currently being studied by a number of European research groups.

While, however, a wide range of measures are already potentially available to monitor the process of psychoanalytic therapy, many of these are too complex or cumbersome to permit routine use. Hence researchers are also working on instruments which would allow the easy collection of a minimal psychoanalytic data set, including measures of both process and outcome. For example, to measure therapeutic process, the European Psychoanalytic Collaborative Study on Process and Outcome has adapted a check-list (the Periodical Rating Scale) that psychoanalysts complete monthly to indicate the manifest and latent content of sessions (Stoker et al. 1996). The checklist includes items related to the patient's general attitude, specific conscious and unconscious concerns, object relations, transference manifestations and reports of the analyst's style of intervention and the patient's reaction to these interventions. The check-list has been shown to have higher inter-rater reliability when used with transcribed sessions, and in a small-scale study was shown to predict treatment outcome. The report of anxiety, guilt and idealisation in the transference was associated with successful treatments, whereas reports of shame, humiliation and existential anxiety were associated with failed treatments (Fonagy in preparation).

A similar simplified approach could be taken to the measurement of psychoanalytic outcome. The minimum psychoanalytic data set could include baseline and annually collected outcomes data from analyst and patient; relatively simple outcome measures are already available for this. It is useful to have some measurement techniques which overlap with those employed by non-psychoanalytic therapists. This is fairly easy in the symptom domain; self-report measures such as SCL-90-R (Derogatis 1983) and the Beck depression inventory (Beck *et al.* 1961) are commonly used in psychotherapy research. Similarly, the global assessment of functioning ratings could readily represent the therapist's perspective. Barkham and colleagues (Barkham *et al.* in press) have developed a new self-report questionnaire, with considerable promise for a simple generic measure of outcome, for the standard assessment of adult psychosocial treatments in the British health-care system. A similar, relatively easy to use clinician-completed measure of outcome is provided by the Functional Analysis of Care Environments, which is in use at fifty British hospitals and which yields operationalised ratings of psychiatric symptoms, interpersonal relationships, activities of daily living and physical health (Clifford 1998).

Measures already exist, therefore, which would enable a rudimentary investigation of the outcome of psychoanalytic treatment. Baseline, annual, and end-of-treatment information could be collected on all patients undertaking psychoanalysis under supervision. These data, if drawn from a substantial sample and if collected with reasonable rigour, could represent the first step towards answering key questions concerning the nature of the psychoanalytic process.

The hope for the future

There can be no excuse for the thin evidence base of psychoanalytic treatment. In the same breath that psychoanalysts often claim to be at the intellectual origin of other talking cures (for example systemic therapy and cognitive behaviour therapy), they also seek shelter behind the relative immaturity of the discipline to explain the absence of evidence for its efficacy. Yet the evidence base of these 'derivatives' of psychoanalytic therapy has been far more firmly established than evidence for psychoanalysis itself. Of course, there are reasons given for this – reasons such as the long-term nature of the therapy, the subtlety and complexity of its procedures, the elusiveness of its self-declared outcome goals, and the incompatibility of direct observation with the need for absolute confidentiality. None of these reasons stands up to careful scrutiny, however. For example, recording the analytic process appears to be possible without the total destruction of the client's trust (Thomä and Kächele 1987). Further, systematic observation lends rigour to the entire enterprise, a rigour that may be a crucial common factor underlying many effective treatments (Fonagy 1999). Audio-taping is far from being a pre-requisite of data gathering in this area. A more likely reason for the absence of psychoanalytic outcome research lies in the fundamental incompatibilities in the world-view espoused by psychoanalysis and most of current social science.

In a recent paper Paul Whittle (in press) describes a 'chasm' between psychoanalysis and psychology. While the method of psychoanalysis was developed to fill gaps in self narrative and self awareness, inevitable because of the limitations of conscious reflection, psychology has a minimalist theory building tradition that Whittle elegantly describes as 'cognitive asceticism'. The kind of narrative making that psychoanalysis entails is so core to human function, so central to the experience of personal meaning (Bruner 1990), that a discipline that has the systematic elaboration of such narratives at its core will probably remain forever vital to the study of the nature of human-kind. The absence of parsimony in psychoanalytic theorisation is defensible because the content of mind is irreducible and because any assertion of a singular reality, at least as far as human nature is concerned, is inherently suspect.

So can we think of psychoanalysis as offering an alternative epistemology to the one we habitually use in psychological research? I believe that such an attitude implicitly consigns psychoanalysis to its current inadequate mode of functioning. And seeing psychology and psychoanalysis at opposite ends of an epistemological continuum runs the risk of shielding the discipline from appropriate criticisms concerning its profound limitations. Psychoanalysis needs to change. Gathering further evidence for psychoanalysis through outcome studies is important, not simply to improve support for existing practices but far more to generate a change of attitudes in psychoanalytic practitioners which is essential to ensure a future for psychoanalysis and psychoanalytic therapies.

There are at least five necessary components to this attitude change

1. the incorporation of data-gathering methods beyond the anecdotal methods that are now widely available in social and biological science
2. moving psychoanalytic constructs from the global to the specific which will facilitate cumulative data gathering
3. routine consideration of alternative accounts for behavioural observations
4. increasing psychoanalytic sophistication concerning social and con-textual influences on behaviour
5. ending the splendid isolation of psychoanalysis by undertaking active collaboration with other disciplines.

Rather than fearing that fields adjacent to psychoanalysis might destroy the unique insights offered by long-term intensive individual therapy, psycho-analysts must embrace the rapidly evolving 'knowledge chain', focused at different levels of the study of brain–behaviour relationships. As Kandel (1998, 1999) pointed out, this may be the only route to the preservation of the hard-won insights of psychoanalysis.

Chapter 16

Applying the evidence in psychological therapies

Anthony D Roth

In an ideal world we would know which of the psychological therapies are most effective for which patients and for which problems. Moreover, we would also understand which 'ingredients' of therapy are effective at bringing about change. In this way each psychotherapeutic encounter could be truly evidence based and matched to the needs of the individual patient. In reality we are far from being able to make statements of such specificity. Some of the reasons for this are detailed elsewhere (Roth and Fonagy 1996, Roth and Parry 1997). The primary problem is that the evidence base does not map directly to practice; efficacy (the results obtained by an intervention in a research context) and clinical effectiveness (the results of the same intervention in standard clinical practice) are not the same thing. This follows from the fact that researchers and clinicians have rather different concerns. Researchers are interested in examining hypotheses about outcomes from therapy, or about the mechanisms which underpin these outcomes. For this reason they are concerned to maximise the internal validity of their studies, something that cannot be achieved without careful structuring of their interventions. The well-designed randomised controlled trial (RCT) is favoured by researchers precisely because, at least in theory, it achieves very high levels of control over potential sources of error variance. While this maximises the capacity for hypothesis testing, it makes it much harder to generalise from the RCT to the consulting room for a number of reasons. Not least of these is the fact that this research design is constructed to contrast outcomes from one therapy as against another, and as a consequence it inevitably minimises the contribution of individual therapists and patients. Although it is possible to devise studies that examine therapist and patient factors as main effects (rather than through *post hoc* analysis), in practice such studies are relatively rare. The consequence is that although we can make some general comments about the average expected outcome from a therapy, individual therapists will implement the same therapy in somewhat different ways, and individual patients will show a variation in their response to the same intervention. Psychological therapy is not administered in the manner of medication or surgery; it develops out of an interaction between the therapist's capacity to engage the patient in implementing therapy, and the patient's capacity to use the therapy. This means that any interpretation of research needs to acknowledge the degree of uniqueness in each therapeutic encounter; equally clinicians need to find some way of understanding the degree of commonality between outcomes in their clinic patients and those treated in research trials.

An earlier generation of psychotherapy research frequently combined patients with a range of presenting problems, something rarely seen within the current literature. For good reason, largely related to considerations of internal validity, most researchers favour the examination of outcomes in research populations chosen for their diagnostic homogeneity. Most trials restrict themselves to patients with a single diagnosis, and seek to exclude any significant comorbidity. This is not the place to rehearse arguments about the wisdom of this approach (Roth and Fonagy (1996) offer a synoptic critique), but it is worth noting that it is an approach which has limitations beyond the philosophical. Comorbid presentations are very common in the general population. For example, an epidemiological survey in the UK (Office of Population Censuses and Surveys 1995) found that mixed anxiety and depression was much more common than depression alone in the general population. In addition, some diagnoses appear to 'cluster', for example people with generalised anxiety disorder were more likely to have an additional diagnosis of obsessional compulsive disorder or depression, and there was a significant association between a diagnosis of obsessional compulsive disorder and a co-occurring diagnosis of depression, phobia and generalised anxiety disorder (a pattern likely to be recognised by most clinicians). The challenge for researchers would be to conduct a trial which examined outcomes in relation to patients with these commonly occurring clusters of comorbid presentations as main effects (rather than through *post hoc* analysis), while maintaining appropriate levels of internal validity. Such trials would have utility because they would cast some light on a common clinical problem arising from comorbidity. For example, treating a patient with mixed depression and anxiety requires some thought about titrating research information about treatment outcomes in depression and in anxiety, in the absence of robust scientific information about how this is best done.

For some conditions applying research findings is complicated by the simple fact that there is not enough research available to draw reliable conclusions. An inspection of the Cochrane database of RCTs shows, for example, that while there are many good quality trials looking at outcomes in depression or panic disorder, there are very few RCTs examining outcomes in anorexia nervosa. To some degree this may reflect a very practical problem. Individuals who are depressed are, unsurprisingly, relatively easy to identify and to recruit. However, certain presentations are relatively uncommon or are usually seen in specialist settings, and this may limit the opportunity for research. The relative paucity of research in some key areas limits our capacity to make reliable statements about expected outcomes, because reviews become based on a limited number of trials. This leads to individual studies achieving an inappropriate weighting in the evaluation of efficacy, with the result that conclusions about efficacy are potentially unstable, the addition of just a few more trials can shift the balance of our conclusions markedly.

Beyond diagnosis, other factors routinely encountered by clinicians also tend to be under-represented in research. There is for example little *direct* exploration of the impact of social factors on outcome, even though material deprivation and the consequences of social exclusion will inevitably impact on the management of many patients seen in public health settings. It is also worth noting that most clients in research trials are white; as a consequence questions about the applicability of psychological therapies across ethnic groups and cultures are very hard to answer.

The majority of trials ask questions about comparative outcome from 'brand names' of therapy. This focus has led to the almost universal use of manualisation (in one form or another) in most research trials; therapists are restricted to a repertoire of specified techniques, and their ability to adhere to them and deliver therapy in line with requirements is monitored carefully. In contrast, much clinical practice is an admixture of theoretical and technical eclecticism, with the consequence that knowing that a technique has proved effective under research conditions does not guarantee that it will work in the hand of clinicians. Outcomes from research trials are usually better than those obtained in clinical practice (Weiss and Weisz 1990), and it is sensible to wonder whether at least part of the explanation for this lies in the greater rigour and focus of therapeutic practice within research. However, this level of prescription is usually seen as inappropriate in clinical practice, where the emphasis on tailoring practice to the patient is seen as a virtue, and linked to notions of clinical freedom. How far this is a reasoned approach could be questioned, but it is the case that while evidence for the benefits of adapting technique to the individual is not compelling, there are also reasons for being cautious about the virtues of manualisation. For example, exclusion criteria for many research trials can select out the very complexities that force clinicians to become more adaptive in their approach, which implies that there may be limits to the appropriateness or feasibility of a 'cookbook' approach. Indeed there is some evidence that therapists judged as more competent are able to deviate appropriately from technical recommendations with more difficult patients (Rounsaville *et al.* 1988), and that these individuals produce greater improvement in their patients (O'Malley *et al.* 1988).

While questions of outcome are important to clinicians, in daily practice they will be more concerned with questions of mechanism, i.e. what are the processes that underpin outcomes? Unfortunately much of what we know about many process–outcome relationships rests on *post hoc* analysis of studies originally designed to ask questions about outcome from specific therapies. Not all studies permit sensible analysis, but some trials have been multiply re-examined for information about process factors. The National Institute of Mental Health multi-centre trial for depression (well described in Elkin 1994) is a good example of this. While initially analysed in relation to outcomes from the therapies employed in the trial, numerous papers on process issues have now appeared; indeed some are cited in this chapter because of the quality of the information they contain. Because of its size, information from this trial is likely to influence thinking about therapy process. Some caution about extrapolation is required however, since most process variables have fairly small effect sizes, and without a broad research base there is a considerable risk of mistaking sample variation for real effects. A recent review (McKay and Barkham 1998, commissioned as part of the evidence base for a clinical guideline) was explicitly briefed to report on a variety of potentially significant process issues. Not only was there relatively little data on which to base comments, but much of the process information that was obtained rested on multiple examination of a relatively small pool of studies, reducing the power and hence the quality of the evidence.

The consequence of *post hoc* analysis is that we know relatively little about some important topics. For example, what is the impact of therapist factors such as their skilfulness? Does training make a difference to outcome? These are not easy questions to answer; there is evidence that more skilful application of a therapy is associated with better outcomes, though the degree to which training confers this skill is less clear (Roth and Fonagy 1996). Which patient factors are pertinent to outcome? In outline we know that motivation, readiness for change, and psychological mindedness are likely to improve outcome (Orlinsky *et al.* 1994), but more specific predictions are harder to make. What is clear is that a positive therapeutic alliance is a significant and necessary underpinning to any therapy, and numerous studies (Horvarth and Symonds 1991) and analyses of major outcome trials (Krupnick *et al.* 1996; Castonguay *et al.* 1996) have now demonstrated a reliable relationship between alliance level and outcome. This description does not of course account for mechanism, though (through very different methodologies) there is increasing interest in exploring the therapeutic manoeuvres that form and sustain the alliance (see, for example, Bennett 1999).

Even where there is direct concern to collect process information, the methodologies we currently employ may not be appropriately sensitive. Stiles and Shapiro (1994) pointed out that treating process ingredients as additive and static variables may be profoundly misleading, either because the behaviour of therapists (and indeed patients) is likely to be mutually responsive to that of the other, or because therapists may deliver certain important ingredients at high levels regardless of patient characteristics or outcomes. Thus therapists may be warm towards their clients in a rather non-specific manner, with the consequence that it might be quite hard to demonstrate an association between warmth and outcome using statistics which assume linear associations. In addition, some process relationships may be quite complex, requiring some sophistication both to discover and to interpret. An example of this would be Blatt *et al.*'s (1996) finding that patient perfectionism impacts on the capacity to form a therapeutic alliance, but only in those patients moderate in their level of perfectionism did this link to outcome.

The search for the 'effective ingredients' of therapy remains an important, though an elusive challenge. All therapies appear to have a number of common factors, unsurprising given that the roots of most approaches lie in engaging patients in the task of self-examination, in the context of a mutually trusting and reasonably honest interaction. Beyond this many therapists make strong claims for the specific benefits of their techniques; indeed the development of new models and their therapeutic applications continues apace. In practice, however, there is surprisingly little evidence for the differential efficacy of one therapy over another (Wampold *et al.* 1997). Process studies of therapy also suggest that the overlap between techniques may be as significant as their differences. In an analysis of the National Institute of Mental Health study of psychological therapy for depression, referred to above, Ablon and Jones (1999) used a Q-sort technique to examine which types of interactions were most characteristic of the two therapies employed: cognitive behaviour therapy and interpersonal psychotherapy. While the therapies have very different rationales, in practice there was a large degree of overlap in terms of what therapists actually did, and the ways in which patients responded. Of course, some differences were also detected between therapies, congruent with their different theoretical emphases. While it is possible to argue that the effective ingredients of each therapy lie with these differences in technique, it seems more reasonable to suggest that most effective therapies will demonstrate some overlap, and that there should be some caution in making too strong a claim about the uniqueness of one approach over another.

There have been studies which 'dismantle' the ingredients of therapy, removing or modifying elements which are thought to be mutative and exploring the resulting outcomes. In some areas this can be an important approach, especially where strong claims are made for the specificity of a particular technique. For example, advocates of eye movement and desensitisation therapy initially maintained that its success in helping patients with post-traumatic stress disorder was related to the therapist tracking their hands across the patient's field of vision while the patient speaks about (and hence re-experiences) their traumatising experience. However, it is evident that such hand movements may not be necessary (Renfey and Spates 1994), and while this finding may not be fatal to advocates of this model as a whole, it does relocate eye movement and desensitisation therapy closer to more conventional therapies in terms of the mechanism underpinning its efficacy. However, there are obvious limitations to the strategy of dismantling. For example, by design most pain-management programmes include a number of components, including input from medical staff, from psychologists and from physiotherapists. Overall it is clear that cognitive behaviour therapy is an effective technique for patients with chronic pain (Morley *et al.* 1999), but any desire to separate out the successful elements of the package may be detrimental if, as is likely, each component may bring about change in more than one outcome, and components interact to produce the overall effect.

Much of the above discussion suggests that information from outcome and process–outcome research translates uneasily to standard practice. An obvious strategy for improving matters would be to conduct more research on the effectiveness of therapy as conducted in routine settings. Unfortunately interpretation of data collected in the field is often limited by considerations of internal validity. Ideally information about effectiveness would be derived from large field trials across a number of settings, in order to overcome the usual statistical problems associated with small-scale open trials or case series. In practice this requires the use of a common metric across clinical settings, and by implication the co-operation of clinicians of disparate orientations and opinions. For now, it remains true that studies of clinical effectiveness within the published literature are fairly rare (Shadish *et al.* 1997).

Notwithstanding the above enumeration of difficulties, there are some conclusions to be drawn from the literature. Certainly there is good evidence for the efficacy of psychological therapies. The evidence relates to outcomes in relation to major mental health conditions, and this suggests that psychological therapies should be considered as a standard part of the repertoire of treatments. It remains true that some therapies are better researched than others, and this places some limits on comments about the comparative efficacy of the therapies. None the less, where good quality research exists, evidence for differential efficacy of therapies is not strong (for example, in depression there is good evidence for the efficacy of cognitive behaviour therapy, interpersonal psychotherapy and of short-term psychodynamic methods). However, there is some evidence for differential efficacy in relation to some disorders, and where this exists it should be noted (for example, the strength of the evidence suggests that obsessional compulsive disorder is best treated using behavioural and cognitive-behavioural methods).

As a generalisation, outcomes from therapy are likely to be moderate, though clinically significant, across a range of conditions. As is to be expected, treatment targets will reflect the nature of the condition being treated; in some conditions (such as some of the anxiety disorders) a complete remission can be expected, while in others improvements in functioning may be more realistic (as is the case for many individuals with schizophrenia). The likelihood of remission–relapse cycles is also an important consideration in thinking about outcomes. For example, individuals with a history of depression are likely to relapse over time if not given further treatment, and this suggests that follow-up maintenance treatments (whose efficacy has been demonstrated, for example Frank *et al.* 1991) might well be considered as an alternative either to brief interventions or to long-term treatment. 'Brand names' of therapy are only partially predictive of outcome, and it is worth recognising that the therapeutic alliance is important to successful treatment. Clearly therapists are not all the same: what works in the hands of one therapist might not work in the hands of another. Equally, patients are not all the same: what works for one patient might not work for another. All of this leads to a cautionary statement – 'evidence-based practice' is more than the direct application of psychotherapy research. In the US the American Psychological Association has attempted to identify 'empirically supported therapies' (Chambless and Hollon 1998). This model is superficially attractive because it appears to resolve some of the ambiguity surrounding our current state of knowledge. However, for all the reasons given above, this certainty is more apparent than real, and the empirically supported therapy approach has created an acrimonious and, at points, divisive debate between researchers, clinicians and purchasers of health care. In the UK a rather different approach has been taken, with a recognition that clinical guidelines are needed to help to weigh evidence, and in some cases to weigh the absence of evidence. The role of professional and clinical judgement in titrating research findings against experience is critical here; without some attempt to test guidelines against conditions found in the field they will have little credence or respect among the majority of clinicians. Guidelines are recommendations, not prescriptions, and can and should be varied by clinicians, not at whim but on the basis of clinical judgement. Of course the possibility remains that even the most carefully written guideline prove ineffective for the most basic of reasons, because no one reads them or uses them. Clearly the dissemination and implementation of guidelines is a critical process, and there needs to be an audit of impact incorporated into the process of distribution. In this way the evidence base can be applied in a manner which takes into account the strengths and the limitations of psychotherapy research, and meets the needs of clinicians for easy interpretation of a very large literature. Ultimately, of course, it should also meet the needs of patients who need the treatment that is, as far as can be ascertained, the most likely to benefit them. And this, of course, is the most compelling reason why we should be concerned with applying the evidence.

Chapter 17

Evidence in social care: the policy context

Peter Huxley

The policy context

This book will appear in the UK during one of the greatest periods of change in health and social-care services. After many years of argument and debate about the relative merits of a generic approach to social care, and the relative merits of integrating mental health services into mainstream health services, a double integration is taking place. Mental health services are being provided by new, specialist, larger provider organisations (mental health trusts), and their services increasingly are being commissioned by primary care. At the same time permissive mechanisms have been put into place to enable the integration of social care into these specialist mental health organisations. New partnership arrangements under Section 31 of the Health Act 1999 will enable local authorities and NHS bodies to improve services to mental health service users through the transferring of functions and the pooling of resources. The partnership arrangements are designed to eliminate the rigid division of health from social care which is very familiar in some parts of the world, for example in Russia where there are entirely separate ministries (of health and of social protection). In other places, notably some public mental health services in the US, the idea of mental health care that does not incorporate social care is unheard of.

The present moves towards the integration of services in the UK raise many concerns and anxieties, especially among those social-care staff (mainly social workers) who are becoming part of the new organisations. They are concerned about the loss of the social perspective and concerned that social-work values should not be subsumed and lose their influence in the new context. Social workers particularly are concerned that they will have fewer opportunities than their health-service colleagues for life-long learning, research and development, and for their own continuing professional development. They fear that the medical model of care might reduce the social model in status, or obscure it altogether. A fundamental difference between the two models of care is their approach to evidence-based practice. In the health service it is commonplace (Cape 2000), and the mental health

National Service Framework presents the supporting evidence (rated for quality) for its standards. Reynolds (2000), accepting that the relationship between research and practice tends to be an uneasy one, and the link erratic and unsystematic, nevertheless argues that evidence-based practice can help overcome the gap between research and practice. It can do this by making a distinction between research that is of direct significance to practice and that which is not, by providing simple rules for evaluating research evidence, and by providing a framework for making practice decisions based on applying research findings in individual cases.

In contrast, in social care, there is a limited, albeit growing realisation of the need to base decision making on supporting evidence. However, as I discuss in more detail on pp. 195–6, this awareness is not located within an entirely accepting culture. How can these differences between the health and social-care approach to the nature of evidence, and the different pace of acceptance of an evidence-based approach in social services, be addressed?

In this chapter, I want to describe what I think the current stage and pace of development of the evidence-based approach is in the social-care field (within a mental health setting), consider how this has arisen, review our present state of knowledge and arrive at a conclusion about the best way forward.

Where are we, and how did we get here?

Social care, as a practical branch of the social sciences, has been caught in the cross pressures of the debate between (broadly speaking) the scientific paradigm and hermeneutics. It has been said that the social sciences have been in a state of crisis since their inception (Hammersley 1993). Chapter 1 by Derek Bolton considers this debate in greater detail than is required here. It is useful to note, for our present purpose, that Bolton argues that the previously antipathetic positions are struggling towards some form of accommodation. He says that the present task 'is to accommodate mind and meaning within a transformed scientific paradigm'.

As Bolton reminds us, in the scientific paradigm, there is an objective evidence base, knowledge of causes (controlling for confounding variables) and generality. In contrast, hermeneutics involves subjective, unreplicable, intuitive claims to knowledge, understanding meaning or reasons, and a preoccupation with particular cases. All of the latter are the stuff of social work and social care – but then these are also the stuff of psychiatry. However, and in my experience, while a majority of psychiatrists, psychologists and economists find that they can make use of the scientific paradigm, many social-care professionals do not appear to find it easy to do so. While this generalisation may be less sustainable at the beginning of the twenty-first century than it was in the 1960s for example, it may be helpful to look at some of the reasons, both good and less good, why this might be the case.

Bolton notes that the scientific paradigm continues to expand into social policy (and social care) with increasing demands to produce the evidence upon which policies and practice are based.

This is not the place to dwell on the mistakes of the past in the creation, appreciation and use of evidence in social work and social-care education. Exactly how we arrived at the present position is a matter of opinion, as is the extent to which things might be changing. The 'present position' itself is contestable, and the following may appear somewhat of a caricature to some readers.

The current position is as follows.

- There is not the same emphasis on evidence-based practice in social care as in health care, or it is developing at a much slower pace.
- Very little research design and quantitative methodology are taught in social-work education compared to psychology for example.
- There are no research competence requirements within basic training (there are within the infrequently obtained advanced award) that require a trained practitioner to have the skills to make critical appraisals of evidence within the scientific or other paradigms.
- Training retains a strong emphasis on individuality, subjective appraisal and understanding (of both individuals and cultures).
- The opportunity for practitioners to undertake empirical research in the field is limited by an absence of a formal requirement for them to do so, and the space and time to do it.
- The culture of social-care organisations is rarely supportive of research activity in the way that health-service culture is.
- There are fewer specific funding options for people in social-care careers to develop their personal research skills, or to follow a research career path, compared to all health professionals.

Some of the possible underlying reasons why the lack of evidence-based culture exists in most social-care organisations are as follows.

- Decision making at a practice level is partly determined by the legal framework in which it takes place, and although this does depend often on the production of 'evidence' to support the legal case, this is individual behavioural evidence.
- Because there is a relative lack of scientific paradigm teaching in pre-basic, basic, and post-basic training, and no requirement for it in a continuing professional development context, there is a basic lack of knowledge and competence in this approach among practitioners and middle and senior managers.
- Decision making at management and committee level, while based on the presentation of arguments and 'facts', is not a rational process and

outcomes are determined politically. This can undermine the case for an evidence-based approach.

- The tradition of what constitutes evidence in the social-care field is different and emphasises understanding and subjective meaning, and interventions based on theoretical schema rather than the use of highly developed bodies of empirical knowledge.
- The materials (journals and professional journals) routinely made available to social-care practitioners and managers contain far more descriptive work than material from empirical trials. Very few practitioners and managers get the time to read research findings, and when they do this is usually in an easily digestible form – one that often fails to refer to the quality of evidence under consideration.
- Practitioner and manager participation in research is usually as providers of information or completers of forms, and in many cases the feedback of results is minimal or non-existent, and rarely involves a systematic consideration of practice or policy implications.
- The tradition of sharing knowledge by word of mouth of current knowledge or of plans for future research that takes place in many health settings, including those not associated closely with university departments, is very uncommon in social-care agencies. This may be, of course, because research and development is not the task of the worker, and may be the task of a separate part of the organisation. What has become an internalised function within most clinicians has not become an internalised function within the social-care professional – such things are the province of others.
- There is less research funding available for social-care as opposed to health-care research, and as a result there are far more health professionals involved in the research process (determining areas to be researched, peer reviewing bids, and making up national and regional advisory bodies). There are more fellowships available for health-care professionals. Those social-care funding bodies that do exist tend to have particular priorities that do not always include mental health, such as housing or children.
- There certainly used to be a widespread belief, partly a self-fulfilling prophecy, that the scientific paradigm is completely inappropriate in this field. While some authors (Pawson and Tilley 1997) suggest that the evidence supports this view, the generally held opinion that the scientific paradigm is not appropriate perhaps owes more to the other factors outlined above.

There are, of course, exceptions to these influences, in particular social-care research activity in the fostering and adoption field. In mental health care one could argue that the massive imbalance in resource availability and influence on strategic research agendas towards 'health' is of itself a major disincentive for social-care researchers wishing to join the field.

Differences in the conception of evidence and the tendency to reject the scientific paradigm are sometimes played out in the field through the debate about methods, in particular whether qualitative approaches are more suited to the generation of evidence in social care. Brian Williams in Chapter 11 argues that qualitative research can provide a high level of evidence in answering some questions such as 'what exists?', conceptualising findings and providing more precise definitions of key issues, but cannot provide a high level of evidence in others.

It might be better to describe the state of social work and social care over the last 40 years as moving from a position in which there was a strong and adverse reaction to positivism, and an outright rejection of the scientific paradigm, to one in which, for various reasons, its potential uses and limitations are better appreciated. It is useful for addressing certain issues and less useful for addressing others. There are pressures to accept the need for better quality evidence, but also a realisation that the best evidence is achieved by the most appropriate method in a particular context. This is a theme that runs throughout this book. As I have indicated above (see pp. 193–4) the confluence of health and social care in the mental health field will throw these issues into sharp relief. On the one side, health care, there will need to be a recognition that the priority and resource given to social-care education, research and development will have to be augmented, and on the other side, social care, there will need to be a recognition that better quality evidence will need to be created and within this agenda there will be an appropriate place for the scientific paradigm.

The form in which the scientific paradigm is adopted in future social-care research, and the way in which it could be used to lead to a progressive body of scientific knowledge, may well resemble the 'scientific realism' approach of Pawson and Tilly (1997). The key feature of scientific realism, and part of its attraction in the social-care field, is that it stresses the mechanics of explanation. 'Social interventions (or programmes) work (that is, they have a successful outcome – O) only insofar as they introduce the appropriate ideas and opportunities (mechanisms – M) to groups in the appropriate social and cultural conditions (contexts – C)' (Pawson and Tilly 1997, p. 57). The authors argue that there will always be contextual variation within and between programmes, a corresponding variation in the effectiveness of causal mechanisms triggered, and a consequential variation in patterns and outcomes, giving realist research the task of modelling the different ways in which Ms, Cs and Os come together. Exploring and explaining the way in which these mechanisms work has in the past often been described as investigating the contents of the 'black box'. An attractive feature of scientific realism is that, within limits, it supports the idea of the accumulation of evidence over time, a central aspect of which is called 'the quest for the continual betterment of practice' (p. 119). An example of the importance of understanding the contents of the 'black box' comes from the introduction of assertive treatment approaches. When studies produced contradictory findings about the impact of assertive community treatment, it became clear that some of them had failed to adopt the full range of necessary characteristics. As a consequence this led researchers to assess the extent to which the treatment offered conformed to the accepted definition of the treatment. Conformity was described as 'programme fidelity' and scales were introduced to measure it. The 'black box' of social work practice requires a similarly rigorous and experimental investigation.

Evidence that things may be changing already in the social-care field appears to be growing. One of the most notable indications is the creation of an evidence-based practice centre at Exeter University in the UK. Other research and evaluation initiatives took place during the 1980s in Stirling (Social Work Research Centre) and Manchester (Mental Health Social Work Research Unit) but the Exeter centre is the first to specifically address the issue of evidence-based practice. Pressure on social science academics to meet the demands of the Higher Education Funding Council in research income and performance has helped to create a climate in which such an initiative can flourish more easily than in the past. The 'best value' agenda in local authorities may also lead to a greater need to compare the relative effectiveness of different services, and to the abandonment of some that cannot be justified in these terms.

The Campbell Collaboration (established to prepare and maintain systematic reviews of the effects of social and educational interventions) is another example of the recognition, instigated by the Cochrane Collaboration, that there is a need to systematically collect and appraise the available evidence. The fundamental principle of the approach is that 'somebody has probably already done it'. As Brian Sheldon has pointed out (1999) we may not be in quite such a secure position in the social-care field, but as I shall attempt to show below with respect to social care in the mental health field, there may already be more evidence available than we assume. Regular updating of the evidence is central to these collaborations because of the rapid development of the knowledge base and the increased capacity to monitor and aggregate evidence available since the development of personal computers, databases, multivariate analysis techniques (especially for categorical data) and the internet.

What evidence do we have already?

In this section I will first examine some of the evidence gathered by the Centre for Evidence-Based Social Services (CEBSS) researchers about the nature and extent of the use of evidence in social-care practice. I will then consider some of the available evidence from the social-care research field. I do this for a number of reasons. First, it shows that there is a body of knowledge available. Second, this body of knowledge should be, but is not, widely known about in both practice and academic circles. Third, it shows us to some extent the type of evidence that is accepted in the field, and the standards applied to it. Finally, it gives us a rough starting point for a consideration of the areas that need further work, and those where new ground will have to be broken.

The CEBSS operates on the fundamental principle that

> all decisions in our field should be based on the best available research evidence. Research evidence should inform both our understanding of the origins and development of social problems and our knowledge of the likely outcomes of different types of service provision.
>
> (CEBSS 1998, p. 1)

They go on to point out that the evidence is required at different levels. Practitioners need to make informed choices in their work with individuals and families, managers need to make informed choices about which services to develop and what the likely outcomes are, and user and carer organisations need to know what works so that they can participate in decision making.

In the absence of evidence we are presented with opinion-based decision making. Changing from opinion-based decision making to evidence-based decision making will 'involve challenges for both practitioners and the social care organizations in which they work' (CEBSS 1998, p. 1). We should remind ourselves at this point that other professional groups also suffer from opinion-based decision making (as this volume testifies). However, others may not perhaps be able to emulate Blenkner's study of 1954, in which social workers predicted client 'movement' (outcome) with an accuracy of zero (0)! This study serves to illustrate a very significant finding about clinical judgement and its relative strengths and weaknesses. In his influential, but now widely ignored book, Meehl (1954) undertook a systematic review of available evidence about actuarial and clinical prediction and found a consistency, since confirmed by others (Vaillant 1962, Sines 1970), that actuarial prediction is always superior to clinical prediction. It is not hard to see why clinical (here used in the generic rather than medical sense) prediction is less successful. One could argue that the use of evidence enables actuarial findings to influence judgement, and that it is here that it can lead to better understanding and better outcomes.

Summaries of the effectiveness of social-work practice have increasingly demonstrated positive outcomes (Sheldon and Macdonald 1999). There has been an increasing interest in the assessment of both outcomes and the content of interventions, perhaps more so in the US. In spite of these developments, research by practitioners into social-work practice has not been widely developed, despite several initiatives to establish it. Sheldon and Macdonald point to the perennial obstacle when they say 'virtually none of the professional grade staff samples had been able to read anything apart from *Community Care'* (p. 2).

Any improvement in the situation appears to be largely a matter of the creation of the capacity (especially time) to undertake evidence-based practice and practice research. The evidence that this capacity is steadily being built into the system is sadly lacking. Sheldon and Macdonald (1999) surveyed 2,500 workers in a dozen agencies in the UK about the nature and extent of evidence-based practice. They found that

- workers supported the idea of evidence-based practice
- workers were not aware of the available research evidence
- understanding of research terminology was very low
- keeping up to date with research was important but there were organisational barriers to this
- training courses contained few references to research
- it is unusual to be asked 'where is the evidence for that?' in social services.

Protected time for reading or evaluating research was wanted, as well as access to decentralised research material and computerised data sources. Local evidence-based working groups have been established, and twenty-two one-day conferences on the importance of research were conducted. Critical appraisal training was made available, and CaredataWeb Literature database and Caredata abstracts were made available online at the National Institute for Social Work site, www.nisw.org.uk/.

The quality of the material made available in these accessible ways is of considerable importance. There is little point in making evidence available if it is of poor quality. It is essential to use a set of standards, perhaps such as those in the National Service Framework (NSF) (see also Brian Williams in Chapter 11, this volume). Given the unsophisticated nature, in research terms, of the practitioners surveyed by the CEBSS, it is important to give workers the tools to assess the quality of the evidence placed before them; hence critical appraisal training is essential. A random selection of Caredata abstracts shows that a very large proportion (more than four-fifths) of the content reports descriptive studies and expert opinion, and not material at the highest level of evidence; even the reviews identified are 'narrative' reviews rather than systematic reviews, and so the potential for bias is greater.

While this state of evidence perhaps reflects the current state of research performance in the field, it is of questionable value to continue to disseminate vast amounts of evidence at the lowest levels of quality. A Kitemark quality system would help the busy practitioner appreciate the quality of the original report that the summary is describing.

Table 17.1 was constructed from a document prepared by the Cochrane and Campbell Collaborations (2000) and supported by the NHS Research

Table 17.1 Methods in evidence-based mental health care

Type of intervention	Major conclusions
Psychosocial rehabilitation	average reduction of 50% in cost of care because of reduced hospitalisation
Income supplementation	no experimental evidence of effects on health. Only one study examined severe mental illness
Vocational rehabilitation	supported employment has better outcomes than 'train and place' methods
Housing	poor housing, overcrowding, high-rise living and dissatisfaction with housing related to poor mental and physical health
Psychological debriefing	counselling after disasters is not effective and might increase long-term distress
Home-based support	home-based support for pregnant women at high risk of depression improves the mental well being of mother and child
Mental health promotion	cognitive behavioural and social interventions can be effective for children experiencing major life events such as divorce and bereavement
Respite care	temporarily relieves mental health problems experienced by long-term carers, and may delay institutionalisation
Family interventions	alleviate some negative aspects of care giving in relatives of people with mental illness
Re-housing	little reliable research, one controlled trial showed that it improved mental health in people whose problems were attributed to housing
Crisis home care	reduces family burden
Crisis intervention	teams find it difficult to avoid hospital admission during treatment period
Case management	appears to increase hospital re-admission rates and not to improve outcomes
Coordinated care	coordinating psychiatric, psychological and social services improves outcomes in schizophrenia
School suicide prevention	insufficient evidence to support curriculum-based suicide prevention programmes
Social work interventions	successful practice focuses on improving the living environment and creating or supporting social networks
Occupational therapy in social services settings	little evidence about effectiveness in people with mental illness
Family-based therapy	need for more well-designed studies; may be as effective as other models
Family psychosocial interventions	may decrease the frequency of relapse, decrease hospitalisation and encourage compliance, but data are few and equivocal; it may improve social function and levels of expressed emotion

and Development Programme. The document was based on searches of the Database of Abstracts of Reviews of Effectiveness (which contains material from all of the major databases such as PsycINFO), but also a wider search, using systematic review methodology, of other sources, including the Applied Social Sciences Index and Abstracts (ASSIA), the Health Technology database and sociological abstracts. I have summarised a selection of the most relevant data for social care in mental health and excluded those of less direct relevance. Because space is limited in this chapter, I have selected those sources that have produced clear and unequivocal evidence using the best methods and of the highest quality available. I have also, where possible, indicated areas where the evidence is weak or non-existent, to help to develop an agenda for future research in the social-care field in mental health.

A good deal of this evidence has been produced within the last few years and is of the highest quality. However, a number of fairly firm conclusions follow from an examination of the evidence presented here. First, although there may be more evidence than we thought, the overall amount is quite small compared to other areas of inquiry. Second, while there are high-quality reviews in many areas there are other areas where they are lacking and need to be undertaken. Third, the limited number of reviews is partly a product of the limited amount of high-quality research undertaken in the social-care field. A notable absence is the review of the effectiveness of training social-care staff in specific interventions, a point made recently by Sheldon (1999).

What should we do next?

In conclusion, from the social-care perspective, there are a number of ways to improve the evidence base and foster evidence based practice

- reduce the amount of low quality evidence that is currently disseminated
- develop a Kitemark system for the standards of social-care evidence
- if this requires a debate about standards, then have it, and move to adopt an agreed system
- teach critical appraisal and evidence-based practice on qualifying courses and ensure that the mental health content of all social work education is consistent with National Service Frameworks
- develop more easily accessed (for example on the internet) sources of Kitemarked practice-based evidence
- support an increase in the infrastructure that will allow social-care staff to participate in the generation and consumption of high-quality evidence
- support an increase in the proportion of current research funding that goes to social-care research in the mental health field, or create special funds for this

- support an increase in the funding for post-basic education in social care, to develop a cadre of staff capable of conducting research of the highest quality in social-care contexts.

Although I argued earlier that the use of evidence enables actuarial findings to influence judgement, and that it is here that it can lead to better understanding and better outcomes, one actually needs *evidence* that making the evidence available can be used to improve practice and outcomes. Early work in this area was not very encouraging. Stricker (1967) assessed the improvement in a clinician's ability to predict the outcome of a mental health problem, when all the additional evidence from validated predictive tests was made available to them. He reports that the additional data seemed to have a minimal impact on their judgement. Work on the provision and use of practice guidelines and protocols suggests that guidelines have little impact on practitioner behaviour and even less on patient outcomes (Parry 2000). One-off interventions, such as training packages, lose their impact over time and 're-inoculation' is necessary. As well as the development of critical appraisal skills in the social-care workforce, it seems highly probable, therefore, that a programme of updating knowledge and of continuing skills training will be necessary.

Unsurprisingly, Meehl (1954) concluded from his summary of the literature that one would be well advised not to rely on clinical judgement alone unless there is a compelling and dramatic reason to do so. 'I did not have the available evidence to hand' cannot always be regarded as a dramatic and compelling reason to rely on one's clinical judgement or opinion (even in an emergency); not having any evidence one way or the other is less reprehensible, but also in the long run indefensible. Not knowing about the available evidence, or not using it, ought to be regarded as unprofessional, uncaring and at best inefficient, at worst potentially dangerous.

Section 4

The way forward

Chapter 18

A User/Survivor perspective: what's behind the evidence?

Simon Allard

The original title to this chapter was to be 'The user perspective: which evidence should be provided by research?'. I've decided to rename it 'A User/Survivor perspective: what's behind the evidence?' because I wanted to broaden it out to discuss some of the background influences that drive the search for 'evidence'. I will, however, be covering what evidence I feel research should be providing.

When we look for evidence we need to be sure what we are seeking evidence for. We could be seeking evidence to support a policy initiative, we could be looking for what is right, what is true or, in the climate of efficiency, we may be looking for cost-effectiveness. We may be searching for new, alternative ways of doing things to replace traditional methods that have failed us, or for what gives us kudos for groundbreaking work. Or we may simply be looking for what works and what is useful.

Each of these lines of enquiry will start from a different standpoint and, therefore, will affect the ways in which investigations are conducted and the 'evidence' that is produced. That is not to say that these questions are necessarily mutually exclusive but we must be aware of the underlying motivation. Progress is as much about discovering the hidden assumptions and agendas at play in mental health research as the results or 'evidence' produced by it.

I do not reject the value of inquiry or the necessity of it. The importance of careful reflection and investigation into issues relating to mental health is a vital element in our need to understand what it is to be a human being. Life is precious but existence is complex and fraught with pressures. Only through processes of meaningful inquiry can we get nearer to making sense of it and progress our collective ability to overcome or cope with problems. In short, I am not here to dismiss evidence relating to mental health care nor the research that is needed to provide it. However, I feel we need to question the validity of what is presented as 'evidence-based research', and highlight the limitations and dangers of passively accepting the supposed legitimacy of what is so often mere rhetoric. I would also question the agenda behind the increased emphasis on 'evidence-based mental health care'.

So why is 'evidence' a dominant 'driver' in modern mental health? The background to this can be found in the document *Modernising Mental Health Services* (Department of Health 1998b) which 'sets out the Government's vision for safe, sound and supportive mental health services for working age adults'. The document goes on to say in Chapter 2, under the title 'The New Vision for Mental Health Services', that

> People with mental health problems often have complex needs which cross traditional organisational boundaries. A modern mental health service will provide care which is integrated, and which is focused on the individual recognising that different people have different needs and preferences. It will be evidenced-based, and outcome-driven. Services will be there for people when they need them, and where they need them. Services must be safe, sound and supportive. Partnerships will be crucial.
>
> (pp. 22–3)

Remember this last phrase 'partnerships will be crucial', I'll come back to it later.

But first I would just like to go through what is meant by 'safe, sound and supportive'

- *safe* to protect the public and provide effective care for those with mental illness at the time they need it
- *sound* to ensure that patients and service users have access to the full range of services which they need
- *supportive* working with patients and service users, their families and carers to build healthier communities.

Anyway, there we have it, 'a modern mental health service will be evidence-based, and outcome driven . . . and safe, sound and supportive'.

Let's look at the Government agenda for increased emphasis on evidence-based mental health care. At first sight it might seem that policy makers are saying that people with mental health support needs deserve the best in health care and, therefore, the receipt of appropriate service provision must come from clinical and ethical practices of the highest quality. The best way, the government believes, to achieve these laudable aims is to find what works and hence greater 'evidence' is being demanded. This, by implication, requires methodologies in both research and practice to be systematic and scientific. As 'scientific practitioners', clinicians will then be equipped with the tools and expertise that will best serve the needs of the people who need to access their services. But does this provide a 'true' and complete picture or are there *other agendas* involved?

Safety agenda

Referring back to the 'Modernising Mental Health Services' document (Department of Health 1998b, we heard that mental health services are to be safe, sound and supportive. Let's look at the first part of 'safe' again, 'to protect the public'.

I would agree that the role of government policy, amongst other things, should be to help to create a safe society for its members, for *all* its members especially the most vulnerable. However, one could well doubt this judging by the following statement

> Care in the community has failed because, while it improved the treatment of many people who were mentally ill, it left far too many walking the streets, often at risk to themselves and a nuisance to others.
>
> (Frank Dobson, the former Secretary of State
> for Health, in the foreword to the aforementioned
> Modernising Mental Health Services)

The message that comes across is that the public needs protecting against people with a diagnosis of mental illness because community care has put the public at a significant risk. I would like to take issue with this on two counts. First, are people with such diagnoses not also members of the public? And second, the statement has a false and discriminatory basis.

The title of the chapter I was originally given was 'The user perspective: which evidence should be provided by research?' Well, my answer would be evidence that prevents senior government ministers from making statements that present a completely skewed picture of reality. At a recent debate at the Maudsley on compulsory community treatment orders, Dr Frank Holloway rejected the argument that community care had failed. He argued that the proportion of homicides committed by people with a mental illness diagnosis had been falling over the last 40 years, and that there was firm evidence for this. So on the contrary, this showed that community care was a resounding success and as such ought to be applauded. The 'safety of the public' statements were not informed by 'evidence-based research' but were actions, I believe, based on political motivation. Because of the media-fuelled public view of people with a mental illness diagnosis being dangerous it seems politically expedient to continue to support that stigmatising view by calling for greater restrictions on the civil rights of a particular section of society.

I am labouring this point to show that this *non*-evidence-based stigmatising attitude of the government towards people with mental health support needs could bias the direction in which funding for research is allocated (i.e. less funding for research into what really works for people, especially community-based therapeutic support systems, and more towards supporting measures for social control and coercion). There is a very real danger that these moves could reduce mental health professionals to becoming agents of social control, especially in view of the proposed introduction of compulsory community treatment orders.

When I was a child I was told the Little Red Riding Hood story and I remember the exchange between Little Red Riding Hood and the Wolf.

Little Red Riding Hood: Why do you have such big teeth, Grandma?
Wolf: All the better to eat you with, my dear!

With psychiatrists as agents of social control, the modern psychiatric equivalent might be

Patient: Why do you inject me with those powerful neuroleptic drugs, doctor?
Doctor: All the better to keep you from being a nuisance to others, my dear!

I highlight these subtexts to 'evidence-gathering' to show what Users/Survivors, dedicated mental health professionals and researchers are all up against. 'Evidence' should be the servant to good-quality mental health care but not subject to government manipulation or a tool for the profit-oriented marketing strategies of pharmaceutical companies.

Let's retrace our steps and look at some basic definitions.

Research

There are two definitions of research in the dictionary (Oxford Interactive Encyclopaedia 1997).

1. A search or investigation undertaken to discover facts and reach new conclusions by the critical study of a subject or by a course of scientific inquiry.
2. Systematic investigation into and study of materials, sources, etc., to establish facts, collate information, etc.; surveying of opinions or background information relevant to a project etc.

I believe that all research is biased to some extent and so the 'evidence' provided by such inquiry is going to reflect that bias (whether that be through social, economic or political motivations). The most costly research is financially backed by pharmaceutical companies and others with a vested interest in shoring up the medical-model basis to 'mental health care'. Such research so often gives greater ammunition (in the form of 'evidence') to those practitioners and policy makers who see individuals as a bundle of symptoms that can be 'cured' by complying with prescribed treatment regimes.

What is 'evidence'?

The dictionary definition has three basic versions (Oxford Interactive Encyclopaedia 1997).

1. An indication, a sign.
2. Something serving as proof.
3. Facts or testimony in support of a conclusion, statement or belief.

If we look at the last definition 'Facts or testimony in support of a conclusion, statement or belief' it refers to 'facts'. But facts do not speak for themselves, they are subject to varying interpretations depending on who is doing the interpreting.

When it comes to looking for facts regarding what can loosely be called the 'human condition', we're likely to run into problems. The nature of human existence brings with it complexities that defy being reduced to simple formulae. Yet 'finding out about the world' has concerned great thinkers for centuries and has produced a litany of epistemological debates. This thirst for knowledge is still with us today and it exists across all disciplines. In the field of mental health, this has traditionally been left to only a small number of people – primarily those involved in psychiatry and psychology. However, Users and Survivors have entered the fray and have much to offer the debate. Many of us want to rewrite the rules of inquiry and have *our* 'value systems' formally incorporated into the design processes of how 'evidence' is collected and what evidence is produced.

Good research should be transparent and easily read, digested and replicated. However, 'evidence' is about data reduction and not everything gets included in the published version. There will inevitably be some bias as to what gets included and what gets left out, and anything can be produced and supported by statistics. The evidence is often viewed as though it was arrived at through objective methods and the data and results of research point to fairly straightforward conclusions. The presence and length of the 'Discussion' sections of research papers in psychiatry and psychology show that this is not the case. These sections are needed precisely because the relationship between data and conclusions is uncertain, ambiguous and subject to various interpretations.

Evidence is not 'context independent'. That is, evidence is valued differently in different contexts by different people and what is important to one group may not be seen as important by another. What interests us is different to what interests biological and medical researchers.

Research methodologies need to develop suitable outcome measures from which the benefits experienced by Users/Survivors from any given study can be evaluated. Suitable outcome measures will need to take into account the value systems of Users/Survivors and relate to our lived experiences. There is, therefore, the need to undertake more 'applied' research in order for the evidence to be relevant to our lives. It should be based on real people with real lives in real situations, somewhat along the lines of an anthropological approach.

The User/Survivor Advisory Group to the London Mental Health Strategies for Action document states

> We value research into the different aspects of human suffering and survival. But we want this research to be from the perspective of people who experienced the turmoil. Our testimonies and our suggestions as to what would really help have been recorded for many years now. It is time for our perspectives and ideas to be taken seriously.
> (User/Survivor Advisory Group 1999, p. 7)

What evidence is valued by Users/Survivors? Users/Survivors (like most people) want 'evidence' of what will make our lives better. For Users/Survivors this requires a broader and better evidence base than is currently available. While we've got much in common with each other, Users/Survivors are not one homogeneous mass all necessarily wanting the same things. We are individuals with individual needs and desires, and believe that our personal testimonies are valid and should be taken into account during research processes. But I would like to suggest what I believe are fairly common themes.

Based on our various experiences, Users/Survivors are critical of conventional, exclusively medical approaches towards dealing with distress. Drug regimes are not a panacea for all 'ills'. Many people are calling for research evidence on medication-reduction programmes and methods of support for coming off neuroleptics and antidepressants. There appears to be no current research that looks at the effects of stopping medication within a controlled withdrawal regime.

Perhaps psychiatric and psychological research could look at other health areas such as pain management and cardiovascular disease to witness how approaches in these areas have altered dramatically when patients take control over their own health regime by including programmes of exercise and diet. This is done through partnerships between practitioner and client, based on concordance rather than compliance. This model of working could offer mental health professionals alternatives to resorting to coercive measures in response to non-compliance with medication, and validate the patient's conscious, rational decision to stop their own medication. The potentially powerful therapeutic working relationship ensuing from this could well make statements such as 'non-compliance is not an option' redundant. While this would not work for all people, I would argue that this is an area that deserves researching for the benefit of client and practitioner alike. It would probably be a substantially cheaper treatment option in the long term as well.

The experience of 'voice-hearing' in particular is an area that deserves to be researched in order to find alternative coping strategies to medication. It may well be worth reminding ourselves that a significant number of people who 'hear voices' never use or do not need to use psychiatric services. The existence of non-patient voice hearers is still a mystery to many psychiatrists.

It would be good to see research evidence that shows how many people make their madness a positive aspect of their lives (i.e. the positive outcomes of living with madness). Life does go beyond psychiatry but traditional research tends to only look at what happens in mental health settings rather than outside in the bigger world. The current focus around resolving chemical imbalances provides the driving force behind much research based on the medical paradigm which narrows the bigger picture and merely pathologises our behaviour.

There is a growth in survivor-led research and many more Users/Survivors want to be included in developing the outcome measures of research programmes so as to reflect our views of what benefits us. Our value systems include things such as our self-defined quality of life, independence, empowerment, dignity, respect, greater control over our own lives and increased self-esteem and ultimately, the right to be treated as valued individuals. These may be highly qualitative (and may need to be refined for research purposes), but quantitative measures alone seriously limit what can be known about a person.

It is necessary to find out how services can be improved, but it is only part of the picture of survivor-led research. Research should be about people and processes, not just outcomes. Survivor-led research values the relationship between researcher and subject, and the relationship between knowledge and experience. The prejudiced attitude to people's experiences in much traditional research reveals its limited scope for producing evidence that is of value to people with mental health support needs.

Added to this list is the potential benefit of complementary therapies which are gaining greater importance as tools to assist mainstream medicine. Many Users/Survivors have gained from such treatments and would welcome more research evidence in this area.

I would also like to see much more culturally based research carried out, especially involving the people who belong to the various diverse communities.

And the list goes on.

So to conclude

Is the way forward through 'emancipatory' research (i.e. only survivors involved) or should we be funding 'participatory' research (i.e. survivors and 'experts' joining forces)? I would say there is a call for both types of research.

Responsibility has been an implicit theme throughout this chapter. It is incumbent upon all of us who work in the field of mental health to strive towards what benefits the people who need mental health support systems. I believe that the intended beneficiaries of our work are people with mental health support needs and, therefore, the representation of their interests is to be the central focus of what we do and how we do it. If we were all to genuinely uphold this principle, together we could substantially alter the landscape of mental health care and support systems.

In terms of research evidence, the starting point must be to listen to what we, as Users/Survivors, have to say about what is important to us. If research processes did this as a matter of course, then I believe the evidence produced, if acted upon, could make a truly enormous and positive contribution to so many people's lives and the evidence would speak for itself.

Chapter 19

The policy perspective: what evidence is influential?

Eddie Kane

Introduction

The relationship between research and policy making is often uncomfortable. There is no off-the-shelf methodology or process to guide researchers and policy makers towards a synthesis of evidence, values and resource imperatives.

For some time it has been proposed that one of the key drivers for clinical and management decision making should be good-quality evidence. The imperative to base health and related policy decisions to a much greater degree on evidence derived from research rather than on values and resource considerations is a more recent phenomenon.

During the 1970s and 1980s some key health policy decisions seemed to be based principally on values and resources. There often appeared to be relatively little focus on research evidence. In the new millennium it seems unlikely that this approach is sustainable. Public expectations of services and healthy longevity have changed markedly. Pressure is being applied to clinicians to develop evidence-based protocols and standardise interventions so that resource usage can be based on evidence for beneficial changes to the health of the population. Policy makers will not escape demands for the same rules to apply to them. There is some evidence in mental health policy making that the tide is turning in the direction of a better balance between values, resource considerations and evidence. In England the National Service Framework for Mental Health (Department of Health 1999) subsequently reinforced by the NHS National Plan (Department of Health 2000) is a good example of synthesising a value-based policy position with evidence to underpin expected outputs, investment decisions and implementation.

What is policy and who makes it?

Policies are developed to create changes and improvements in services, and in the health services policy making aims to

- improve the health of populations
- change funding or accountability structures.

The scope of a policy change could include

- improving direct patient care
- achieving better value for money
- changing the accountability for delivery
- empowering a new group of decision makers
- introducing a new funding or resource-raising structure
- setting targets for health improvement
- increasing the involvement of people who use services in decision making (Gray 1997).

Collating evidence to shape policy seems an attractive way of making progress and establishing robust, politically defensible, patterns of care and resourcing. However, finding good quality, influential evidence that stands the sort of aggressive and often non-scientific scrutiny it is likely to receive is not always easy in the mental health field. This is one of the reasons frequently given by policy makers for falling back onto policy making driven principally by their values tempered by resource availability. Even where robust evidence is available it often appears to have little direct impact on policy formulation.

It is important to recognise that policy making is not conducted at one level. It occurs either as a primary or modifying activity at national, regional and local level. There is no doubt that nationally articulated policy approaches are filtered and translated at various levels of the health commissioning and delivery systems.

The groups involved in the policy-making process include

- government ministers
- regional levels of government and regional officers of central government
- local authorities
- health authorities, NHS trusts and primary care groups and trusts
- local practitioners and managers.

It is not always the same evidence that is influential at these various levels, and neither is it always clear why action to introduce or revise policy is taken at a particular point in time. Therein lies one of the most significant reasons why evidence-based policy making does not yet have the impact that its advocates promote. The question of what evidence is powerful, why, when, at what level, and whether the various types of evidence can be constructed in a multi-layered and coherent whole, is critical to establishing an evidence-based policy framework for mental health.

The policy-making process

There is little evidence that policy making is a clear, linear process moving from issue description to remedy reflecting how things actually happen. It is unlikely that such a linear approach is regularly possible in the turbulent environments in which decisions at national, regional and local levels are made. Policy making in the real world is a process with a number of stages. It may occasionally be linear or it may loop backwards and forwards. A number of commentators, including Hogwood and Gunn, describe a staged process as a framework for analysing how policy is made. The stages are neither definitive, nor are they a description of what happens in every instance. They do, however, provide a way of viewing the complex real-world policy-making process that is essential to an understanding of what evidence is influential for all policy makers (Hogwood and Gunn 1984).

The depth and rigour of these stages will vary according to the issue and the environment in which it is being considered. Some issues will involve detailed and complex analysis drawing on sophisticated quantitative techniques, others will need a politician to make a rapid decision based on limited information. Furthermore the analysis, which is employed at each stage, will vary depending on who is involved, at what organisational level they operate and what related, or often unrelated, issues they are dealing with at the time. Identifying the particular models or sets of related assumptions, which influence policy makers at any level, is essential when trying to understand the real-world policy-making process. To the detached observer or academic analyst the assumptions made by policy makers may seem incoherent or inconsistent but they may still be perspectives which can and do influence practical policy making. The stages that Hogwood and Gunn and others describe vary, but they include the following six processes.

Finding, filtering and defining issues

This stage focuses on the identification of an issue or an opportunity that suggests to policy makers that action is needed. This puts an issue onto someone's agenda for discussion and action, and is often the point when another previously pressing issue is excluded. Areas of research, which may inform this stage, include social exclusion indicators, needs assessments, and forecasts of the impact of various technologies, including drugs and other interventions.

At this juncture the process can move immediately to political and administrative processes with little specific or detailed analytical work being done before action is taken. Alternatively it may be identified as an issue which would benefit from fundamental and objective analysis before any action is taken. This objective analysis is often absent in real-world policy making, which probably explains why a good deal of policy making moved to the default position of action without evidence. For example the decision that 'boot camps' for young offenders should be introduced to the UK was taken even though evidence was available from the US indicating that they failed in one of their prime objectives, i.e. the prevention of re-offending. Further refinement and definition is almost certainly required at this stage. The reality is that most issues and opportunities are not single strand, and teasing apart the various elements and, where possible, measuring and identifying their dimensions may be important.

Setting directives and priorities

This stage involves answering at least two questions

1.   what is the precise objective of this particular policy?
2.   how will we know when we have achieved that objective?

It is important to try and understand what the impact of the policy is likely to be, since there is almost always a gap between the expected and desired future. Although the idea of impact assessment is becoming increasingly accepted as a useful construct, there is still relatively little evidence that it is carried out systematically, particularly across departments and authorities with policy-making responsibilities. This lack of precision is also evident when looking at the way in which the various 'must dos' in the health service are prioritised. For many years mental health policy making at all levels has been characterised by large numbers of objectives competing for limited resources with either few or, even worse, competing levels of priority being given to various policy strands by different organisations in the chain of decision making. There have been significant improvements, for example health and social-care policy advice being brought together in the Department of Health, and the strong steer in the NHS National Plan towards care trusts as the model of choice unifying the delivery of local health and social-care services. Despite this drive towards minimising and clarifying priorities there is still a long way to go.

Forecasting and option review

It is important to try to forecast which issues or opportunities may develop over time. It is useful to examine the alternative possible futures taking different assumptions about the development of both the issue and the responding policy, and to understand that there are usually several routes to achieve an objective or set of objectives. Policy makers at all levels are frequently criticised for adopting policies which are based chiefly on the values of individuals who are then willing to support a particular way forward. At best this will mean that only one of a range of options available is being considered when a more independent analysis may identify alternatives.

Nevertheless, experience tends to point to advocacy being a stronger determinant of option choice than independent analysis.

Implementation and monitoring

When an option is chosen to address the problem or exploit the opportunity the process of implementation and monitoring needs to be addressed. The complexity of potential problems varies widely. For example, government ministers need to gain their opposite number's support in areas which have a cross-departmental impact. There also needs to be a buy-in to the policy at ground level where the detail or the spirit of the policy is implemented. The National Service Framework for Mental Health is a good example of a policy designed to get broad stakeholder support for radical change in mental health services. It also tried to ensure that, as far as possible, the key government-level values that services should be 'safe, sound and supportive' were translated through evidence and practical examples to a level identifiable by individual clinicians, service users and carers. Once the supporting implementation programme is underway some level of monitoring is needed. The level of monitoring varies tremendously from very unstructured to specific and analytical. The implementation of mental health policy based around the National Service Framework for Mental Health has, and will increasingly have, precise specification of the operational standards expected. The imposition of control and consistency of implementation, at least in part, is an attempt to ensure consistency of experience for service users.

Evaluation

Evaluation may be built into policy implementation from the outset, or it may come about as a result of someone questioning the validity or value of the particular approach. The possibility of conducting real outcome evaluation, as opposed to output evaluation which is focussed on implementation and monitoring, depends on the degree to which the desired outcomes were clear from the outset. If the outcomes were not clear it is difficult to determine whether the policy is delivering as intended, and whether there is any objective basis for whether to continue to give the policy priority and, perhaps more importantly, continuing to resource it or even invest further. A cursory read through the journals that focus on mental health shows that policy evaluation, when taken from different perspectives, yields different views of the success or otherwise of particular strands of policy. Whilst to some extent this is a function of people starting from fairly fixed positions on a particular topic and articulating what often amounts to little more than prejudices, it also points to the fact that a good deal of policy making in past years which is now being evaluated had little or no clarity and precision about the actual outcome expected.

Maintenance, succession or termination

The results of evaluation, even where there is difficulty in defining the original expected outcomes, should lead at least to a perspective which would allow policy makers to determine whether the current position should be maintained, developed or terminated. It is important, particularly in the area of mental health policy, that a clear decision is made as a result of an evaluation. Too often in the past, policy decisions which were either not having a beneficial impact or were not being implemented have lain 'on the books', followed by some clinicians and ignored by others. It is encouraging to note that in the mental health arena there is an increasing intent to make much more explicit the need to examine the interrelationship of existing policies with proposed new ones, and to make decisions to confirm, modify or terminate existing policy streams where they do not support or where they actually conflict with a new direction of travel.

Is evidence influential?

To address this key question it is important to be clear about what is meant in this context by evidence. Evidence can be simply classified into two distinct types

Type 1 evidence has most, but not always all, of the following features:

- it has a primacy of *CONTENT*, i.e. it focusses on numerical, statistical and clinical data
- it originates with academically defined problems
- it is rooted in the context of previous work
- it is provided by conventional academic research
- it is typical of the traditional approach to biomedical research.

Type 2 evidence has most, but not always all, of the following features:

- it focusses on understanding the *CONTEXT*, i.e. the environment in which the data were produced
- it originates in the experience of tackling complex multi-faceted problems in a shifting social or cultural context
- it recognises that complex problems in complex environments may require new approaches
- it values experiential learning history.

The two evidence types should not be viewed in any hierarchy, they have equal value and impact on the policy-making process overall. The differentiation comes in the way in which they combine to impact at different points and on different people in a particular policy-making process.

These two types of evidence often combine and become particularly influential in one or more of the following ways

- providing a framework of reference or background context that impacts on the policy makers to persuade or predispose them towards a particular choice of topic or area for action
- providing the basis for point-by-point development of a policy based on clear, robust and widely accepted empirical grounds
- providing consumer or user information, which is available to particular interest groups that are able to use it to bring pressure to bear for policy development or change in a given area.

Five broad categories of issue appear to be drivers for action in all of these groups, they are

- political, professional and ethical values
- availability and constraint of resources
- failures and crises
- canvassed views of selected focus groups
- representation from pressure groups.

These issue categories can be found at the heart of almost all recent and proposed changes to mental health policy and legislation in the UK. They are used to explain and underpin a series of objectives which include

- improving direct patient care
- responding to consumer or user opinion
- changing accountability for service delivery
- setting targets for health improvement
- achieving better value for money
- introducing new funding or resourcing structures
- empowering a new group of decision makers
- increasing the involvement of people who use services
- improving professional accountability.

It is essential for researchers to appreciate the driving power of these categories and issues to policy makers at all levels if their work is to be influential. Guiding policy makers towards the decisions that will ensure that policy can both deliver value-based positions and be robust, relevant and beneficial to professionals and service users alike, means that a number of critical aspects have to be covered. The evidence should

- be presented in a way which is accessible to the target audience
- clarify or identify an issue of concern or an area for action

- have a clear cost–benefit analysis
- have a methodology which is owned and understood by the target audience
- be based on collaborative work in multi-dimensional studies with large cohorts.

Clearly not all research will or can cover each one of these aspects. However, the likelihood of evidence being influential, and the benefits of research being realised for the wider community, are reduced the further the presentation of research evidence moves from this construct.

There has been relatively little significant investigation into the extent to which research evidence influences the policy-making process. A study by the Institute for Social Research at the University of Michigan interviewed 204 top US policy makers. The study found a very positive attitude towards seeking out and using research data in the formation of policy. However, the actual reported level of utilisation was, in fact, low. Even more striking was the fact that 44 per cent of the interviewees reported instances when they purposely disregarded relevant information in making policy decisions. The study found that it was rare for policy formulation to be determined by a point-by-point reliance on empirically grounded data. Policy makers were influenced by research evidence in the way that they thought about issues. They integrated the information with their own values and experience, merging the two to form a frame of reference or perspective against which the social implications of alternative policies were evaluated (Caplan *et al.* 1975). Thus research evidence was both sought and not used at the point-by-point, concrete level, but it was influential at a conceptual level. The study went on to examine the major factors contributing to the use and non-use of research evidence. It concluded by advancing the 'two communities theory': the two communities being researchers and policy makers, who are characterised by conflicting values, rewards and language. Lack of contact and lack of trust were put forward as major explanations for variations in utilisation, particularly at a local policy-making level.

Even in long-running research programmes with established good relationships between researchers and commissioners, it is difficult to ascertain whether research evidence has had an effect on policy. A study in 1999 explored the interface between researchers and service commissioners in the NHS (Harries *et al.* 1999). The study involved a literature review and case studies of social research projects initiated by NHS health authority managers and general practitioners. They identified the relationship between researchers and commissioners of research as critical and the importance of trust developed over time in that relationship as fundamental if research evidence was to have maximum impact. The relationship was characterised as needing to be honest, flexible and open in order to negotiate changing priorities on the side of the commissioners and changes in methods or direction on the part of the research team. The health authority commissioners in the study also identified indirect benefits from research, including new ways of looking at policy questions and building new alliances particularly with service users and providers. Nevertheless, this study found it difficult to establish the degree to which the research programmes reviewed had influenced policy making at any level, and even more difficult to establish the degree to which there had been any impact on the lives of service users.

The process of research is often presented and perceived as a logical, linear process bringing order to chaos. This perception underpins much of the support for evidence-based policy making, medicine and management. Policy making, whilst often having its base in particular political value systems, is also frequently characterised as being built on systematic analysis of clear and robust options. Even a cursory examination of examples of both streams of endeavour demonstrates a mismatch between the ideal and the reality. Both policy making and research are driven by subjective judgements. These will include judgements on the brief, the choice of methodology, commissioning prescriptions for research projects, short-term political events, and priorities for policy making alongside financial and resource realities for both. It is not surprising then that the two communities of policy making and research do not yet link together easily to create evidence-based policies, translated by rational management processes into the delivery of accessible and effective mental health care (Bulmer 1986; Booth and Gowe 1988).

Conclusions

There is an intuitive appeal in promoting evidence-based policy making which, as with evidence-based medicine (although not without its critics), has been hailed as the key to improving clinical standards. The implementation of such an approach is not without its problems and needs some compromise in attitudes between researchers and policy makers. The most constant feature of the environment in which policy makers and practitioners operate is its turbulence. Arguably, change and organisational disruption are the most dependable features of work in mental health services. The challenge for researchers, and for those who seek to use the evidence that their work offers, is to come to terms with the reality of service and organisational change, and to identify opportunities and methods of increasing the impact of their work on the formulation and development of policy in that environment.

There is an increasing interest, at each of the levels of policy making identified, in trying to agree areas for action, policy initiation or development based on evidence rather than relying solely on strongly held value positions. If that interest is to be fostered and focussed researchers should be encouraged to design studies that take into account

1.   how and by whom the results will be used
2.   the need to persuade decision makers to use the evidence derived from the work (Sheldon *et al.* 1998).

The research community needs to do more to systematically identify promising implementation techniques and build consensus with policy makers on areas where more research is necessary. There is little to demonstrate that passive dissemination of research evidence and information generally has anything other than a random background effect on policy makers, at best influencing their frame of reference (Bero *et al.* 1998). Well-structured systematic reviews based on collaborative work with large cohorts that show consistent, clearly communicated results are more likely to be influential and persuade policy makers to take action or promote further research.

In turn policy makers have a responsibility to ensure that their work takes proper account of the available evidence. The investment choices that are made and the performance monitoring systems that are developed should be much more focussed on ensuring consistency of delivery against well-evidenced policy directions and decisions. The challenge is to move away from relationships between researchers and policy makers that are characterised by lack of either trust or shared goals, to one that is coherent and mutually supportive. This does not mean constraining proper value-based political action nor weakening scientific rigour. Instead it points to ensuring that policy is supported by evidence and that research is conducted in a way that gives it real-time relevance and consequently promotes its benefits to the maximum number of people.

If the results of research are to be of practical use then they have to be timely, comprehensive and practical. Some researchers fear that their findings will be misused if they move closer to policy makers. This is a somewhat short-sighted view. The chances of their findings being simplified and distorted are much more likely if neither the original researcher nor some interpreter has taken the trouble to offer the key findings and caveats in a comprehensible format. It is also probable that without a closer relationship between researchers and policy makers the research findings will not reach anyone in a position to promote them and ensure that they have some influence.

Good quality, well-presented and comprehensible research evidence cannot make politically difficult decisions any easier, indeed it often makes them more difficult since the compromises that produce coalitions of interest are more difficult to manufacture in the face of clear evidence to follow one course rather than another. However, simply because some decisions may be easier in the absence of evidence does not mean their adverse consequences will be avoided. The promotion of compromise is not the principle aim of policy makers at whatever level, and predicting the substantive consequences of decisions is increasingly taking on a higher profile. Even where the evidence available to policy makers indicates that all available options are unpalatable, sharing robust evidence is more likely to make one of those options more acceptable to those who have to take the decision and to those who are affected by it. To disregard or rubbish well-presented, robust evidence, or to fail to collect information about the complexity of choices a policy maker is facing, is to weaken the current and future influence of policy makers and researchers and the trust that their respective constituencies invest in them. The relationship between researchers and policy makers will occasionally be tense but that tension can be creative and beneficial. What we must move from is the lack of contact and trust that have resulted in important evidence being ignored, dismissed or not even sought. Policy makers and researchers at every level need to grasp the opportunities and move forward together for the benefit of service users and the wider community.

Acknowledgements

Professor Charles Easmon for his invaluable help in development of the Type 1 and 2 classification of evidence and Dr Sian Rees for her constructive advice on early drafts.

Chapter 20

The researcher's perspective: which type of evidence can be delivered?

Sir David Goldberg

The evidence that can certainly be delivered by researchers is that which is consonant with the political imperatives of the government that happens to be in power, or which shows that there is an alternative way of doing things that is both better and cheaper than the traditional way. We were able to produce an evaluation that met both of these criteria when we demonstrated that psychiatric care in a district general hospital was superior to care in a mental hospital, and was also cheaper (Goldberg 1979; Jones *et al.* 1979). Schmiedebach, in Chapter 2 of this volume, argues that there are three types of evidence, and political evidence is presumably an example of his first type, i.e. evidence based upon social, religious and cultural contents, and on personal convictions. The health-services researcher offers Schmiedebach's third type of evidence, i.e. evidence from scientific research that shows that having the treatment is effective. Here the concept of 'treatment' is extended well beyond the effectiveness of a new drug, and extends to the effectiveness of a way of organising clinical services. The situation is not quite as clear as Schmiedebach describes because research aimed at understanding the causes of mental illness is not really as dead as he suggests, and is in fact still funded in most developed countries both by governments through their research councils and by charitable bodies. However, Schmiedebach is quite right in asserting that his third type of evidence has assumed progressively greater importance in the last half of the twentieth century.

Those engaged in health-services research like to suppose that their findings lead to progressive changes in the way in which services are delivered. However, this is to make a naïve mistake. Services develop mainly through Type-1 evidence: political imperatives are shaped by pressure on the health minister from his political party, from the media of the day, and from advice given him from within his department. Health services research is very much a subsidiary activity – a way of finding out whether the service changes suggested by Type-1 evidence are really as effective as had been hoped, or whether some other way of organising services is both cheaper and better.

When the better way of doing things is also more expensive, we know how much the extra quality costs. There are examples of this in drugs to treat cancer and AIDS, and within our own field the choices between newer anti-depressants and established ones, and between atypical neuroleptics and conventional anti-psychotics, are cases in point. Whether evidence can be delivered depends in part on

- whether the 'evidence' is credible
- the availability of resources
- the extent to which ministers feel under pressure to respond.

However, the most that can be hoped of most studies is that they will result in minor, largely cosmetic, policy changes that have been determined by Type-1 evidence.

However, this is not to sound too despairing a note. The 'case management approach' has largely been replaced by 'assertive community treatment' because of the numerous studies showing that only the latter is really effective. More recently, 'supervision registers' are suffering a similarly ignominious fate. Where new drugs are concerned, problems are rather more complicated, as Marshall shows in Chapter 7 of this volume. Reluctance of journal editors to publish the results of randomised controlled trials (RCTs) showing negative results, and pressure from powerful drug companies to market their latest nostrum, have resulted in a situation where newer, far more expensive drugs are preferred to older cheaper drugs, despite rather poor evidence of greater effectiveness. Marshall, in Chapter 7, draws our attention to many of the sources of bias that can effect the results of RCTs; one might also mention that those prepared to give informed consent to be randomised to a treatment are also a highly biased sample of those seeking treatment, yet one is rarely given information about the way in which they are different. The anthropological studies described by Bartlett in Chapter 12 are presumably liable to many of the same sorts of bias, as the researcher sifts through the huge amount of fieldwork data to find the few nuggets that will be reported.

Finzen, in Chapter 3, points out that milieu therapies grew out of the previous century's moral treatment; but today one can use scientific methods to investigate the efficacy of various milieus. It is also the case that hypotheses derived from understanding problems may be investigated by formal scientific methods if such hypotheses can be captured in an operational form. George Brown's investigations (Brown and Harris 1978) of the causal processes involved in the aetiology of depressive illness are a case in point of this important procedure. The demonstration of the effectiveness of psychological therapies – all of them derived from understanding – by scientific methods is of course another. As Philip Graham points out (Graham 1998), a good clinician always begins in an 'understanding' mode, and introduces explanatory, scientific thinking at that stage in the interaction when different management decisions need to be made.

In Chapter 4 James and Burns assert that we have been 'intoxicated by innovation'. It would be good if we were. One of the more depressing aspects of life in the NHS with a steadily diminishing budget is that there are seldom resources to be spared for true innovation – the finance officer feels happy if the budget can be balanced without removing too many essential services. Most innovation that does occur is supported by central research money, and is highly welcome: it provides Kane's 'type A' evidence (see Chapter 19), or Bolton's scientifically rigorous data (see Chapter 1). It has been usual for local health authorities to find extra resources when such central monies have been made available.

'Evidence-based medicine', which is today's politically correct slogan, may turn out to be a passing fad, and will quickly die a death if it becomes apparent that it is being made the excuse for denying patients suitable treatments. It is typically providing data about the average patient, and the standards it requires may be more rigorous than individual patients find reasonable. The individual patient needs 'patient-based evidence', which relates known data about the effectiveness of various treatments to that particular individual.

One of our problems is that topics are chosen for research by those who may not understand that some problems are unresearchable, and that other topics that are thought important are unjustly neglected. However, in future the voice of users should at least ensure that RCTs focus on better outcome measures, although as Finzen, in Chapter 3, rightly points out, typically RCTs exclude social factors that always contribute to the efficacy of treatment.

It would not be appropriate to end with a pessimistic thought. Health services research is today far more focused on the needs of users and carers than it has ever been in the past, and that can only be a good thing. Like democracy, RCTs are the least bad form of investigation that we have, but they do need to be supplemented by other sources of evidence if their findings are to be used to best effect.

Chapter 21

Evidence in the twenty-first century: the way forward

Stefan Priebe and Mike Slade

The first section of this book dealt with how the concept of evidence in mental health care developed over time, and what impact it has had on policy decisions. In the second and third sections, current methodologies and applications of the concept of evidence in practice were described. The authors adopted very different perspectives and expressed views that are partly inconsistent with each other. The resulting picture of the present 'state of the art' appears heterogeneous and inconclusive. Several authors chose to discuss the strengths of randomised controlled trials (RCTs), which may reflect the dominant role of RCTs in current research and their popularity in the scientific community. However, limitations of RCTs were also outlined, and alternative approaches suggested. Specifically, it was argued that 'evidence-based mental health care' does not mean 'RCT-based mental health care'. Randomised controlled trials are a valuable tool in the armoury, but not the only one. What conclusions can be drawn about what should be done differently for improving the evidence base in mental health care? How will research in this field progress in the future?

There is good reason to be cautious with prognoses and recommendations. With regard to clinical work, research evidence suggests that the prognoses of psychiatrists and psychologists on how their patients may fare in the future have surprisingly little predictive validity (see, for example, Kaiser *et al.* 1998) and that treatment recommendations are frequently ignored (see Lehman and Steinwachs 1998a). When we consider the future of research we enter mere speculation.

A number of distinct research methodologies and types of evidence have been described in this book, and others (for example neuroanatomy, sociology and ethics) could also have been included. It seems unlikely that any one approach will soon emerge as the clear winner and make all the others redundant, unless one feels that RCTs and meta-analyses are in that position already. Thus, different approaches will continue to co-exist, be applied by various research schools and compete for the same funding options. One way forward might be to identify which types of research question can be best answered by which methodological approach. Issues and problems would have to be specified that can be most appropriately addressed by one of the defined methods, for example an individual case study, a qualitative study, or a mega-trial in the form of a multi-centre RCT. To some extent this has already happened, but a full consensus about the most appropriate application and the limits of each of the current technologies does not exist. Such a consensus is unlikely to emerge by arguing the relative merits of each approach, since they are based on different premises. Non-partisan and multi-disciplinary research will be needed. Alternatively, progress may be made by integrating different methodological approaches, and calls for such integration seem popular. If each of the methods has its merits, but cannot provide all the desired evidence on its own, why not simply combine them in multi-method studies? We are sure that increasingly this will be tried and possibly lead to qualitatively improved methods and new insights. However, there is the danger that insufficiencies of defined approaches may not be overcome by simply putting them together. Integration is likely to pose additional problems beyond those associated with each individual approach. As a German saying goes 'two one-legged people don't make a runner'.

Any suggestion about what should be done depends on how the current situation is judged. One might feel that the different technologies are now sufficiently advanced that if the methods were applied to all the unsolved questions in mental health care, plenty of conclusive and informative evidence will be yielded. We would argue that the situation is not quite as rosy, and that each approach still has serious shortcomings. In our view, the challenge is not just to apply existing technologies in bigger trials and in a more rigorous fashion than in the past. We feel that current approaches have serious limitations, and see a need for further endeavours and innovative ideas to find and create more appropriate research methods. This has clear implications for research funding. More money should be spent on advancing research concepts and methodologies rather than on mega-trials. Such basic research has to have a long-term perspective. It might not appeal to all funding bodies, which are often interested in paying for research that produces quick and practically relevant results. We dare predict that the next decades will witness the development of new and more appropriate methodologies, and the sooner we have them the better.

In most industrialised countries, mental health services are under increasing pressure to document activities and to provide data on the outcomes of their patients. The response to this pressure may vary between nations, but there is little doubt that more and more data will be routinely accumulated in mental health services. Some of the data may be used for evaluation and research. The idea to use routine data for research purposes is not new and has been advocated in the literature over the last two decades under the banner of 'outcome management' (Ellwood 1988; Salvador-Carulla 1999; Huxley 1998). So far, the results have not been overwhelming and numerous obstacles have been identified. Yet the quality and completeness of routine data is arguably improving, and better systems for collecting and analysing routine data may open up new research options. Routine data systems, such as the Basis-Dokumentation in Germany or the Minimum Data Set in the UK, which are to be rolled out in the foreseeable future, have not primarily been set up to address detailed research questions. The question is whether they nevertheless provide helpful evidence and whether they can be used for hooking on additional modules of data sets that are designed for research. Although there is still some way to go, we believe that routine data sets will ultimately pay off for research. Individual and aggregated data will be obtained within the same system and used for different purposes: aggregated data for evaluation of services and research, individual data for outcome management on a clinical level and, occasionally, also for research. Outcome management, a technical term, involves the regular assessment of outcome variables such as patients' quality of life and satisfaction with treatment. The results are then fed back into the care process for monitoring progress, adjusting treatment decisions and strengthening the patient's role. Experience has shown that data must be of clinical and immediate use if staff and patients are to be motivated to collect them in sufficient quality. Outcome management provides a framework for that.

The use of routinely collected data and data systems for research would be beneficial in more than one way. It would save research funding, because in research projects only additional data collection would have to be paid for. It would also produce bigger and more complete data sets with substantially improved external validity. Finally, it would help to assess outcomes over long periods of time, rather than the 2 or 3-year period that follow-ups in research studies are usually funded for. Currently, results of those medium-term follow ups are extrapolated to longer term care, and this might be misleading.

As far as research into mental health care services is concerned, the current popular approach is to compare individual outcomes of patients allocated to differently configured services, with the allocation preferably following an RCT design. The findings suggest an association between the structural organisation of a service and treatment outcome. The nature of the association and mediating factors are frequently regarded as a black box that one knows little about. However, organisational structures rarely have a direct impact on treatment outcomes. The mediating factors, most notably the clinical practice in the given service and the quality of therapeutic relationships, more directly account for variance in outcome. It may be predicted that opening that black box will be a major challenge to research, no matter whether more qualitative or more quantitative methods are applied. One might want to distinguish between studies that investigate how elements of the service structure influence clinical practice and how they influence relationships in the service. Different studies, mostly with experimental designs, will examine how components of clinical practice and patterns of interactions impact on individual outcome. This conceptual distinction seems essential for a better understanding of what definable service characteristics and ingredients make a difference to clinical practice, and what interaction patterns and processes are to be modified for improving outcome (Priebe 2000). Process-oriented research will almost certainly require new methods for assessing what is going on in the health-care services, by moving beyond what clinicians and patients say they do to look at what they really do and how they communicate. These methods will have to disentangle the complexity of therapeutic processes that current research designs can hardly capture. If such research is successful and eventually leads to an understanding of how and why treatment processes work, the current emphasis on establishing statistical associations between interventions and outcome might be redundant. This would, in a sort of circle or spiral, bring us back to the underlying research paradigm of early phases in psychiatry (see Schmiedebach, Chapter 2, this volume).

One practical route into such research might be specific studies on the so-called non-specific factors in mental health care. Since the 1960s there has been sporadic interest in non-specific factors in psychiatry, but by and large they have not been extensively studied and are often dismissed as confounding factors, the effect of which has to be controlled for. Researching these factors might go some way to explaining why and how patients do or do not change when interacting with mental health professionals in services. Of course, the findings of such research may turn some of the non-specific factors into specific ones, because there will be a specific theory about their action. More generally, the best prospect for evidence-based mental health treatment, service and policy planning may be an integration of research examining what is common across groups and what is different across individuals, where the unit of analysis might be patients (as is currently most common), but might also be service configurations, team configurations, values, funding priorities, etc. Unlike the current focus on group commonalities, such an integration would not result in easily summarised findings. However, the resulting information might be of more relevance to those seeking to translate research into practice. Indeed, we would argue that at the level of making decisions regarding the treatment for individual patients, the vision that a full understanding of treatment processes may replace a prediction of outcome on the basis of statistical probability may be over optimistic for a long time to come, but is nevertheless more relevant to clinical practice than knowing the 'true' number-needed-to-treat.

Social factors may also impact on the collection and use of evidence. Most authors in this book, including ourselves, used the term 'evidence' in short when they actually meant evidence for the efficacy or effectiveness of an intervention and service. The underlying assumption that mental health care primarily aims at being therapeutically effective may be particularly undisputed in a publicly funded health-care system. In privately funded health care – and not just mental health care – this is less obvious, and services do not only aim at being effective, they also have to be attractive to patients and purchasers. In fact, the attractiveness of a service is essential for its economic survival. How effective the service is and how well it can publicise its effectiveness is only one of several aspects of its attractiveness. For instance, in western Europe and America there are many psychotherapists propagating approaches that do not pretend to be evidence based at all. Despite the lack of evidence, or perhaps because of it, they are attractive and find sufficient numbers of customers who are willing to pay for it. The notion of evidence may have to be widened in the future, if it is to retain its dominant position. Evidence may have to be provided for health services that appeal to the community and which satisfy demand in the society, regardless of their medical or psychological pedigree. The concept of post-modernism (Laugharne, Chapter 6 this volume) may provide a framework for understanding the remit and social context of mental health care in the future. It is conceivable that the current understanding of evidence will become less important and that research as a social process will either have objectives other than providing 'true evidence', or will occur in settings other than academic and scientific institutions. The provision of evidence is one of the main objectives of researchers, and justifies their professional status, influence and income. A changed notion of evidence or its disappearance as a socially important concept is likely to go hand-in-hand with a change in how research is institutionalised and funded. This change, however, will not be unique or specific to mental health care. If it happens it will affect wide areas of research and academia, of which mental health research is only one part.

The overall accessibility of different forms of media and electronic communication will provide the basis for a much wider, faster and more public communication about evidence, leading to new definitions of what constitutes evidence, and new sorts of evidence which different groups in society will want and accept. If there have ever been mental health researchers working in an ivory tower, they will probably have to leave it in the future and engage in a more intensive dialogue with funders and interest groups. On the one hand, national and other boundaries to worldwide communication are disappearing; on the other, local context may become more important both for the conditions and environment of research and as a subject of studies. That context as well as individual differences, cultural, political and temporal factors – the latter meaning influences on how the validity of findings might change over time – will have to be taken into account. We will probably need to develop new paradigms of enquiry for adequately considering all these factors.

Any research aiming to provide evidence needs funding. Some potential funders, mainly, but not only, the pharmaceutical industry, have a vested interest in what they want to see evidence for as a result of their funding. A level playing field for different approaches in mental health care will be difficult to achieve in this situation. Even more important to the scientific community may be attempts to control publication bias. Conflict of interest should be declared, as already happens in some forward-thinking journals. However, ways also have to be found to control for incomplete reporting of data and spin in publication strategies, such as multiple reporting of findings of one and the same drug trial (see Slade and Priebe, Chapter 10, this volume). Bureaucratic procedures may have to be put in place for achieving this, such as pre-submission of study protocols to journals so that the reported results can be checked against the original protocol. The cost of additional rigidity, however, may be outweighed by the gain in credibility and acceptance of study results. The current notion of evidence in its widest sense depends on information shared by the scientific community and communicated with users, stakeholders and the public. Publication of results in whatever form is an essential part of this process. As far as possible, it should be protected against fraud and spin (see Marshall, Chapter 7, this volume). Strong disincentives should be put in place for professional malpractice in research and dissemination of findings.

If one reads psychiatric and psychological textbooks written a hundred or so years ago, some passages may still apply, and indeed sound like they were written yesterday. Many other parts, however, appear hopelessly outdated and, sometimes, even funny. There is no reason to assume that future readers of present textbooks and current evidence will not be similarly amused. The pace of change has arguably increased in industrialised societies, and it might not take long before what we now take as granted and obvious will be regarded as outdated, and in many cases as wrong. This humbling notion may underline that societies and the generation of knowledge within them is always changing and in transition. Without ignoring the achievements of research in mental health care, we may well see ourselves at the beginning of an exciting path into unknown territory leading to better mental health care based on proper 'evidence'.

References

Ablon, J.S. and Jones, E.E. (1999) Psychotherapy process in the National Institute of Mental Health treatment of depression collaborative research program. *Journal of Consulting and Clinical Psychology* **67**: 64–75.

Ackerknecht, E.H. (1957) *Kurze Geschichte der Psychiatrie*. Stuttgart: Enke Verlag.

Ackner, B. (1957) Insulin treatment of schizophrenia: A controlled study. *Lancet* **2**: 607–11.

Adams, C., Freemantle, N. and Lewis, G. (1996) Meta-analysis. In *Mental Health Service Evaluation*, H.-C. Knudsen and G. Thornicroft (eds). Cambridge: Cambridge University Press, pp. 176–94.

Adams, C.E., Power, A., Frederick, K. and Lefebvre, C. (1994) An investigation of the adequacy of MEDLINE searches for randomized controlled trials (RCTs) of the effects of mental health care. *Psychological Medicine* **24**: 741–8.

Alderman, N. (1996) Central executive deficit and response to operant conditioning methods. *Neuropsychological Rehabilitation* **6**: 161–86.

Alderman, N. and Burgess, P. (1990) Integrating cognition and behaviour: a pragmatic approach to brain-injury rehabilitation. In *Cognitive Rehabilitation in Perspective*, R.L.I. Wood and I. Fussey (eds). Basingstoke: Taylor and Francis.

Alderman, N. and Burgess, P. (1994) A comparison of treatment methods for behaviour disorders following herpes simplex encephalitis. *Neuropsychological Rehabilitation* **4**: 31–48.

Alderman, N. and Knight, C. (1997) The effectiveness of DRL in the management and treatment of severe behaviour disorders following brain injury. *Brain Injury* **11**: 79–101.

Alderman, N. and Ward, A. (1991) Behavioural treatment of the dysexecutive syndrome: reduction of repetitive speech using response cost and cognitive overlearning. *Neuropsychological Rehabilitation* **1**: 65–80.

Alderman, N., Fry, R.K. and Youngson, H.A. (1995) Improvement of self-monitoring skills, reduction of behaviour disturbance and the dysexecutive syndrome: comparison of response cost and a new programme of self-monitoring training. *Neuropsychological Rehabilitation* **5**: 193–221.

Alderman, N., Knight, C. and Morgan, C. (1997) Use of a modified version of the Overt Aggression Scale in the measurement and assessment of aggressive behaviours following brain injury. *Brain Injury* **11**: 503–23.

Alderman, N., Bentley, J. and Dawson, K. (1999a) Issues and practice regarding behavioural outcome measurement undertaken by a specialised service provider. *Neuropsychological Rehabilitation* **9**: 385–400.

Alderman, N., Davies, J.A., Jones, C. and McDonnell, P. (1999b) Reduction of severe aggressive behaviour in acquired brain injury: case studies illustrating clinical use of the OAS-MNR in the management of challenging behaviours. *Brain Injury* **13**: 669–704.

Alexander, D.R., Barnes, F.G.L., Brander, J., *et al.* (1926) The value of malaria therapy in dementia paralytica. Preliminary report from the London County Mental Hospitals Service. *British Medical Journal* **2**: 603.

Allebeck, P. (1989) Schizophrenia: a life-shortening disease. *Schizophrenia Bulletin* **15**: 81–9.

Altman, D.G. (1994) The scandal of poor medical research. *British Medical Journal*, *308*, 283–4.

Altman, D.G. and Bland, J.M. (1999) Statistics notes. Treatment allocation in controlled trials: why randomise? *British Medical Journal* **318**: 1209.

American Medical Association (1990) Office of Quality Assurance. *Attributes to Grade the Development of Practice Parameters.* Chicago, IL: American Medical Association.

American Psychiatric Association (1979) *Diagnostic and Statistical Manual of Mental Disorders*, 3rd edition. Washington, DC: American Psychiatric Press.

American Psychiatric Association (1987) *Diagnostic and Statistical Manual of Mental Disorders*, 3rd edition (revised). Washington, DC: American Psychiatric Press.

American Psychiatric Association (1994) *Diagnostic and Statistical Manual of Mental Disorders*, 4th edition. Washington, DC: American Psychiatric Press.

American Psychiatric Association (1996) *Practice Guidelines*. Washington, DC: American Psychiatric Press.

American Psychiatric Association (1997) Expert consensus guidelines are released for treatment of bipolar disorder: *American Family Physician* **55**: 1447–9.

Anderson, E.M. and Lambert, M.J. (1995) Short-term dynamically oriented psychotherapy: a review and meta-analysis. *Clinical Psychology Review* **15**: 503–14.

Anderson, J. and Adams, C. (1996) Family interventions in schizophrenia. *British Medical Journal* **313(7056)**: 505–6.

Andrews, G., Slade, M. and Peters, L. (1999) Classification in psychiatry. ICD-10 versus DSM-IV, *British Journal of Psychiatry* **174**: 3–5.

Anstadt, T., Merten, J., Ullrich, B. and Krause, R. (1997) Affective dyadic behavior, core conflictual relationship themes, and success of treatment. *Psychotherapy Research* **7**: 397–419.

Arbeitkreis O. P. D. (ed.) (1996) *Operationalisierte Psychodynamische Diagnostik: Grundlagen und Manual.* Berne and Stuttgart: Hans Huber.

Ardener, E. (1975) Belief and the problem of women. In *Perceiving Women*, S. Ardener (ed.). London: Dent.

Asaph, J.W., Janoff, K., Wayson, K., *et al.* (1991) Carotid endarterectomy in a community hospital: a change in physicians' practice patterns. *American Journal of Surgery* **161**: 616–18.

Asch, D. and Hershey, J. (1995) Why some health policies don't make sense at the bedside. *Annals of Internal Medicine* **122**: 846–50.

Astin, J.A. (1998) Why patients use alternative medicine; results of a national study. *Journal of the American Medical Association* **279**: 1548–53.

Audini, B., Marks, I.M., Lawrence, R.E., Connolly, J. and Watts, V. (1994) Home-based versus out-patient/in-patient care for people with serious mental illness. Phase II of a controlled study. *British Journal of Psychiatry* **165**: 204–10.

Baars, B. (1986) *The Cognitive Revolution in Psychology*. New York: Guildford Press.

Baastrup, P.C., Poulsen, J.C., Schou, M., Thomsen, K. and Amdisen, A. (1970) Prophylactic lithium: double-blind discontinuation in manic-depressive and recurrent-depressive disorder. *Lancet* **2**: 326–30.

Bachrach, L. (1984) *The Homeless Mentally Ill and Mental Health Services: an Analytical Review of the Literature*. Washington: US Department of Health and Human Services, Churchill Livingstone.

Bacon, F. (1620) *Novum Organum Scientiarium*. T. Fowler (ed.) (1878), Oxford: Oxford University Press.

Baldessarini, R.J. (1970) Frequency of diagnoses of schizophrenia versus affective disorders from 1944 to 1968. *American Journal of Psychiatry* **127**: 757–63.

Barbour, R.S. and Kitzinger, J. (eds) (1998) *Developing Focus Group Research*. London: Sage.

Barham, P. and Hayward, R. (1991) *From Mental Patient to the Community*. London: Routledge.

Barker, D. and Rose, G. (1979) *Epidemiology in Medical Practice*, second edition. London: Churchill Livingstone.

Barkham, M., Margison, F., Leach, C. *et al.* (in press) Service profiling and outcomes benchmarking using the CORE-OM: Towards practice-based evidence in the psychological therapies. *Journal of Consulting and Clinical Psychology*.

Baron, R. and Kenny, D. (1986) The moderator-mediator variable distinction in social psychological research. *Journal of Personality and Social Psychology* **41**: 1173–82.

Barratt, R.J. (1988a) Interpretations of schizophrenia. *Culture, Medicine and Psychiatry* **12**: 357–88.

Barratt, R.J. (1988b) Clinical writing and the documentary construction of schizophrenia. *Culture, Medicine and Psychiatry* **12**: 265–99.

Barry, P. and Riley, J.M. (1987) Adult norms for the Kaufman Hand Movements Test and a single-subject design for acute brain injury rehabilitation. *Journal of Clinical and Experimental Neuropsychology* **9**: 449–55.

Bateman, A. and Fonagy, P. (1999) The effectiveness of partial hospitalization in the treatment of borderline personality disorder – a randomised controlled trial. *American Journal of Psychiatry* **156**: 1563–9.

Bateman, A. and Fonagy, P. (submitted) Follow-up of psychoanalytically oriented partial hospitalisation treatment of borderline personality disorder. *American Journal of Psychiatry*.

Bateson, G., Jackson, D., Haley, J. and Weakland J. (1956) Towards a theory of schizophrenia. *Behavioural Science* **1**: 251–64.

Bauer, M.S., Callahan, A.M., Jampala, C. *et al.* (1999) Clinical practice guidelines for bipolar disorder from the Department for Veterans Affairs. *American Journal of Psychiatry* **60**: 9–21.

Bayle, A.L.J. (1822) *Recherches sur l'arachnitis chronique*. Paris: Thèse No. 247.

Beaumont, G. (1983) Neuropsychology and the organisation of behaviour. In *Physical Correlates of Behaviour*, A. Gale and P. Edwards (eds). London: Academic Press.

Beck, A.T. (1976) *Cognitive Therapy and the Emotional Disorders*. New York: International Universities Press.

Beck, A.T., Ward, C.H., Mendelson, M., Mock, J. and Erbaugh, J. (1961) An inventory for measuring depression. *Archives of General Psychiatry* **4**: 561–71.

Beck, A.T., Rush, A.J., Shaw, B.F. and Emery, G. (1979) *Cognitive Therapy of Depression.* New York: Guildford Press.

Becker, T., Knapp, M., Knudsen, H.C. *et al.*, and the EPSILON Study Group (2000) Aims, outcomes measures, study sites and the patient sample. EPSILON Study 1. In 'Reliable outcome measures for mental health service research in five European countries', G. Thornicroft, T. Becker and M. Knapp (eds). *British Journal of Psychiatry* **177(39)**: S1–S7.

Bennett, D.E., (1998) *Deriving a model of therapist competence from good and poor cases in the therapy of borderline personality disorder.* Unpublished doctoral dissertation, UK: University of Sheffield.

Bero, L.A., Grilli, R., Grimshaw, J.M., Harvey, E., Oxman, A.D. and Thomson, M.A. on behalf of the Cochrane (1998) Effective Practice and Organisation of Care Review Group. Closing the gap between research and practice: an overview of systematic reviews and interventions to promote the implementation of research findings. *British Medical Journal* **317**: 465–8.

Berrios, G.E. (1996) Early electroconvulsive therapy in Britain, France and Germany: a conceptual history. In *150 Years of British Psychiatry. Volume II: the Aftermath*, H. Freeman and G.E. Berrios (eds). London: Atlantic Highlands, Athlone, pp. 3–15.

Bion, W.R. (1967) Notes on memory and desire. *Psychoanalytic Forum* **2**: 272–3, 279–80.

Birley, J.L.T. (1990) DSM III: from left to right or from right to left? *British Journal of Psychiatry* **157**: 116–18.

Black, N. (1996) Why we need observational studies to evaluate the effectiveness of health care. *British Medical Journal* **312**: 15–18.

Blackburn, I.M., Bishop, S., Glen, A.I.M., Whalley, L.J. and Christie, J.E. (1981) The efficacy of cognitive therapy in depression: a treatment trial using cognitive therapy and pharmacotherapy, each alone and in combination. *British Journal of Psychiatry* **139**: 181–9.

Blatt, S.J., Quinlan, D.M., Zuroff, D.C. and Pilkonis, P.A. (1996) Interpersonal factors in brief treatment of depression: further analyses of the National Institute of Mental Health, Treatment of Depression Collaborative Research Program. *Journal of Consulting and Clinical Psychology* **64**: 162–71.

Bleiberg, E., Fonagy, P. and Target, M. (1997) Child psychoanalysis: critical overview and a proposed reconsideration. *Psychiatric Clinics of North America* **6**: 1–38.

Blenkner, M. (1954) Predictive factors in the initial interview in family casework, *Social Service Review* **28**: 65–73.

Bolton, D. (1984) Philosophy and psychiatry. In *The Scientific Principles of Psychopathology*, P. McGuffin, M. Shanks and R. Hodgson (eds). London and New York: Academic Press, pp. 739–62.

Bolton, D. and Hill, J. (1996) *Mind, Meaning, and Mental Disorder: The Nature of Causal Explanation in Psychology and Psychiatry.* Oxford: Oxford University Press.

Booth, T. and Gowe, R. (1988) *Developing Policy Research.* London:

Bourne, H. (1953) The insulin myth. *Lancet* **2**: 964–9.

Bowden, C.L., Brugger, A.M., Swann. A.C. *et al.* (1994) Efficacy of divalproex versus lithium and placebo in the treatment of mania. *Journal of the American Medical Association* **271**: 918–24.

Bowling, A. (1991) *Measuring Health. A Review of Quality of Life Measurement Scales*. Buckingham: Open University Press.

Bowling, A. (1995) *Measuring Disease. A Review of Disease-specific Quality of Life Measurement Scales*. Buckingham: Open University Press.

Bowling, A. (1997) *Research Methods in Health. Investigating Health and Health Services*. Buckingham: Open University Press.

Breuer, J. and Freud, S. (1895) Studies in hysteria. In *The Standard Edition of the Complete Psychological Works of Sigmund Freud*, vol. 2. London: Hogarth Press, 1978.

Brown, G.W. and Harris, T.O. (1978) *Social Origins of Depression: A Study of Psychiatric Disorder in Women*. London: Tavistock.

Brown, G.W. and Harris, T.O. (1986) Establishing causal links: The Bedford College studies of depression. In *Life Events and Psychiatric Disorders*, K. Katschinig (ed.). Cambridge: Cambridge University Press.

Brown, G.W., Monck, E.M., Carstairs, G.M. and Wing, J.K. (1962) Influence of family life on the course of schizophrenic illness. *British Journal of Preventive and Social Medicine* **16**: 55–68.

Bruner, J. (1990) *Acts of Meaning*. Cambridge MA: Harvard University Press.

Bryant, M., Simons, A. and Thase, M. (1999) Therapist skill and patient variables in homework compliance: Controlling an uncontrolled variable in cognitive therapy outcome research. *Cognitive Therapy and Research* **23**: 381–99.

Bucci, W. (1997) *Psychoanalysis and Cognitive Science: A Multiple Code Theory*. New York: Guilford Press.

Bucci, W. and Miller, N. (1993) Primary process analogue: The Referential Activity measure. In *Psychodynamic Treatment Research*, N. Miller, L. Luborsky, J. Barber and J. Docherty (eds). New York: Basic Books, pp. 381–406.

Bulmer, M. (1986) *Social Science and Social Policy*. London: Allen and Unwin.

Burgess, P.W. (1997) Theory and methodology in executive function research. In *Methodology of Frontal and Executive Function*, P. Rabbitt (ed.). Hove: Psychology Press, pp. 81–116.

Burgess, P.W., Alderman, N., Evans, J.J., Emslie, H. and Wilson, B.A. (1998) The ecological validity of tests of executive function. *Journal of the International Neuropsychological Society* **4**: 547–58.

Burns, T., Creed, F., Fahy, T., Thompson, S., Tyrer, P. and White, I. (1999) Intensive versus standard case management for severe psychotic illness. A randomised trial. *Lancet* **353**: 2185–9.

Burke, W.H. and Lewis, F.D. (1986) Management of maladaptive social behavior of a brain-injured adult. *International Journal of Rehabilitation Research* **9**: 335–42.

Burke, W.H., Zencius, A.H., Weslowski, M.D. and Doubleday, F. (1991) Improving executive function disorders in brain-injured clients. *Brain Injury* **5**: 241–52.

Burns, B.L. and Santos, A.B. (1995) Assertive community treatment: an update of randomized trials. *Psychiatric Services* **46**: 669–75.

Burns, T. (1997) Case management, care management and care programming. *British Journal of Psychiatry* **170**: 393–5.

Burns, T. and Priebe, S. (1996) Mental health care systems and their characteristics: a proposal. *Acta Psychiatrica Scandinavica* **94**: 381–5.

Burns, T. and Priebe, S. (1999) Mental health care failure in England: myth and reality. *British Journal of Psychiatry* **174**: 191–2.

Burns, T., Fahy, T., Thompson, S. *et al.* (1999a) Intensive case management for severe psychotic illness. *Lancet* (letter) **354**: 1385–6.

Burns, T., Creed, F., Fahy, T., Thompson, S., Tyrer, P. and White, I. (1999b) Intensive versus standard case management for severe psychotic illness: a randomised trial. *Lancet* **353**: 2185–9.

Burns, T., Fiander, M., Kent, A. *et al.* (2000) Effects of case load size on the process of care of patients with severe psychotic illness. Report from the UK700 trial. *British Journal of Psychiatry* **177**: 427–33.

Burtt, E.A. (1932) *The Metaphysical Foundations of Modern Physical Sciences.* London: Routledge and Kegan Paul.

Cade, J.F.J. (1949) Lithium salts in the treatment of psychotic excitement. *Medical Journal of Australia* **36**: 349–52.

Campbell, D.T. and Stanley, J.C. (1966) Experimental and quasi-experimental designs for research on teaching. In *Handbook of Research on Teaching*, N.L. Gage (ed.). Chicago: Rand-McNally.

Cape, J. (2000) Clinical effectiveness in the UK: Definitions, history and policy trends. *Journal of Mental Health* **9**: 3237–46.

Capgras, J. and Reboul-Lachaux, J. (1923) L'illusion des 'sosies' dans un delire systematise chronique. *Bulletin de la Société Clinique Médicine Mentale* **11**: 6–16.

Caplan, Nathan, *et al.* (1975) *The Use of Social Knowledge in Policy Decisions at the National Level.* University of Michigan: Institute for Social Research.

Carstairs, G.M. and Kapur, R.L. (1976) *The Great Universe of Kota: Stress, Change and Mental Disorder in an Indian Village.* Berkeley: University of California Press.

Castel, R. (1976) *L'Ordre Psychiatrique. l'Âge d'or de l'Alienisme.* Paris: Les Éditions de Minuit.

Castonguay, L.G., Goldfried, M.R., Wiser, S. and Raue, P.J. (1996) Predicting the effect of cognitive therapy for depression: A study of unique and common factors. *Journal of Consulting and Clinical Psychology* **64**: 497–504.

CEBSS (1998) What is evidence-based social care? In *Evidence-Based Social Care, Newsletter of the Centre for Evidence Based Social Services*, Issue 1. Exeter: Centre for Evidence Based Social Services.

Chadwick, P.D. and Lowe, C.F. (1990) Measurement and modification of delusional beliefs. *Journal of Consulting and Clinical Psychology* **58(2)**: 225–32.

Chalmers, I., Dickersin, K. and Chalmers, T.C. (1992) Getting to grips with Archie Cochrane's agenda. *British Medical Journal* **305**: 786–8.

Chalmers, I., Enkin, M. and Keirse, M.J. (1993) Preparing and updating systematic reviews of randomized controlled trials of health care. *Millbank Quarterly* **71**: 411–37.

Chambless, D.L. and Gillis, M.M. (1993) Cognitive therapy of anxiety disorders. *Journal of Consulting and Clinical Psychology* **61(2)**: 248–60.

Chambless, D.L. and Hollon, S.D. (1998) Defining empirically supported therapies. *Journal of Consulting and Clinical Psychology* **66(1)**: 7–18.

Chassan, J.B. (1967) *Research Design in Clinical Psychology and Psychiatry.* New York: Appleton-Century-Crofts.

Cierpka, M., Bucheim, P., Freyberger, H.J. *et al.* (1995) Die erste Version einer Operationalisierten Psychodynamischen Diagnostik (OPD-1). *Psychotherapeutics* **40**: 69–78.

Clarke, L. (1993) The opening of doors in British mental hospitals in the 1950s. *History of Psychiatry* **4**: 527–51.

Clarke, M.J. and Stewart, L.A. (1994) Obtaining data from randomised controlled trials: how much do we need for reliable and informative meta-analyses? *British Medical Journal* **309**: 1007–10.

Clarkin, J.F., Yeomans, F. and Kernberg, O.F. (1998) *Psychodynamic Psychotherapy of Borderline Personality Organisation: A Treatment Manual.* New York: Wiley.

Clifford, J. (1986) *Partial Truths in Writing Culture: the Poetics and Politics of Ethnography.* J. Clifford and G.E. Marcus (eds). Berkeley: University of California Press.

Clifford, J. (1988) *The Predicament of Culture: Twentieth Century Ethnography, Literature, and Art.* London: Harvard University Press.

Clifford, P. (1998) *The Use of an Extended Medical Record in the Measurement of Outcomes: the Reliability and Validity of the Functional Assessment of Care Environments (FACE).* London: Report to the UK Department of Health.

Cochrane, A.L. (1979) 1931–1971: a critical review, with particular reference to the medical profession. In *Medicine for the Year 2000.* London: Office of Health Economics, pp.1–11.

Cochrane and Campbell Collaborations (2000) *Evidence from systematic reviews of research relevant to implementing the 'wider public health' agenda: An update and development of 'Evidence from systematic reviews of research relevant to the forthcoming White Paper on Public Health (1 May 1998).* UK Cochrane Centre, NHS Research and Development Programme, Middle Way, Summertown Pavilion, Oxford OX2 7LG.

Cochrane Collaboration (1995) *Cochrane Collaboration Handbook*, updated July 1995. Oxford: Cochrane Collaboration.

Cohen, A., Dolan, B. and Eastman, N.L.G. (1996) Research on the supervision registers: inconsistencies in local research ethics committee responses. *Journal of Forensic Psychiatry* **7(2)**: 413–19.

Coid, J. (1994) Failure in community care: psychiatry's dilemma. *British Medical Journal* **308(6932)**: 805–6.

Cole, J.O., Goldberg, S.C., and Klerman, G.L. (1964) Phenothiazine treatment in acute schizophrenia. *Archives of General Psychiatry* **10**: 246–61.

Coleman, W. (1987) Experimental physiology and statistical inference: the therapeutic trial in nineteenth-century Germany. In *The Probalistic Revolution, vol. 2: Ideas in the Science*, L. Krüger, G. Gigerenzer and M.S. Morgan (eds). Cambridge, MA: MIT Bradford, pp. 201–26.

Colthart, M. (1991) Cognitive psychology applied to the treatment of acquired language disorders. In *Handbook of Behavior Therapy and Psychological Science: an Integrative Approach*, P.R. Martin (ed.). New York: Pergamon Press.

Concise Oxford Dictionary (1993) Oxford: Oxford University Press.

Conner, M. and Norman, P. (eds) (1998) *Predicting Health Behaviour.* Buckingham: Open University Press.

Cook, D.J., Guyatt, G.H., Ryan, G. *et al.* (1993) Should unpublished data be included in meta-analyses? Current convictions and controversies. *Journal of the American Medical Association* **269**: 2749–53.

Cook, D.J., Sackett, D.L. and Spitzer, W.O. (1995) Methodologic guidelines for systematic reviews of randomised control trials in health care from the Potsdam Consultation on Meta-Analysis. *Journal of Clinical Epidemiology* **48**: 167–71.

Cookson, J.C. (1997) Lithium: balancing risks and benefits. *British Journal of Psychiatry* **171**: 120–4.

Cookson, J.C. (in press) The use of antipsychotic drugs and lithium in mania. *British Journal of Psychiatry* Supplement.

Cookson, J.C. and Duffelt, R. (1994) The treatment of schizophrenia outside hospital. *Clinician* **12**: 53–66.

Cookson, J.C. and Sachs, G.S. (2000) Lithium: clinical use in mania and prophylaxis of affective disorders. In *Schizophrenia and Mood Disorders: the New Drug Therapies in Clinical Practice*, P.F. Buckley and J.L. Waddington (eds). Oxford: Butterworth Heinemann, pp. 155–78.

Cope, D.N. (1994) Traumatic brain injury rehabilitation outcome studies in the United States. In *Brain Injury and Neuropsychological Rehabilitation, International Perspectives*, A.L. Christensen and B.P. Hazzell (eds). Hillsdale, NJ: Lawrence Erlbaum Associates Inc.

Coppen, A., Noguera, R., Bailey, J. *et al.* (1971) Prophylactic lithium in affective disorders: controlled trial. *Lancet* **2**: 275–9.

Counsell, C.E., Clarke, M.J., Slattery, J. and Sandercock, P.A. (1994) The miracle of DICE therapy for acute stroke: fact or fictional product of subgroup analysis? *British Medical Journal* **309**: 1677–81.

Crapanzano, V. (1986) Hermes' dilemma: the masking of subversion. In *Ethnographic Description in Writing Culture; the Poetics and Politics of Ethnography*, J. Clifford and G.E. Marcus (eds). Berkeley: University of California Press.

Creed, F., Black, D., Anthony, P. *et al.* (1990) Randomised controlled trial of day patient versus inpatient psychiatric treatment. *British Medical Journal* **300** 6731, 1033–7.

Creed, F., Black, D., Anthony, P. *et al.* (1991) Randomised controlled trial of day and in-patient psychiatric treatment. 2: Comparison of two hospitals. *British Journal of Psychiatry* **158**: 183–9.

Creed, F., Mbaya, P., Lancashire, S., Tomenson, B., Williams, B. and Holme, S. (1997) Cost effectiveness of day and in-patient psychiatric treatment. *British Medical Journal* **314**: 1381–5.

Creed, F., Burns, T. and Butler, T. (1999) Comparison of intensive and standard case management for patients with psychosis. Rationale of the trial. *British Journal of Psychiatry* **174**: 74–8.

Creer, C. and Wing, J. (1974) *Schizophrenia at Home*. Surbiton, Surrey: National Schizophrenia Fellowship.

Crits-Christoph, P., Cooper, A. and Luborsky, L. (1988) The accuracy of therapists' interpretations and the outcome of dynamic psychotherapy. *Journal of Consulting and Clinical Psychology* **56**: 490–5.

Crossley, D. (1993) The introduction of leucotomy: a British case history. *History of Psychiatry* **4**: 553–64.

Crowther, R., Marshall, M., Bond, G.R. and Huxley, P. (2000) Vocational rehabilitation for people with severe mental disorders. In preparation.

Cundall, R.L., Brooks, P.W. and Murray, L.G. (1972) A controlled evaluation of lithium prophylaxis in affective disorders. *Psychological Medicine* **2**: 308–11.

Danziger, K. (1987) Statistical method and the historical development of research practice in American psychology. In *The Probalistic Revolution, vol. 2: ideas in the sciences*, L. Krüger, G. Gigerenzer and M.S. Morgan (eds). Cambridge, MA: MIT Bradford, pp. 35–47.

Davanloo, H. (1980) *Short-term dynamic psychotherapy*. New York: Jason Aronson.

Davis, J.R., Turner, W., Rolinder, A. and Cartwright, T. (1994) Natural and structured baselines in the treatment of aggression following brain injury. *Brain Injury* **8**: 589–97.

Dean, C., Philips, J., Gadd, E.M., Joseph, M. and England, S. (1993) Comparison of community based service with hospital based service for people with acute, severe psychiatric illness. *British Medical Journal* **307**: 473–6.

Department of Health (1984) *NHS Management Inquiry*. London: HMSO.

Department of Health (1993) *The Health of the Nation, Key Area Handbook, Mental Illness*. London: Department of Health.

Department of Health (1998) *The New NHS: Modern and Dependable*. London: HMSO.

Department of Health (1998b) *Modernising Mental Health Services: Safe, Sound and Supportive*. London: HMSO.

Department of Health (September 1999) *National Service Framework for Mental Health – Modern Standards and Service Models*. London: Department of Health.

Department of Health (2000) *NHS National Plan*. London: HMSO: CM.4818-1-2000.

Derogatis, L.R. (1983) *SCL-90R: Administration, Scoring and Procedures – Manual II*. Towson, MD: Clinical Psychometric Research Inc.

Desjarlais, R., Eisenberg, L., Good, B. and Kleinman, A. (1995) *World Mental Health: Problems and Priorities in Low-income Countries*. Oxford: Oxford University Press.

Detre, T. (1997) Managed Care and the Future. *Archives of General Psychiatry* **54**: 201–4.

Dick, P., Cameron, L., Cohen, D., Barlow, M. and Ince, A. (1985) Day and full time psychiatric treatment: a controlled comparison. *British Journal of Psychiatry* **147**: 246–9.

Dijksterhuis, E.J. (1961) *The mechanization of the world-picture*, C. Dikshoorn (trans.). Oxford: Oxford University Press.

DiMascio, A., Weissman, M.M., Prusoff, B.A. *et al.* (1979) Differential symptom reduction by drugs and psychotherapy in acute depression. *Archives of General Psychiatry* **36(13)**: 1450–6.

Dobson, K.S. (1989) A meta-analysis of the efficacy of cognitive therapy for depression. *Journal of Consulting and Clinical Psychology* **57(3)**: 414–19.

Dörner, K. (1993) The role of psychiatry in solving the social question 1790–1990. In *Proceedings of the 1st European Congress on the History of Psychiatry and Mental Health Care*, L. de Goei and J. Vijslaar (eds). Rotterdam: Erasmus, pp. 331–7.

Drake, R.E. and Sederer, L.I. (1986) The adverse effects of intensive treatment of chronic schizophrenia. *Comprehensive Psychiatry* **27(4)**: 313–26.

Drury, V., Birchwood, M., Cochrane, R. and MacMillan, F. (1996a) Cognitive therapy and recovery from acute psychosis: a controlled trial. I. Impact on psychotic symptoms. *British Journal of Psychiatry* **169(5)**: 593–601.

Drury, V., Birchwood, M., Cochrane, R. and MacMillan, F. (1996b) Cognitive therapy and recovery from acute psychosis: a controlled trial. II. Impact on recovery time. *British Journal of Psychiatry* **169(5)**: 602–7.

Duggan, L., Fenton, M., Dardennes, R.M. *et al.* (1999) Olanzapine for schizophrenia (Cochrane Review) In *The Cochrane Library*, issue 3. Oxford: Update Software.

Egger, M. and Smith, G.D. (1998) Bias in location and selection of studies. *British Medical Journal* **316**: 61–6.

Egger, M., Smith, G.D., Schneider, M. and Minder, C. (1997) Bias in meta-analysis detected by a simple, graphical test. *British Medical Journal* **315**: 629–34.

Eisenberg, L. (1984) Rudolf Ludwig Karl Virchow: Where are you now that we need you? *American Journal of Medicine* **77**: 524–32.

Elkin, I. (1994) The NIMH Treatment of Depression Collaborative Research Programme: Where we began and where we are. In *Handbook of Psychotherapy and Behaviour Change*, fourth edition, A.E. Bergin and S.L. Garfield (eds). New York: Wiley, pp. 114–39.

Elkin, I., Shea, M.T., Watkins, J.T. *et al.* (1989) National Institute of Mental Health Treatment of Depression Collaborative Research Program. General effectiveness of treatments. *Archives of General Psychiatry* **46(11)**: 971–82.

Elkin, I., Gibbons, R.D., Shea, M.T. *et al.* (1995) Initial severity and differential treatment outcome in the National Institute of Mental Health Treatment of Depression Collaborative Research Program. *Journal of Consulting and Clinical Psychology* **63(5)**: 841–7.

Ellis, A. (1962) *Reason and Emotion in Psychotherapy*. New York: Lyle-Stuart.

Ellrodt, G., Cook, D., Lee, J. *et al.* (1997) Evidence-based disease management. *Journal of the American Medical Association* **278**: 1687–92.

Ellwood P. (1988) Outcomes management – a technology of patient experience. *New England Journal of Medicine* **318**: 1549–56.

Emmelkamp, P.M.G. (1982) *Phobic and Obsessive Compulsive Disorders: Theory, Research and Practice*. New York: Plenum Press.

Engstrom, E.J. (1997) Kulturelle Dimensionen von Psychiatrie und Sozialpsychologie: Emil Kraepelin und Willy Hellpach. In *Kultur und Kulturwissenschaften um 1900*, vol. 2, R. vom Bruch, F.W. Graf and G. Hübinger (eds). Stuttgart: Steiner, pp. 164–89.

Evans, M.D., Hollon, S.D., DeRubeis, R.J. *et al.* (1992) Differential relapse following cognitive therapy and pharmacotherapy for depression. *Archives of General Psychiatry* **49(10)**: 802–8.

Evans-Pritchard, E.E. (1940) *The Nuer*. Oxford: Clarendon Press.

Evans-Pritchard, E.E. (1951) *Social Anthropology*. London: Routledge and Kegan Paul.

Eysenck, H.J. (1994) Meta-analysis and its problems. *British Medical Journal* **309**: 789–92.

Falloon, I.R. and Pederson, J. (1985) Family management in the prevention of morbidity of schizophrenia: the adjustment of the family unit. *British Journal of Psychiatry* **147**: 156–63.

Falloon, I.R., Boyd, J.L., McGill, C.W. *et al.* (1982) Family management in the prevention of exacerbations of schizophrenia: a controlled study. *New England Journal of Medicine* **306, 24**: 1437–40.

Fals-Stewart, W., Marks, A.P. and Schafer, J. (1993) A comparison of behavioral group therapy and individual behavior therapy in treating obsessive-compulsive disorder. *Journal of Nervous and Mental Disease* **181(3)**: 189–93.

Feinstein, A. and Horwitz, R. (1997) Problems in the 'evidence' of 'evidence based medicine'. *American Journal of Medicine* **103**: 529–35.

Feldman, R. (1993) Evidence. In *A Companion to Epistemology*, J. Dancy and E. Sosa (eds). Oxford, *Malden*, Mass.: *Blackwell* (Blackwell Companions to Philosophy)

Finzen, A. (1998) *Das Pinelsche Pendel. Die Dimension des Sozialen im Zeitalter der Biologischen Psychiatrie*. Bonn: Edition das Narrenschiff im Psychiatrie-Verlag.

Flexner, A. (1910) Report for the Carnegie Foundation for the Advancement of Teaching.

Foa, E.B., Steketee, G., Grayson, J.B. and Latimer, P.R. (1984) Deliberate exposure and blocking of obsessive-compulsive rituals: immediate and long-term effects. *Behaviour Therapy* **15**: 450–72.

Foley, S.H., Rouansaville, B.J., Weissman, M.M., Sholomskas, D. and Chevron, E.S. (1989) Individual versus conjoint interpersonal psychotherapy for depressed patients with marital disputes. *International Journal of Family Psychiatry* **10**: 29–42.

Fonagy, P. (1995) Playing with reality: the development of psychic reality and its malfunction in borderline patients. *International Journal of Psycho-Analysis* **76**: 39–44.

Fonagy, P. (1999) Achieving evidence-based psychotherapy practice: A psychodynamic perspective on the general acceptance of treatment manuals. *Clinical Psychology: Science and Practice*. **6**: 442–4.

Fonagy, P. and Moran, G.S. (1991) Studies of the efficacy of child psychoanalysis. *Journal of Consulting and Clinical Psychology* **58**: 684–95.

Fonagy, P. and Target, M. (1996) Predictors of outcome in child psychoanalysis: A retrospective study of 763 cases at the Anna Freud Centre. *Journal of the American Psychoanalytic Association* **44**: 27–77.

Fonagy, P., Edgcumbe, R., Target, M., Miller, J. and Moran, G. (unpublished manuscript) *Contemporary Psychodynamic Child Therapy: Theory and Technique*.

Fonagy, P., Gerber, A., Higgitt, A. and Bateman, A. (in preparation) *The comparison of intensive (5 times weekly) and non-intensive (once weekly) treatment of young adults*.

Fonagy, P., Steele, H., Moran, G., Steele, M. and Higgitt, A. (1991) The capacity for understanding mental states: The reflective self in parent and child and its significance for security of attachment. *Infant Mental Health Journal* **13**: 200–17.

Fonagy, P., Moran, G.S., Edgcumbe, R., Kennedy, H. and Target, M. (1993) The roles of mental representations and mental processes in therapeutic action. *The Psychoanalytic Study of the Child* **48**: 9–48.

Fonagy, P., Kachele, H., Krause, R. *et al.* (1999) *An Open Door Review of Outcome Studies in Psychoanalysis*. London: International Psychoanalytical Association.

Fonagy, P., Gerber, A., Higgitt, A., and Bateman, A. (2001). The comparison of intensive (5 times weekly) and non-intensive (once weekly) treatment of young adults. In P. Fonagy, H. Kachele, R. Kraus, E. Jones, R. Perron, J. Clarkin, A.J. Gerber and E. Allison (eds), *An open door review of outcome studies in psychoanalysis* (2nd edn), pp. 128–132. London: International Psychoanalytical Association.

Ford, R., Beadsmoore, A., Ryan, P., Repper, J., Craig, T. and Muijen, M. (1995) Providing the safety net case management for people with a serious mental illness. *Journal of Mental Health* **1**: 91–7.

Forster, E. (1930) Selbstversuch mit Meskalin. *Deutsche Zeitschrift für Nervenheilkunde* **127**: 1–14.

Fortes, M. (1945) *The Dynamics of Clanship Among the Tallensi*. London: Oxford University Press (for the International African Institute).

Foucault, M. (1961) Madness and civilisation: a history of insanity in the Age of Reason. Translated by R. Howard of Folie et d—raison: histoire de la folie a l'age *classique* (Paris: Librairie Plon, 1961) London: Tavistock (reprinted by Routledge 1997).

Foucault, M. (1965) *Madness and Civilization. A History of Insanity in the Age of Reason.* London, Sydney and Wellington: Tavistock.

Foucault, M. (1967) *Madness and Civilization. A History of Insanity in the Age of Reason.* London: Tavistock Publications.

Fowler, D. and Morley, S. (1989) The cognitive-behavioural treatment of hallucinations and delusions: a preliminary study. *Behavioural Psychotherapy* **17**: 267–82.

Frank, E., Kupfer, D.J., Wagner, E.F., McEachrn, A.B. and Cornes, C. (1991) Efficacy of interpersonal therapy as a maintenance treatment of recurrent depression. *Archives of General Psychiatry* **48**: 1053–9.

Freedman, N., Hoffenberg, J.D., Vorus, N. and Frosch, A. (1999) The effectiveness of psychoanalytic psychotherapy: the role of treatment duration, frequency of sessions, and the therapeutic relationship. *Journal of the American Psychoanalytic Association* **47**: 741–72.

Freud, S. (1895) Project for a scientific psychology. In *The Standard Edition of the Complete Psychological Works of Sigmund Freud*, volume 1. London: Hogarth Press, 1978, pp. 283–397.

Freud, S. (1904) Freud's psycho-analytic procedure. In *The Standard Edition of the Complete Psychological Works of Sigmund Freud*, volume 7, J. Strachey (ed). London: Hogarth Press, pp. 247–54.

Freud, S. (1905) On psychotherapy. In *The Standard Edition of the Complete Psychological Works of Sigmund Freud*, volume 7, J. Strachey (ed.). London: Hogarth Press, pp. 255–68.

Freud, S. (1916–17) Analytic therapy. Lecture XXVIII in 'Introductory lectures on psycho-analysis'. In *The Standard Edition of the Complete Psychological Works of Sigmund Freud*, volume 17, J. Strachey (ed.). London: Hogarth Press, pp. 448–63.

Freud, S. (1933) New introductory lectures on psychoanalysis. In *The Standard Edition of the Complete Psychological Works of Sigmund Freud*, volume 22, J. Strachey (ed.). London: Hogarth Press, pp. 1–182.

Freud, S. (1937) Analysis terminable and interminable. In *The Standard Edition of the Complete Psychological Works of Sigmund Freud*, volume 23, J. Strachey (ed.). London: Hogarth Press, pp. 209–53.

Garcia, J.G. and Lam, C. (1990) Treating urinary incontinence in a head-injured adult. *Brain Injury* **4**: 203–7.

Garety, P.A., Kuipers, L., Fowler, D., Chamberlain, F. and Dunn, G. (1994) Cognitive behavioural therapy for drug-resistant psychosis. *British Journal of Medical Psychology* **67(3)**: 259–71.

Geddes, J. (1996) On the need for evidence-based psychiatry. *Evidence Based Medicine* **1(7)**: 199–200.

Geddes, J. and Lawrie, S.M. (1996) Obstetric complications and schizophrenia: a meta-analysis. *British Journal of Psychiatry* **167**: 786–93.

Geddes, J., Reynolds, S., Steiner, D. and Szatmari, P. (1997) Evidence based practice in mental health. New journal acknowledges an approach whose time has come. *British Medical Journal* **315**: 1483–84.

Geddes, J.R., Verdoux, H., Takei, N. *et al.* (1999) Schizophrenia and complications of pregnancy and labor: an individual patient data meta-analysis. *Schizophrenia Bulletin* **25(3)**: 413–23.

Geddes, J.R., Wilczynski, N., Reynolds, S., Szatmari, P. and Streiner, D.L. (1999a) Evidence-based mental health – the first year. *Evidence-Based Mental Health* **2**: 3–5.

Geddes, J., Freemantle, N. Harrison, P. and Bebbington, P. (2000) Atypical antipsychotics in the treatment of schizophrenia: systematic overview and meta-regression analysis. *British Medical Journal* **321(7273)**: 1371–6.

Geddes, L. and Harrison, P. (1997) Closing the gap between research and practice. *British Journal of Psychiatry* **171**: 220–5.

Geertz, C. (1983) *Local Knowledge: Further Essays in Interpretive Anthropology.* New York: Basic Books.

Geertz, C. (1993) *The Interpretation of Cultures.* London: Fontana.

Gerstmann, J. (1928) *Die Malariabehandlung der Progressiven Paralyse.* Wien: Springer.

Gilbody, S. and Song, F. (2000) Publication bias and the integrity of psychiatry research. *Psychological Medicine* **30**: 253–8.

Goethe, J.W. (1792–1796) *Wilhelm Meisters Lehrjahre.* Ein Roman, Berlin: Unger JF 1795–1796. Zitiert nach der Artemis-Gedenkausgabe der Werke Goethes.

Goffman, E. (1961) *Asylums: Essays on the Social Situation of Mental Patients and Other Inmates.* Anchor Books (reprinted by Pelican, Harmondsworth, 1968).

Goldberg, D.P. (1979) The costs and benefits of psychiatric care. In *The Social Consequences of Psychiatric Disorders*, L. Robins and J.K. Wing (eds). New York: Brunner/Mazel.

Goldberg, D. (1991) Cost effectiveness studies in the treatment of schizophrenia: a review. *Social Psychiatry and Psychiatric Epidemiology* **26**: 139–42.

Goldfried, M.R. and Wolfe, B.E. (1996) Psychotherapy practice and research. Repairing a strained alliance. *American Psychologist* **51(10)**: 1007–16.

Goldner, E.M. and Bilsker, D. (1995) Evidence-based psychiatry. *Canadian Journal of Psychiatry* **40**: 97–101.

Goodwin, F.K. and Jamison, K.R. (1990) *Manic-Depressive Illness.* Oxford: Oxford University Press.

Goodwin, F.K., Murphy, D.C., and Bunney, W.F. (1969). Lithium carbonate treatment in depression and mania: a longitudinal double-blind study. *Archives of General Psychiatry* **21**: 486–96.

Gottesman, I.I. and Bertelsen, A. (1989) Confirming unexpressed genotypes for schizophrenia. Risks in the offspring of Fischer's Danish identical and fraternal discordant twins. *Archives of General Psychiatry* **46**: 867–72.

Graham, P. (1998) *Cognitive Behaviour Therapy for Children and Families.* Cambridge, New York, NY: Cambridge University Press.

Gray, A., Marshall, M. and Lockwood, A. (1997) The costs of social services case management: findings from a randomised controlled trial. *British Journal of Psychiatry* **170**: 47–52.

Gray, J.A.M. (1999) Postmodern medicine. *Lancet* **354**: 1550–3.

Gray, J.M. and Robertson, I. (1989) Remediation of attentional difficulties following brain injury: three experimental single case studies. *Brain Injury* **3**: 163–70.

Greco, P.J., Eisenberg, J.M. (1993) Changing physician practices. *New England Journal of Medicine* **329**: 1271–4.

Greenhalgh, T. (1997) How to read a paper: Getting your bearings. *British Medical Journal* **315**: 243–6.

Greenwood, R.J. and McMillan, T.M. (1993) Models of rehabilitation programmes for the brain-injured adult: I. Current provision, efficacy, and good practice. *Clinical Rehabilitation* **7**: 248–55.

Gregoire, G., Derderian, F. and Le Lorier, J. (1995) Selecting the language of the publications included in a meta-analysis: is there a Tower of Babel bias? *Journal of Clinical Epidemiology* **48**: 159–63.

Griesinger, W. (1868–69) Physiopsychologische Selbstbeobachtung. *Archiv für Psychiatrie und Nervenkrankheiten* **1**: 201–3.

Griffiths, R. (1988) *Agenda for Action: A Report to the Secretary for State for Social Services*. London: HMSO.

Guarnieri, P. (1994) The History of Psychiatry in Italy: A Century of Studies. In *Discovering the History of Psychiatry*, M.S. Micale and R. Porter (eds). New York and Oxford: University Press, pp. 248–59.

Gunn, J., Maden, A. and Swinton, M. (1991) Treatment needs of prisoners with psychiatric disorders. *British Medical Journal* **303**: 338–40.

Guyatt, G., Sackett, D., Sinclair, J. *et al.* (1995) Users' guide to the medical literature: IX: A method for grading health care recommendations. *Journal of the American Medical Association* **274**: 1800–4.

Haddock, G., Morrison, A.P., Hopkins, R., Lewis, S. and Tarrier, N. (1998) Individual cognitive-behavioural interventions in early psychosis. *British Journal of Psychiatry* **34(suppl. 3)**: 305–11.

Hall, J. (1979) Assessment procedures used in studies on long-stay patients. *British Journal of Psychiatry* **135**: 330–5.

Hall, J.N. (1980) Ward rating scales for long-stay patients: a review. *Psychological Medicine* **10**: 277–88.

Halligan, P.W. and Marshall, J.C. (eds) (1996) *Method in Madness: Case Studies in Cognitive Neuropsychiatry*. Hove: Psychology Press.

Hammersley, M. (1983) *Ethnography: Principles in Practice*. London: Routledge.

Hammersley, M. (1992) *What's Wrong with Ethnography?* London: Routledge.

Hammersley, M. (ed.) (1993) *Social Research: Philosophy, Politics and Practice*. London: Sage.

Hare, E. (1983) Was insanity on the increase? *British Journal of Psychiatry* **142**: 451.

Hargreaves, W.A., Glick, I.D., Drues, J., Showstack, J.A. and Feigenbaum, E. (1977) Short versus long hospitalization: a prospective controlled study. VI: Two-year follow-up results for schizophrenics. *Archives of General Psychiatry* **34(3)**: 305–11.

Harries, U., Elliot, H. and Higgins, A. (1999) Evidence-based policy making in the NHS: exploring the interface between research and the commissioning process. *Journal of Public Health Medicine* **21(1)**: pp. 29–36.

Harris, E.C. and Barraclough, B. (1998) Excess mortality of mental disorders. *British Journal of Psychiatry* **173**: 11–53.

Hart, E. and Bond, M. (1996) *Action Research for Health and Social Care*. Buckingham: Open University Press.

Hay, P.J. (2000) Psychotherapy for bulimia nervosa and binging. *Cochrane Database of Systematic Reviews*, vol. Issue Issue **1**.

Haynes, R.B., Sackett, D.L., Gray, J.A., Cook, D.J. and Guyatt, G.H. (1996) Transferring evidence from research into practice: 1. The role of clinical care research evidence in clinical decisions. *Evidence-Based Medicine* **1(7)**: 196–7.

Haynes, R.B., Sackett, D.L., Gray, J.A., Cook, D.L. and Guyatt, G.H. (1997) Transferring evidence from research into practice: 2. Getting the evidence straight. *Evidence-Based Medicine* **2(1)**: 4–6.

Head, H. (1926) *Aphasia and Kindred Disorders*. Cambridge: Cambridge University Press.

Hegel, M.T. and Ferguson, R.J. (2000) Differential reinforcement of other behavior (DRO) to reduce aggressive behavior following traumatic brain injury. *Behavior Modification* **24**: 94–101.

Heinicke, C.M. and Ramsey-Klee, D.M. (1986) Outcome of child psychotherapy as a function of frequency of sessions. *Journal of the American Academy of Child Psychiatry* **25**: 247–53.

Hersen, M. and Barlow, P.H. (1984) *Single Case Experimental Designs: Strategies for Studying Behaviour Change*, second edition. New York: Pergamon.

Herz, M.I., Endicott, J., Spitzer, R.L. and Mesnikoff, A. (1971) Day versus in-patient hospitalization: a controlled study. *American Journal of Psychiatry* **10**: 1371–82.

Hirsch, S.R., Gain, R., Rohde, P., Stevens, B.C. and Wing, J.K. (1973) Outpatient maintenance of chronic schizophrenic patients with long-acting fluphenazine: Double-blind placebo trial. *British Medical Journal* **1**, 633–637.

Hobson, R.F. (1985) *Forms of Feeling: The Heart of Psychotherapy*. New York: Basic Books.

Hoffmann, K., Isermann, M., Kaiser, W. *et al.* (2000) Quality of life in the course of deinstitutionalisation – Part IV of the Berlin deinstitutionalisation study (in German). *Psychiatrische Praxis* **27**: 183–8.

Hogarty, G.E., Anderson, C.M., Reiss, D.J. *et al.* (1986) Family psychoeducation, social skills training, and maintenance chemotherapy in the aftercare treatment of schizophrenia. I. One-year effects of a controlled study on relapse and expressed emotion. *Archives of General Psychiatry* **43(7)**: 633–42.

Høglend, P. (1993) Personality disorders and long-term outcome after brief psychodynamic psychotherapy. *Journal of Personality Disorders* **7**: 168–81.

Hogwood, B.W. and Gunn, L.A. (1984) *Policy Analysis for the Real World*. Oxford: Oxford University Press.

Hollon, S.D., DeRubeis, R.J., Evans, M.D., Wiemer, M.J., Garvey, M.J., Grove, W.M. and Tuason, V.B. (1992) Cognitive therapy and pharmacotherapy for depression. Singly and in combination. *Archives of General Psychiatry* **49(10)**: 774–81.

Holloway, F. (1991) Case management for the mentally ill: looking at the evidence. *International Journal of Social Psychiatry* **31**: 2–13.

Holloway, F. and Carson, J. (1998) Intensive case management for the severely mentally ill: controlled trial. *British Journal of Psychiatry* **172**: 19–22.

Horton, A.M.C. and Howe, R.H. (1981) Behavioural treatment of the traumatically brain-injured: a case study. *Perceptual and Motor Skills* **53**: 349–50.

Horvath, A.O. and Symonds, B.D. (1991) Relation between working alliance and outcome in psychotherapy: a meta-analysis. *Journal of Counseling Psychology* **38**: 139–49.

Hume, D. (1777) *An Enquiry Concerning Human Understanding*. Oxford: Oxford University Press, 1902.

Hume, D. (1978) *A Treatise of Human Nature*. Oxford: Oxford University Press.

Hunter, R. and Macalpine, I. (1963) *Three Hundred Years of Psychiatry: 1535–1860*. London: Oxford University Press.

Huxley, P. (1998) Outcome management in mental health: a brief review. *Journal of Mental Health* **7(3)**: 273–84.

Institute of Medicine (1992) Committee on Clinical Practice Guidelines. *Guidelines for Clinical Practice: from Development to Use*, M.J. Field and K.N. Lohr (eds). Washington, DC: National Academy Press.

Irwig, L., Tosteson, A.N., Gatsibusm, C. *et al.* (1994) Guidelines for meta-analyses evaluating diagnostic tests. *Annals of Internal Medicine* **120**: 667–76.

Jackson, A. (ed.) (1987) *Anthropology at Home*. London: Tavistock.

Jackson, H., McGorry, P., Edwards, J. *et al.* (1998) Cognitively-oriented psychotherapy for early psychosis (COPE), preliminary results. *British Journal of Psychiatry* **172(suppl. 33)**: 93–100.

Jaspers, K. (1923) *Allgemeine Psychopathologie*. Berlin: Springer Verlag. English translation by J. Hoenig and M.W. Hamilton, *General Psychopathology*. Manchester: Manchester University Press.

Johnson, A.L. (1983) Clinical trials in psychiatry. *Psychological Medicine* **13**: 1–8.

Johnson, S., Salvador-Carulla, L. and EPCAT Group (1998) Description and classification of mental health services: a European perspective. *European Psychiatry* **13**: 333–41.

Johnstone, L. (1997) Psychiatry: are we allowed to disagree? *Clinical Psychology Forum* **100**: 31–4.

Jones, E.E., Cumming, J.D. and Pulos, S. (1993) Tracing clinical themes across phases of treatment by a Q-set. In *Psychodynamic Treatment Research: a Handbook of Clinical Practice*, N. Miller, L. Luborsky, J. Barber and J. Docherty (eds). New York: Basic Books, pp. 14–36.

Jones, K. (1993) *Asylums and After: a Revised History of the Mental Health Services from the Early Eighteenth Century to the 1990s*. London: Athlone.

Jones, R., Goldberg, D.P. *et al.* (1979) Cost-benefit analysis and the evaluation of psychiatric services. *Psychol Med* **7**: 701–701.

Joyce, A.S. and Piper, W.E. (1993) The immediate impact of transference interpretation in short-term individual psychotherapy. *American Journal of Psychotherapy* **47**: 508–26.

Juni, P., Witschi, A., Bloch, R. and Egger, M. (1999) The hazards of scoring the quality of clinical trials for meta-analysis (see comments). *Journal of the American Medical Association* **282**: 1054–60.

Kaiser, W., Isermann, M., Hoffmann, K. and Priebe, S. (1998) Entlassungen in vollstationäre Einrichtungen – Ergebnisse einer Umfrage. Postskriptum zu Teil III der Berliner Enthospitalisierungsstudie (Discharge of patients to full-time institutional settings. Results of a survey. Postscript to Part III of the Berlin Deinstitutionalization Study). *Psychiatrische Praxis* **26**: 22–4.

Kandel, E.R. (1998) A new intellectual framework for psychiatry. *American Journal of Psychiatry* **155**: 457–69.

Kandel, E.R. (1999) Biology and the future of psychoanalysis: a new intellectual framework for psychiatry revisited. *American Journal of Psychiatry* **156**: 505–24.

Karp, D.A. (1992) Illness ambiguity and the search for meaning. *Journal of Contemporary Ethnography* **21(2)**: 139–70.

Kazdin, A.E. (1984) Statistical analyses for single case experimental design. In *Single Case Experimental Designs: Strategies for Studying Behaviour Change*, second edition, M. Hersen and P.H. Barlow (eds). New York: Pergamon.

Kearney, S. and Fussey, I. (1991) The use of adapted leisure materials to reinforce correct head positioning in a brain-injured adult. *Brain Injury* **5**: 295–302.

Keck, P.E., McElroy, S.L., Strakowski, S.M., *et al.* (1996) Factors associated with maintenance anti-psychotic treatment of patients with bipolar disorder. *Journal of Clinical Psychiatry* **57**: 147–51.

Kemp, R., Kirov, B., Everitt, B., Hayward, P. and David, A. (1998) Randomised controlled trial of compliance therapy. *British Journal of Psychiatry* **172**: 413–19.

Kendler, K.S. (1990) Toward a scientific psychiatric nosology: strengths and limitations. *Archives of General Psychiatry* **149**: 112–17.

Kessler, R.C., McGonagle, K.A., Zhao, S. *et al.* (1994) Lifetime and 12-month prevalence of DSM-III-R psychiatric disorders in the United States: results from the National Comorbidity Survey. *Archives of General Psychiatry* **51**: 8–19.

Khan, A., Warner, H.A. and Brown, W.A. (2000) Symptom reduction and suicide risk in patients treated with placebo in antidepressant clinical trials. *Archives of General Psychiatry* **57**: 311–17.

Kingdon, D.G. and Turkington, D. (1991) The use of cognitive behavior therapy with a normalizing rationale in schizophrenia. Preliminary report. *Journal of Nervous and Mental Disease* **179(4)**: 207–11.

Kitcher, P. (1999) Sigmund Freud. In *The MIT Encyclopedia of the Cognitive Sciences*, R.A. Wilson and F.C. Keil (eds). Cambridge, MA: The MIT Press, pp. 328–9.

Kleijnen, J., Gotzsche, P., Kunz, R.A., Oxman, A.D. and Chalmers, I. (1997) So what's so special about randomisation? In *Non-Random Reflections on Health Services Research*, A. Maynard and I. Chalmer (eds). London: British Medical Journal Publications, pp. 93–107.

Kleinman, A. (1977) Culture, depression and the 'new' cross cultural psychiatry. *Social Science and Medicine* **11**: 3–11.

Kleinman, A. (1986) *Social Origins of Distress and Disease: Depression, Neurasthenia and Pain in Modern China*. New Haven, CT: Yale University Press.

Kleinman, A. (1987) Anthropology and Psychiatry: the Role of Culture in Cross-Cultural Research on Illness. *British Journal of Psychiatry* **151**: 447–54.

Klerman, G.L., Weissman, M.M., Rouansaville, B.J. and Chevron, E.S. (1984) *Interpersonal Therapy of Depression I*. New York: Basic Books.

Kluiter, H. (1997) Inpatient treatment and care arrangements to replace or avoid it – searching for an evidence-based balance. *Current Opinion in Psychiatry* **10**: 160–7.

Kluiter, H. and Wiersma, D. (1996) Randomised controlled trials of programmes. In *Mental Health Service Evaluation*, H.C. Knudsen and G. Thornicroft (eds). Cambridge: Cambridge University Press, pp. 259–80.

Korn, E.L. and Baumrind, S. (1991) Randomised clinical trials with clinician-preferred treatment. *Lancet* **337**: 149–53.

Kottgen, C., Sonnichsen, I., Mollenhauser, K. and Jurth, R. (1984) Group therapy with families of schizophrenia patients: results of the Hamburg Camberwell family interview study III. *International Journal of Family Psychiatry* **5**: 84–94.

Kovacs, M., Rush, A.J., Beck, A.T. and Hollon, S.D. (1981) Depressed outpatients treated with cognitive therapy or pharmacotherapy. A one-year follow-up. *Archives of General Psychiatry* **38(1)**: 33–9.

Koyré, A. (1968) *Metaphysics and Measurement: Essays in the Scientific Revolution*. London: Chapman and Hall.

Krause, B. (1989) *The Sinking Heart: A Punjabi Communication of Distress.*

Krause, R. (1997) *Allgemeine psychoanalytische Krankheitslehre. Grundlagen.* Stuttgart, Germany: Kohlhammer.

Krupnick, J.L., Sotsky, S.M., Simmens, S. *et al.* (1996) The role of the therapeutic alliance in psychotherapy and pharmacotherapy outcome: findings in the National Institute of Mental Health Treatment of Depression Collaborative Research Program. *Journal of Consulting and Clinical Psychology* **64**: 532–9.

Kuhn, T. (1962) *The Structure of Scientific Revolutions.* Chicago: University of Chicago Press.

Kuipers, E., Garety, P., Fowler, D. *et al.* (1997) The London East Anglia randomised control trial of cognitive behaviour therapy for psychosis. I: effects of the treatment phase. *British Journal of Psychiatry* **171**: 319–27.

Kunz, R. and Oxman, A.D. (1998) The unpredictability paradox: review of empirical comparisons of randomised and non-randomised clinical trials. *British Medical Journal* **317**: 1185–90.

L'Abbe, K.A., Detsky, A.S. and O'Rourke, K. (1987) Meta-analysis in clinical research. *Annals of Internal Medicine* **107**: 224–33.

Laing, R.D. (1960) *The Divided Self.* Harmondsworth: Penguin.

Laing, R.D. (1960) *The Divided Self.* London: Tavistock.

Lau, J., Joannidis, J.P.A. and Schmid, C.H. (1998) Summing up evidence: one answer is not always enough. *Lancet* **351**: 123–7.

Laugharne, R. (1999) Evidence-based medicine, user involvement and the postmodern paradigm. *Psychiatric Bulletin* **23**: 641–3.

Leach, E.R. (1954) *Political Systems of Highland Burma.* Cambridge, MA: Harvard University Press.

Lebow, J.L. (1983) Research assessing consumer satisfaction with mental health treatment: a review of findings. *Evaluation and Program Planning* **6**: 211–21.

Leff, J. (1988) *Psychiatry Around the Globe: A Transcultural View.* London: Gaskell.

Leff, J., Kuipers, L., Berkowitz, R., Eberlein-Vries, R. and Sturgeon, D. (1982) A controlled trial of social intervention in the families of schizophrenic patients. *British Journal of Psychiatry* **141**: 121–34.

Leff, J., Kuipers, L. and Sturgeon, D. (1985) A controlled trial of social intervention in the families of schizophrenic patients: two-year follow up. *British Journal of Psychiatry* **146**: 594–600.

Lehman, A.F. (1996) Measures of quality among persons with severe and persistent mental disorders. In *Mental Health Outcome Measures*, G. Thornicroft and M. Tansella (eds). Heidelberg: Springer, pp. 75–92.

Lehman, A.F., Steinwachs, D.M. and the Co-Investigators of the PORT Project (1998a) An issue: translating research into practice: the schizophrenia Patient Outcomes Research Team (PORT) treatment recommendations. *Schizophrenia Bulletin* **24**: 1–10.

Lehman, A.F., Steinwachs, D.M. and the Co-Investigators of the PORT Project (1998b) Patterns of usual care for schizophrenia: initial results from the schizophrenia Patient Outcomes Research Team [PORT] client survey. *Schizophrenia Bulletin* **24**: 11–20.

Lewis, A. (1967) *The State of Psychiatry.* London: Routledge and Kegan Paul.

Lewis, S. (1995) A search for meaning: making sense of depression. *Journal of Mental Health* **4**: 369–82.

Licht, R.W. (1998) Drug treatment of mania: a critical review. *Acta Psychiatrica Scandinavica* **97**: 387–97.

Licht, R.W., Gouliea, G., Vesterfaarl, P. *et al.* (1994) Treatment of manic episodes in Scandinavia; the use of neuroleptic drugs in a clinical routine setting. *Journal of Affective Disorders* **32**: 179–85.

Littlewood, R. (1986) Russian Dolls and Chinese Boxes: an Anthropological Approach to the Implicit Models of Comparative Psychiatry. In Transcultural Psychiatry, J. Cox (ed.). London: Croom Helm.

Littlewood, R. (1990) From categories to contexts: a decade of the new cross-cultural psychiatry. *British Journal of Psychiatry* **156**: 308–27.

Littlewood, R. and Lipsedge, M. (1985) Culture Bound Syndromes. *In Recent Advances in Clinical Psychiatry 5*, K. Granville-Grossman (ed.). Edinburgh: Churchill Livingstone.

Littlewood, R. and Lipsedge, M. (1988) Psychiatric illness among British Afro-Caribbeans. *British Medical Journal* **296**: 950–1.

Locke, J. (1690a) *An Essay Concerning Human Understanding*, P.H. Nidditch (ed.). Oxford: Oxford University Press, 1975.

Locke, J. (1690b) *Two Treatises on Government*, P. Laslett Nidditch (ed.). Cambridge: Cambridge University Press, 1960.

Lomas, J., Enkin, M., Anderson, G.M., *et al.* (1991) Opinion leaders versus audit and feedback to implement practice guidelines. Delivery after previous cesarian section. *Journal of the American Medical Association* **265**: 2202–7.

Lonigan, C.J., Elbert, J.C. and Johnson, S.B. (1998) Empirically supported psychosocial interventions for children: an overview. *Journal of Clinical Child Psychology* **27**: 138–45.

Loudon, J.B. and Waring, H. (1976) Toxic reactions to lithium and haloperidol. *Lancet* **2**: 1088.

Lyotard, J.F. (1984) *The Postmodern Condition: a Report on Knowledge*. Manchester: Manchester University Press.

MacFarlane, W., Dushay, R., Stasny, P., Deakins, S. and Link, B. (1996) A comparison of two levels of family-aided assertive community treatment. *Psychiatric Services* **47**: 744–50.

Maden, A., Taylor, C., Brook, D. and Gunn, J. (1995) *Mental Disorder in Remand Prisoners*. A report commissioned by the Directorate of Prison Health Care, Home Office unpublished report. Cited in *Special Hospitals Service Authority*, London: Service for Security Care, Home Office.

Maggs, R. (1963) Treatment of manic illness with lithium carbonate. *British Journal of Psychiatry* **109**: 56–65.

Maidment, I. (2000) St John's Wort in the treatment of depression. *Psychiatric Bulletin* **24**: 232–4.

Main, M. and Hesse, P. (1990) Lack of resolution of mourning in adulthood and its relationship to infant disorganisation: some speculations regarding causal mechanisms. In *Attachment in the Preschool Years*, M. Greenberg, D. Cicchetti and E.M. Cummings (eds). Chicago: University of Chicago Press, pp. 161–82.

Maj, M., Pirozzi, R., Magliano, L., Bartoli, L. (1998) Long-term outcome of lithium prophylaxis in bipolar disorder: a 5-year prospective study of 402 patients at a lithium clinic. *American Journal of Psychiatry* **155**: 30–5.

Malan, D.H. (1963) *A Study of Brief Psychotherapy*: New York: Plenum Press.

Malan, D.H. (1976) *The Frontiers of Brief Psychotherapy*. New York: Plenum Press.

Malinowski, B. (1919) Kula: The circulating exchange of valuables in the archipelagos of Eastern New Guinea. *Man* **20**: 97–105.

Malinowski, B. (1967) *A Diary in the Strict Sense of the Term*. London: Routledge and Kegan Paul.

Mander, A.J. and Loudon, J.B. (1988) Rapid recurrence of mania following abrupt discontinuation of lithium. *Lancet* **ii**: 15–17.

Mann, J. (1973) *Time-limited Psychotherapy*. Cambridge, MA: Harvard University Press.

Markowitz, J.C., Klerman, G.L. and Perry, S.W. (1992) Interpersonal psychotherapy of depressed HIV-positive outpatients. *Hospital and Community Psychiatry* **43(9)**: 885–90.

Marks, I.M., Connolly, J., Muijen, M. *et al.* (1994) Home-based versus hospital-based care for people with serious mental illness. *British Journal of Psychiatry* **165**: 179–94.

Marmor, J. (1975) *Psychiatrists and their Patients: a National Study of Private Office Practice*. Washington, DC: The Joint Information Service of the American Psychiatric Association and the National Association for Mental Health.

Marriott, S. and Palmer, C. (1996) Clinical practice guidelines: on what evidence is our clinical practice based? *Psychiatric Bulletin* **20**: 363–66.

Marshall, M. (1996) Case management: a dubious practice, *British Medical Journal* **312(7030)**: 523–4.

Marshall, M. (1996) *Case Management for People with Severe Mental Disorders*. In *The Cochrane Library*. London: British Medical Journal Publications.

Marshall, M. and Lockwood, A. (1998) *Assertive Community Treatment for People with Severe Mental Disorders* (Cochrane Review). *The Cochrane Library* [3].

Marshall, M. and Lockwood, A. (1999) *Assertive Community Treatment for People with Severe Mental Disorders* (Cochrane Review). In *The Cochrane Library*, Oxford: Update Software.

Marshall, M., Lockwood, A. and Gath, D. (1995) Social services case-management for long-term mental disorders: a randomised controlled trial. *Lancet* **345**: 409–12.

Marshall, M., Gray, A., Lockwood, A. and Green, R. (1997) *Case Management for Severe Mental Disorders. The Cochrane Collaboration* [2].

Marshall, M., Lockwood, A., Gray, A. and Green, R. (1999) *Case Management for People with Severe Mental Disorders – a Systematic Review* (Cochrane Review) In: The Cochrane Library. Oxford: Update Software.

Marshall, M., Crowther, R., Almaraz-Serrano, A.M. *et al.* (2000) Day hospital versus admission for acute psychiatric disorders (a systematic review of individual patient data). In preparation.

Marshall, M., Lockwood, A., Bradley, C. *et al.* (2000) Unpublished rating scales a major source of bias in randomised controlled trials of treatments for schizophrenia? *British Journal of Psychiatry* **176**: 249–53.

Martinson, R. (1974) What works? Questions and answers about prison reform. *Public Interest* **35**: 22–45.

Mateer, C.A. and Ruff, R.M. (1990) Effectiveness of behavioral management procedures in the rehabilitation of head-injured patients. In *Neurobehavioural Sequelae of Traumatic Brain Injury*, R.L.I. Wood (ed.). New York: Taylor and Francis.

Mattes, J.A., Rosen, B. and Klein, D.F. (1977) Comparison of the clinical effect-iveness of 'short' versus 'long' stay psychiatric hospitalization. II. Results of a 3-year post-hospital follow-up. *Journal of Nervous and Mental Disease* **165(6)**: 387–94.

Maudsley, H. (1868) *Physiologie und Pathologie der Seele*. Würzburg: A. Stubers-Buchhandlung.

Mays, N. and Pope, C. (1995) Qualitative research: rigour and qualitative research. *British Medical Journal* **311**: 109–12.

Mays, N. and Pope, C. (eds) (1996) *Qualitative Research in Health Care*. London: BMJ Books, p. 18.

McCreadie, R.G. and Morrison, D.P. (1985) The impact of lithium in south-west Scotland. *British Journal of Psychiatry* **146**: 70–4.

McGovern, D. and Owen, A. (1999) Intensive case management for severe psychotic illness. *Lancet* **354**: 1384–6.

McGrew, J.H. and Bond, G.R. (1995) Critical ingredients of assertive community treatment: judgments of the experts. *Journal of Mental Health Administration* **22(2)**: 113–25.

McHugo, G.J., Drake, R.E., Teague, G.B. and Xie, H. (1999) Fidelity to assertive community treatment and client outcomes in the New Hampshire dual disorders study. *Psychiatric Services* **50(6)**: 818–24.

McKay, H. and Barkham, M. (1998) *Evidence from Cochrane reviews and published reviews and meta-analyses 1990–1998: report to the National Counselling and Psycho-logical Therapies Clinical Guidelines Development Group*. Psychological Therapies Research Centre, University of Leeds.

McLean, A., Jr, Stanton, K.M., Cardenas, D.D. and Bergerud, D.B. (1987) Memory training combined with the use of oral physostigmine. *Brain Injury* **1**: 145–59.

Mechanic, D. (1998) Emerging trends in mental health policy and practice. *Health Affairs* **17** November/December: 82–98.

Medical Disability Society (1998) *Report of the Working Party on the Management of Traumatic Brain Injury*. London: Royal College of Physicians.

Meehl, P. (1954) *Clinical Versus Statistical Prediction*. Minnesota: University of Minnesota Press.

Meichenbaum, D. (1974) *Cognitive Behaviour Modification*. Morristown, NJ: Gen-eral Learning Press.

Mental Health Foundation (1997) *Knowing Our Own Minds*. London: Mental Health Foundation.

Mental Health Foundation (2000) *Strategies for Living*. London: Mental Health Foundation.

Miles, M.B. and Huberman, A.M. (1984) *Qualitative Data Analysis: a Sourcebook of New Methods*. London: Sage.

Mill, J.S. (1843) *A System of Logic*. London: John W. Parker.

Milrod, B., Busch, F., Cooper, A. and Shapiro, T. (1997) *Manual for Panic-Focused Psychodynamic Psychotherapy*. Washington, DC: American Psychiatric Press.

Milton, J. (1993) *Presenting the Case for Psychoanalytic Psychotherapy Services*.

Mojtabai, R. and Rieder, R. (1998) Limitations of the symptom-oriented approach to psychiatric research. *British Journal of Psychiatry* **173**: 198–202.

Moncrieff, J. (1997) Lithium: evidence reconsidered. *British Journal of Psychiatry* **171**: 113–19.

Monsen, J., Odland, T., Faugli, A., Daae, E. and Eilersten, D.E. (1995a) Personality disorders and psychosocial changes after intensive psychotherapy: a prospective follow-up study of an outpatient psychotherapy project, 5 years after the end of treatment. *Scandinavian Journal of Psychology* **36**: 256–68.

Monsen, J., Odland, T., Faugli, A., Daae, E. and Eilersten, D.E. (1995b) Personality disorders: changes and stability after intensive psychotherapy focussing on affect consciousness. *Psychotherapy Research* **5**: 33–48.

Moran, G., Fonagy, P., Kurtz, A., Bolton, A. and Brook, C. (1991) A controlled study of the psychoanalytic treatment of brittle diabetes. *Journal of the American Academy of Child and Adolescent Psychiatry* **30**: 926–35.

Morley, S., Ecclestone, C. and Williams, A.C. de C. (1999) Systematic review and meta-analysis of randomised controlled trials of cognitive behaviour therapy and behaviour therapy for chronic pains in adults, excluding headache. *Pain* **80**: 1–13.

Mosher, L. (1983) Alternatives to psychiatric hospitalisation: why has research failed to be translated into practice? *New England Journal of Medicine* **309**: 1579–80.

Mueser, K.T. and Berenbaum, H. (1990) Psychodynamic treatment of schizophrenia: is there a future? *Psychological Medicine* **2**: 253–62.

Mueser, K.T., Bond, G.R., Drake, R.E. and Resnick, S.G. (1998) Models of community care for severe mental illness: a review of research on case management. *Schizophrenia Bulletin* **24(1)**: 37–74.

Mufson, L., Moreau, D., Weissman, M.M. *et al.* (1994) Modification of interpersonal psychotherapy with depressed adolescents (IPT-A): phase I and II studies. *Journal of the American Academy of Child and Adolescent Psychiatry* **33(5)**: 695–705.

Muijen, M., Marks, I., Connolly, J. and Audini, B. (1992) Home based care and standard hospital care for patients with severe mental illness: a randomised controlled trial. *British Medical Journal* **304(6829)**: 749–54.

Muir Gray, J.A.- Churchill Livingstone (1997) Evidence Based Healthcare – how to make Health Policy and Management Decisions – Policy Analysis for the Real World – Brian W. Hogwood and Lewis A. Gunn – *Oxford University Press* – 1984.

Müller, Ch. (1998) *Wer hat die Geisteskranken von den Ketten befreit. Skizzen zur Psychiatriegeschichte?* Bonn: Edition Das Narrenschiff im Psychiatrie Verlag.

Mulrow, C.D. (1987) The medical review article: state of the science. *Annals of Internal Medicine* **106**: 485–8.

Mulrow, C.D. (1994) Rationale for systematic reviews. *British Medical Journal* **309**: 597–9.

Mulrow, C.D., Williams, J.W., Jr, Gerety, M.B. *et al.* (1995) Case-finding instruments for depression in primary care settings. *Annals of Internal Medicine* **122**: 913–21.

Murdoch, B.E., Pitt, G., Theordoros, D.G. and Ward, E.C. (1999) Real-time continuous visual biofeedback in the treatment of speech breathing disorders following childhood traumatic brain injury: a case report. *Paediatric Rehabilitation* **3**: 5–20.

Murphy, E., Dingwall, R., Greatbatch, D. *et al.* (1998a) Qualitative research methods in health technology assessment: a review of the literature. *Health Technology Assessment* **2(16)**: 1–276.

Murphy, M.K., Black, N.A., Lamping, D.L. *et al.* (1998b) Consensus development methods, and their use in clinical guideline development. *NHS Health Technology Assessment Programme* **2(3)**.

National Institute of Mental Health. (1985) *Measuring Social Functioning. Mental Health Studies: Concepts and Instruments*. NIMH: Rockville (DHHS Publication No. (ADM) 85–1384).

Nayak, D. (1998) In defense of polypharmacy. *Psychiatric Annals* **28**: 190–6.

Naylor, C.D. (1995) Grey zones of clinical practice: some limits to evidence-based medicine. *Lancet* **310**: 101–3.

Office of Population Censuses and Surveys (1995) *The Prevalence of Psychiatric Morbidity among Adults Living in Private Households*. London: HMSO.

Okely, J. (1996) *Own or Other Culture*. London: Routledge.

Okely, J. and Callaway, H. (eds) (1992) *Anthropology and Autobiography* (edited volume). London: Routledge.

Olfson, M. & Pincus, H.A. (1994) Outpatient psychotherapy in the United States, II: Patterns of utilization. *American Journal of Psychiatry*, **151**, 1289–94.

Olfson, M. and Pincus H.A. (1996) Outpatient mental health care in nonhospital settings: distribution of patients across provider groups. *American Journal of Psychiatry* **153**: 1353–6.

Olfson, M., Pincus, H.A. and Dial, T.H. (1994) Professional practice patterns of US psychiatrists. *American Journal of Psychiatry* **151**: 89–95.

O'Malley, S.S., Foley, S.H., Rounsaville, B.J. *et al.* (1988) Therapist competence and patient outcome in interpersonal psychotherapy of depression. *Journal of Consulting and Clinical Psychology* **56**: 496–501.

Oppenheim, A.N. (1997) *Questionnaire Design, Interviewing and Attitude Measurement*. London: Pinter Publishers Ltd.

Orlinsky, D.E., Grawe, K. and Parks, B.K. (1994) Process and outcome in psychotherapy. In *Handbook of Psychotherapy and Behaviour Change*, fourth edition, A.E. Bergin and S.L. Garfield (eds). New York: Wiley, pp. 270–376.

Owens, D.J. and Batchelor, C. (1996) Patient satisfaction and the elderly. *Social Science and Medicine* **42(11)**: 1483–91.

Oxford Interactive Encyclopedia (CD Rom) (1997) TLC Properties Inc. *The Electronic New Shorter English Dictionary, Encyclopedia Edition 1996*. Oxford: Oxford University Press.

Oxman, A.D., Guyatt, G.H., Singer, J. *et al.* (1991) Agreement among reviewers of review articles. *Journal of Clinical Epidemiology*. **44**: 91–8.

Pardes, H., Sirovatka, P. and Pincus, H.A. (1985) Federal and state roles in mental health. In: *Psychiatry: a Multi-volume Textbook*, J.O. Cavenar Jr (ed.). Philadelphia: Lippincott and Co.

Parry, G. (2000) Developing treatment choice guidelines in psychotherapy. *Journal of Mental Health* **9(3)**: 273–82.

Pasamanick, B., Albini, J.L., Scarpitti, F.R., Lefton, M. and Dinitz, S. (1966) Two years of a home care study for schizophrenics. *Proceedings of the Annual Meeting of the American Psychopathological Association* **54**: 515–26.

Paterson, A. and Zangwill, O.L. (1944) Recovery of spatial orientation in the post-traumatic confusional state. *Brain* **67**: 54–8.

Patton, M.Q. (1990) *Qualitative Evaluation and Research Methods*. London: Sage.

Pawson, R. and Tilley, N. (1997) *Realistic Evaluation*. London: Sage.

Pelosi, A.J. and Jackson, G.A. (2000) Home treatment – enigmas and fantasies. *British Medical Journal* **320(7230)**: 308–9.

Perkins, R. (2000) Solid evidence? *Open Mind* **101(Jan/Feb)**: 6.

Perry, A., Tarrier, N., Morris, R., McCarthy, E. and Limb, K. (1999) Randomised controlled trial of efficacy of teaching patients with bipolar disorder to identify early symptoms of relapse and obtain treatment. *British Medical Journal* **318**: 149–53.

Persel, C.S., Persel, C.H., Ashly, M.J. and Krych, D.K. (1997) The use of non-contingent reinforcement and contingent restraint to reduce physical aggression and self-injurious behaviour in a traumatically brain-injured adult. *Brain Injury* **11**: 751–60.

Peto, R., Collins, R. and Gray, R. (1993) Large-scale randomized evidence: large, simple trials and overviews of trials. *Annals of the New York Academy of Science* **703**: 314–40.

Pharoah, F., Mari, J. and Streiner, D.L. (2000) Family intervention for schizophrenia. *Cochrane Database of Systematic Reviews*, vol. Issue **1**: 2000.

Pharoah, F.M., Mari, J.J. and Streiner, D. (2000) Family intervention for schizophrenia (Cochrane Review) In: *The Cochrane Library*, Issue 4. Oxford: Update Software.

Phelan, M., Slade, M., Thornicroft, G. *et al.* (1995) The Camberwell Assessment of Need: the validity and reliability of an instrument to assess the need of people with severe mental illness. *British Journal of Psychiatry* **167**: 589–95.

Pick, A. (1903) On reduplicative paramnesia. *Brain* **36**: 260–7.

Pincus, H.A. and McQueen, L. (in press) The limits of an evidence-based classification of mental disorders. In *Psychiatric Classification and Values*, Sadler J.Z. (ed.). Washington, DC: American Psychiatric Press.

Pincus, H.A., Pardes, H., Rosenfeld, A.H. (1983) Consensus development conferences: assessing and communicating advances in mental health research. *American Journal of Psychiatry* **140**: 1329–31.

Pincus, H.A., Zarin, D.A. and West, J.C. (1996) Peering into the 'black box': measuring outcomes of managed care. *Archives of General Psychaitry* **53**: 870–7.

Pincus, H.A., Tanielian, T.L., Marcus, S.C., Olfson, M., Zarin, D.A., Thomson, J. and Magus Zits, J. (1998) Prescribing trends in psychotropic medications: primary care, psychiatry, and other medical specialties. *Journal of the American Medical Association* **279**: 526–31.

Pincus, H.A., Zarin, D.A., Tanielian, T.L. *et al.* (1999) Psychiatric patients and treatments in 1997: findings from the American Psychiatric Practice Research Network. *Archives of General Psychiatry* **56**: 441–9.

Pinel, P. (1801) *Traité médico-philosophique sur l'aliénation mentale ou la manie.* Paris: Richard, Caille and Ravier.

Pocock, S.J. (1987) *Clinical Trials: A Practical Approach.* Chichester: Wiley.

Popper, K. (1959) *The Logic of Scientific Discovery.* London: Hutchinson.

Popper, K.R. (1962) *Conjectures and Refutations.* New York: Basic Books.

Popper, K.R. (1963) *Conjectures and Refutations.* London: Routledge and Kegan Paul.

Porter, R. (1993) Hearing the mad. Communication and excommunication. In *Proceedings of the 1st European Congress on the History of Psychiatry and Mental Health Care*, L. de Goei and J. Vijslaar (eds). Rotterdam: Erasmus, pp. 338–52.

Porter, R. and Micale, M.S. (1994) Reflection on psychiatry and its histories. In *Discovering the History of Psychiatry*, M.S. Micale and R. Porter (eds). New York and Oxford: Oxford University Press, pp. 3–36.

Post, R.M., Ketter, T.A., Pazzaglia, P.J. *et al.* (1996) Rational polypharmacy in the bipolar affective disorders. *Epilepsy Research Supplement* **11**: 153–80.

Priebe, S. (1989) Über die Subjektivität der psychiatrischen Diagnose (On the subjectivity of psychiatric diagnosis). *Psychiatrische Praxis* **16**: 86–9.

Priebe, S. (2000) Ensuring and improving quality in community mental health care. *International Review of Psychiatry* **12**: 226–32.

Prien, R.F., Caffey, E.M., Jr., Klett, C.J. (1973) Prophylactic efficacy of lithium carbonate in manic-depressive illness. *Archives of General Psychiatry* **28**: 337–41.

Rack, P. (1982) *Race, Culture and Mental Disorder*. London: Tavistock.

Rees L. (1997) The place of clinical trials in the development of psychopharmacology. *History of Psychiatry* **8**: 1–20.

Reil, J.C. (1808) *Beiträge zur Beförderung einer Curmethode auf Psychischem Wege*. Halle: Curtsche Buchhandlung.

Renfey, G. and Spates, C.R. (1994) Eye movement desensitisation: A partial dismantling study. *Journal of Behaviour Therapy and Experimental Psychiatry* **25**: 231–9.

Reus, V.I. (1993) Rational polypharmacy in the treatment of mood disorders. *Annals of Clinical Psychiatry* **5**: 91–100.

Reynolds, S. (2000) Evidence based practice and psychotherapy research. *Journal of Mental Health* **9(3)**: 257–66.

Reznek, L. (1991) *The philosophical defence of psychiatry*. London: Routledge.

Robertson, I., Gray, J. and McKenzie, S. (1988) Microcomputer-based cognitive rehabilitation of visual neglect: three multiple-baseline single-case studies. *Brain Injury* **2**: 151–63.

Robinson, W.S. (1951) The logical structure of analytic induction. *American Sociological Review* **16(6)**: 812–18.

Roelcke, V. (1999) Laborwissenschaft und Psychiatrie: Prämissen und Implikationen bei Emil Kraepelins Neuformulierung der psychiatrischen Krankheitslehre. In *Strategien der Kausalität: Konzepte der Krankheitsverursachung im 19. und 20. Jahrhundert*, C. Gradmann and T. Schlich (eds). Pfaffenweiler: Centaurus, pp. 93–116.

Rogers, A., Day, J.C., Williams, B., *et al.* (1998) The meaning and management of neuroleptic medication: a study of patients with a diagnosis of schizophrenia. *Social Science and Medicine* **47(9)**: 1313–23.

Rosenhan, D.L. (1981) On being sane in insane places. *Science* **179**: 250–8.

Roth, A. and Fonagy, P. (1996) *What works for whom?* London: Guilford Press.

Roth, A.D. and Parry, G. (1997) The implications of psychotherapy research for clinical practice and service development: lessons and limitations. *Journal of Mental Health* **6(4)**: 367–80.

Rounsaville, B.J., O'Malley, S., Foley, S. and Weissman, M.M. (1988) Role of manual guided training in the conduct and efficacy of interpersonal therapy for depression. *Journal of Consulting and Clinical Psychology* **56**: 681–8.

Ruggeri, M. (1996) Satisfaction with psychiatric services. In *Mental Health Outcome Measures*, G. Thornicroft and M. Tansella (eds). Heidelberg: Springer, pp. 27–51.

Ruggeri, M. and Dall'Agnola, R. (1993) The development and use of Verona Expectations for Care Scale (VECS) and the Verona Service Satisfaction (VSS*)*. *Psychological Medicine* **23**: 511–24.

Ruggeri, M., Biggeri, A., Rucci, P. and Tansella, M. (1998) Multivariate analysis of outcome of mental health care using graphical chain models. *Psychological Medicine* **28**: 1421–31.

Sabshin, M. (1990) Turning points in twentieth century American psychiatry. *American Journal of Psychiatry* **147(10)**: 1267–74.

Sackett, D.L. and Wennberg, J.E. (1997) Choosing the best research design for each question. *British Medical Journal* **315**: 1636–27.

Sackett, D.L., Haynes, R.B., Guyatt, G.H. and Tugwell, P. (1991) *Clinical Epidemiology: A Basic Science for Clinical Medicine.* Toronto: Little Brown.

Sackett, D., Rosenberg, W., Muir Gray, J., Haynes, R. and Richardson, W. (1996) Evidence based medicine: what it is and what it isn't. *British Medical Journal* **312**: 71–2.

Sackett, D.L., Richardson, S., Rosenberg, W. and Haynes, R.B. (1997) *Evidence-based Medicine: How to Practise and Teach EBM.* London: Churchill Livingstone.

Salkovskis, P.M., Forrester, E. and Richards, C. (1998) Cognitive-behavioural approach to understanding obsessional thinking, *British Journal of Psychiatry (Supplement)* **35**: 53–63.

Salvador-Carulla, L. (1996) Assessment instruments in psychiatry: description and psychometric properties. In *Mental Health Outcome Measures*, G. Thornicroft and M. Tansella (eds). Heidelberg: Springer Verlag, pp. 189–206.

Salvador-Carulla, L. (1999) Routine outcome assessment in mental health research. *Current Opinion in Psychiatry* **12**: 207–10.

Sandell, R. (1999) *Long-Term Findings of the Stockholm Outcome of Psychotherapy and Psychoanalysis Project (STOPPP).* Paper presented at the Psychoanalytic Long-Term Treatments Conference: A Challenge for Clinical and Empirical Research in Psychoanalysis, Hamburg, Germany.

Sargent, W. and Slater, E. (1946, 1948, 1963). *An Introduction to Physical Methods of Treatment in Psychiatry.* Edinburgh: Livingstone.

Sartorius, N. (1983) Evaluation in mental health programmes. In *Methodology in Evaluation of Psychiatric Treatment*, T. Helgason (ed.). Cambridge: Cambridge University Press, pp. 59–67.

Sartorius, N. (1997) Evaluating mental health services. A world perspective. In *Making Rational Mental Health Services*, M. Tansella (ed.). Rome: Il Pensiero Scientifico Editore, pp. 239–45.

Sartorius, N. and Harding, N. (1984) Issues in the evaluation of mental health care. In *Evaluation of Health Care*, W.W. Holland (ed.). Oxford: Oxford University Press, pp. 226–42.

Sartorius, N. and Janca, A. (1996) Psychiatric assessment instruments developed by the World Health Organisation. In *Mental Health Outcome Measures*, G. Thornicroft and M. Tansella (eds)., Heidelberg: Springer Verlag, pp. 153–77.

Sartorius, N., Jablensky, A., Korten, G. *et al.* (1986) Early manifestations and first-contact incidence of schizophrenia in different cultures. *Psychological Medicine* **16**: 909–28.

Savage, G. (1886) Documented quote. *Journal of Mental Science* **32**: 301.

Sazbon, L. and Groswasser, Z. (1991) Time-related sequelae of TBI in patients with prolonged post-comatose unawareness (PC-U) state. *Brain Injury* **5**: 3–8.

Schene, A., Tessler, R. and Gamache, G. (1994) Instruments measuring family or care giver burden in severe mental illness. *Social Psychiatry and Psychiatric Epidemiology* **29**: 228–40.

Schinnar, A.P., Rothbard, A.B., Kanter, R. and Jung, Y.S. (1990) An empirical literature review of definitions of severe and persistent mental illness. *American Journal of Psychiatry* **147**: 1602–8.

Schmidt, U., Tanner, M., Dent, J. (1996) Evidence-based psychiatry: pride and prejudice (editorial). *Psychiatric Bulletin* **20**: 705–7.

Schmiedebach, H.-P. (1986) *Psychiatrie und Psychologie im Widerstreit. Die Auseinandersetzung in der Berliner medicinisch-psychologischen Gesellschaft (1867–1899)*. Husum: Matthiesen (Abhandlungen zur Geschichte der Medizin und der Naturwissenschaften, 51).

Schou, M. (1984) Long-lasting neurological sequelae after lithium intoxication. *Acta Psychiatrica Scandinavica* **70**: 594–602.

Schou, M., Juel-Nielson, N., Stromgren, E. and Voldby, H. (1954) The treatment of manic psychoses by administration of lithium salts. *Journal of Neurology, Neurosurgery and Psychiatry* **17**: 250–60.

Schulz, K.F., Chalmers, I., Hayes, R.J. and Altman, D.G. (1995) Empirical evidence of bias. Dimensions of methodological quality associated with estimates of treatment effects in controlled trials. *Journal of the American Medical Association* **273**: 408–12.

Scott, J. (1988) Chronic depression. *British Journal of Psychiatry* **153**: 287–97.

Scott, J.E. and Dixon, L.B. (1995) Assertive community treatment and case management for schizophrenia. *Schizophrenia Bulletin* **21**: 657–68.

Scull, A. (1979) *Museums of Madness. The Social Organization of Insanity in Nineteenth-Century England*. London: Allen Lane.

Scull, A. (1989) *Social Order/Mental Disorder: Anglo-American Psychiatry in Historical Perspective*. London: Routledge.

Shadish, W.R., Matt, G.E., Navarro, A.M. *et al.* (1997) Evidence that therapy works in clinically representative conditions. *Journal of Consulting and Clinical Psychology* **65**: 355–65.

Shapiro, D.A. and Firth, J. (1987) Prescriptive versus exploratory psychotherapy. Outcomes of the Sheffield Psychotherapy Project. *British Journal of Psychiatry* **151**: 790–9.

Shapiro, D.A., Barkham, M., Rees, A. *et al.* (1994) Effects of treatment duration and severity of depression on the effectiveness of cognitive-behavioral and psychodynamic-interpersonal psychotherapy. *Journal of Consulting and Clinical Psychology* **62(3)**: 522–34.

Shapiro, D.A., Rees, A., Barkham, M. *et al.* (1995) Effects of treatment duration and severity of depression on the maintenance of gains after cognitive-behavioral and psychodynamic-interpersonal psychotherapy. *Journal of Consulting and Clinical Psychology* **63**: 378–87.

Shapiro, M.B. (1961) The single case in fundamental clinical psychological research. *British Journal of Medical Psychology* **34**: 255–63.

Shapiro, M.B. (1966) The single case in clinical psychology research. *Journal of General Psychology* **74**: 3–23.

Shapiro, M.B. and Ravenette, A.T. (1959) A preliminary experiment of paranoid delusions. *Journal of Mental science* **105**: 255–62.

Sheldon, B. (1999) Trials and tribulations. In *Evidence Based Social Care*, Issue 4. Exeter: Centre for Evidence Based Social Services.

Sheldon, T.A., Guyatt, G.H. and Haines, A. (1998) When to act on evidence. *British Medical Journal* **17**: 139–42.

Sheldon, B. and Macdonald, G. (1999) *Research and Practice in Social Care; Mind the Gap*. Exeter: Centre for Evidence Based Social Services.

Shepherd, G. (1990) Case management. *Health Trends* **22**: 59–61.

Shiller, A.D., Burke, D.T., Kim, H.J. *et al.* (1999) Treatment with amantadine potentiated motor learning in a patient with traumatic brain injury of 15 years' duration. *Brain Injury* **13**: 715–21.

Shorter, E. (1997) *A History of Psychiatry. From the Era of the Asylum to the Age of Prozac.* New York, Chichester and Brisbane: John Wiley and Sons.

Sidman, M. (1960) *Tactics of Scientific Research: Evaluating Experimental Data in Psychology.* New York: Basic Books.

Sifneos, P. (1979) *Short-term dynamic psychotherapy.* New York: Plenum.

SIGN (1999) *An Introduction to Sign Methodology for the Development of Evidence-based Clinical Guidelines.* Scottish Intercollegiate Guidelines Network.

Simes, R.J. (1986) Publication bias: the case for an international registry of clinical trials. *Journal of Clinical Oncology* **4**: 1529–41.

Sines, O. (1970) Actuarial versus clinical prediction in psychopathology. *British Journal of Psychiatry* **116**: 129–44.

Sitzia, J. and Wood, N. (1997) Patient satisfaction: a review of issues and concepts. *Social Science and Medicine* **45(12)**: 1829–43.

Sledge, W.H., Tebes, J., Rakfeldt, J., Davidson, L., Lyons, L. and Druss, B. (1996) Day hospital/crisis respite care versus in-patient care, part I: clinical outcomes. *American Journal of Psychiatry* **153**: 1065–73.

Sloane, R.B., Staples, F.R. and Schneider, L.S. (1985) Interpersonal therapy versus Nortriptyline for depression in the elderly. In *Clinical and Pharmacological Studies in Psychiatric Disorders*, G.D. Burrows, T.R. Norman and L. Dennerstein (eds). London: John Libbey, pp. 344–6.

Smith, M.L. and Glass, G.V. (1977) Meta-analysis of psychotherapy outcome studies. *American Psychologist* **32**: 752–60.

Solomon, P. (1992) The efficacy of case management services for severely mentally disabled clients. *Community Mental Health Journal* **28**: 163–80.

Spitzer, M. (1998) The history of neural network research in psychopathology. In *Neural Networks and Psychopathology*, D.J. Stein and J. Ludik (eds), pp. 14–33.

St Leger, A.S., Schneiden, H. and Walsworth-Bell, J.P. (1992) *Evaluating Health Services Effectiveness.* Milton Keynes: Open University Press.

Stanton, A.H., Gunderson, J.G., Knapp, P.H. *et al.* (1984) Effects of psychotherapy in schizophrenia: I. Design and implementation of a controlled study. *Schizophrenia Bulletin* **10**: 520–63.

Stein, L.I. and Test, M.A. (1980) Alternative to mental hospital treatment. I. Conceptual model, treatment program, and clinical evaluation. *Archives of General Psychiatry* **37(4)**: 392–7.

Steiner, D. and Norman, G. (1989) *Health Measurement Scales.* Oxford: Oxford University Press.

Sterling, T.D. (1959) Publication decisions and their possible effects on inferences drawn from tests of significance – or vice versa. *Journal of the American Statistical Association* **54**: 30–4.

Stevens, A. and Gabbay, J. (1991) Needs assessment. *Health Trends* **23**: 20–3.

Stevenson, J. and Meares, R. (1992) An outcome study of psychotherapy for patients with borderline personality disorder. *American Journal of Psychiatry* **149**: 358–62.

Stewart, M., Brown, J.B., Weston, W.W. *et al.* (1995) *Patient-centered Medicine: Transforming the Clinical Method.* London: Sage.

Stiles, W.B. and Shapiro, D.A. (1994) Disabuse of the drug metaphor. Psycho-therapy process-outcome correlations. *Journal of Consulting and Clinical Psychology* 942–8.

Stoker, J., Beenen, F. and the Dutch Psychoanalytic Institute. (1996, February) Outline of a quality monitoring and checking system for long-term (4 or 5 times a week) psychoanalytic treatment. Paper presented at the Stuttgart Kolleg.

Stokes, P.E., Shamoian, C.A., Stoll, P.M., and Patton, M.J. (1971). Efficacy of lithium as acute treatmentof manic-depressive illness. *Lancet* 1: 1319–25.

Strauss, A.L. and Corbin, J. (1990) *Basics of Qualitative Research: Grounded Theory Procedure and Techniques*. London: Sage.

Stricker, G. (1967) Actuarial, naïve clinical and sophisticated clinical prediction of pathology from figure drawings. *Journal of Consulting Psychology* 31: 492–4.

Stroup, D.F., Berlin, J.A., Morton, S.C. *et al.* (2000) Meta-analysis of observational studies in epidemiology: a proposal for reporting. Meta-analysis Of Observational Studies in Epidemiology (MOOSE) group. *Journal of the American Medical Association* 283: 2008–12.

Sturmey, P. (1996) *Functional Analysis in Clinical Psychology*. Guildford: John Wiley and Sons.

Sullivan H.S. (1953) *The Interpersonal Theory of Psychiatry*. New York: Norton.

Sullivan, M.D. (1993) Placebo controls and epistemic control in orthodox medicine. *Journal of Medicine and Philosophy* 18: 213–31.

Summerfield, D. (1995) Psychological responses to war and atrocity: the limitations of current concepts. *Social Science and Medicine* 40(8): 1073–82.

Sutton, A.J., Duval, S.J., Tweedie, R.L., Abrams, K.R. and Jones, D.R. (2000) Empirical assessment of effect of publication bias on meta-analyses. *British Medical Journal* 320: 1574–7.

Szasz, T. (1961) *The Myth of Mental Illness: Foundations of a Theory of Personal Conduct*. New York: Harper and Row.

Tansella, M. (1989) Evaluating community psychiatric services. In *The Scope of Epidemiological Psychiatry*, P. Williams, G. Wilkinson and K. Rawnsley (eds). London: Routledge, pp. 386–403.

Tarrier, N., Barrowclough, C., Vaughn, C. *et al.* (1988) The community management of schizophrenia. A controlled trial of a behavioural intervention with families to reduce relapse. *British Journal of Psychiatry* 153: 532–42.

Tarrier, N., Yusupoff, L., Kinney, C. *et al.* (1998) Randomised controlled trial of intensive cognitive behaviour therapy for patients with chronic schizophrenia. *British Medical Journal* 317(7154): 303–7.

Taylor, D. (1996) Through the minefield: how to decide which drug to use and when. *Schizophrenia Monitor* 6: 1–5.

Taylor, R. and Thornicroft, G. (1996) Uses and limits of randomised controlled trials in mental health services research. In *Mental Health Outcome Measures*, G. Thornicroft and M. Tansella (eds). Heidelberg: Springer Verlag, pp. 143–51.

Teague, G.B., Bond, G.R. and Drake, R.E. (1998) Program fidelity in assertive community treatment: development and use of a measure. *American Journal of Orthopsychiatry* 68(2): 216–32.

Thomä, H. and Kächele, H. (1987) *Psychoanalytic practice. I: Principles*. New York: Springer Verlag.

Thompson, C. (1989)*The Instruments of Psychiatric Research*. Chichester: Wiley.

Thompson, L.W., Gallagher, D. and Breckenridge, J.S. (1987) Comparative effectiveness of psychotherapies for depressed elders. *Journal of Consulting and Clinical Psychology* **55**: 385–90.

Thompson, S.G. (1994) Why sources of heterogeneity in meta-analysis should be investigated. *British Medical Journal* **309**: 1351–5.

Thompson, S., *et al.* (1999) Intensive case management for severe psychotic illness (letter). *Lancet* **354**: 1385–6.

Thornicroft, G. and Tansella, M. (1996) *Mental Health Outcome Measures*. Heidelberg: Springer Verlag.

Thornicroft, G. and Tansella, M. (1999) *The Mental Health Matrix: a Manual for Service Improvement*. Cambridge: Cambridge University Press.

Thornicroft, G., Wykes, T., Holloway, F., Johnson, S. and Szmukler, G. (1998a) From efficacy to effectiveness in community mental health services. PRiSM Psychosis Study 10. *British Journal of Psychiatry* **173**: 423–7.

Thornicroft, G., Strathdee, G., Phelan, M. *et al.* (1998b) Rationale and design: PRiSM Psychosis Study 1. *British Journal of Psychiatry* **173**: 363–70.

Thornicroft, G., Becker, T., Holloway, F. *et al.* (1999) Community mental health teams: evidence or belief? *British Journal of Psychiatry* **175**: 508–13.

Thornley, B. and Adams, C. (1998) Content and quality of 2000 controlled trials in schizophrenia over 50 years. *British Medical Journal* **317**: 1181–4.

Thornton, T. (1997) Reasons and causes in philosophy and psychopathology. Feature article with peer commentaries. *Philosophy, Psychology and Psychiatry* **4**: 307–22.

Tonelli, M.R. (1998) Philosophical limits of evidence-based medicine. *Academic Medicine* **73(12)**: 1234–40.

Treadwell, K. and Page, T.J. (1996) Functional analysis: identifying the environmental determinants of severe behavior disorders. *Journal of Head Trauma Rehabilitation* **11**: 62–74.

Tuke, D.H. (1882) *Chapters on the History of the Insane in the British Isles*. London: Kegan Paul, Trench and Co.

Tyrer, P. (1998) Cost-effective or profligate community psychiatry? *British Journal of Psychiatry* **172**: 1–3.

Tyrer, P. (2000) Effectiveness of intensive treatment in severe mental illness. *British Journal of Psychiatry* **176**: 492–8.

Tyrer, P., Morgan, J., Van Horn, E. *et al.* (1995) A randomised controlled study of close monitoring of vulnerable psychiatric patients. *Lancet* **345**: 756–9.

Tyrer, P., Coid, J., Simmonds, S., Joseph, P. and Marriott, S. (1997) Community mental health team management for those with severe mental illnesses and disordered personality. In *Schizophrenia Module of The Cochrane Database of Systematic Reviews*, updated 01 September 1997, Adams C.E., Duggan L., de Jesus Mari J. and White, P. (eds). Available in The Cochrane Library (database on disk and CDROM). *The Cochrane Collaboration*; Issue 4. Oxford: Update Software. Updated quarterly.

Tyron, W.W. (1982) A simplified time-series analysis for evaluating treatment interventions. *Journal of Applied Behaviour Analysis* **15**: 423–9.

US Department of Health and Human Services (1999) *Mental Health: a Report of the Surgeon General*. Rockville MD: US Department of Health and Human Services, Substance Abuse and Mental Health Services Administration, Center for

Mental Health Services, National Institute of Mental Health, National Institutes of Health.

User/Survivor Advisory Group (1999) *Mental Health in London: a Strategy for Action.* Report of the work of the User/Survivor Advisory Group, London Regional Office: Department of Health.

Vaillant, G.E. (1962) The prediction of recovery in schizophrenia. *Journal of Nervous and Mental Disease* **35**: 534–42.

von Cramon, D.Y. and Matthes-von Cramon, G. (1994) Back to work with a chronic dysexecutive syndrome? *Neuropsychological Rehabilitation* **4**: 399–417.

von Wright, G.H. (1971) *Explanation and Understanding.* London: Routledge and Kegan Paul.

Wagner, E.H., Austin, B.T. and Von Korff, M. (1996) Organizing care for patients with chronic illness. *Millbank Quarterly* **74(4)**: 511–44.

Wagner, E.H., Davis, C., Schaefer, J., Von Korff, M. and Austin, B.A. (1999) Survey of leading chronic disease management programs: are they consistent with the literature? *Managed Care Quarterly* **7(3)**: 60–70.

Wagner-Jauregg, J. (1887) Ueber die Einwirkung fieberhafter Erkrankungen auf Psychosen, *Jahrbuch für Psychiatrie* **7**: 94–131.

Wagner-Jauregg, J. (1918/19) Ueber die Einwirkung der Malaria auf die progresssive Paralyse. *Psychiatrisch-neurologische Wochenschrift* **20**: 132–4, 251–5.

Wampold, B.E., Mondin, G.W., Moody, M. *et al.* (1997) A meta-analysis of outcome studies comparing bona-fide psychotherapies: empirically 'all must have prizes'. *Psychological Bulletin* **122**: 203–15.

Weiner, D.B. (1993) The scientific origins of psychiatry in the French Revolution. In *Proceedings of the 1st European Congress on the History of Psychiatry and Mental Health Care*, L. de Goei and J. Vijslaar (eds). Rotterdam: Erasmus, pp. 314–30.

Weiner, D.B. (1994) 'Le geste de Pinel': The history of a psychiatric myth. In *Discovering the History of Psychiatry*, M.S. Micale and R. Porter (eds). New York and Oxford: Oxford University Press, pp. 232–47.

Weiss, B. and Weisz, J.R. (1990) The impact of methodological factors on child psychotherapy outcome research: a meta-analysis for researchers. *Journal of Consulting and Clinical Psychology* **54**: 789–95.

Weissman, M.M. and Markowitz, J.C. (1994) Interpersonal psychotherapy. Current status. *Archives of General Psychiatry* **51(8)**: 599–606.

Weissman, M.M., Prusoff, B.A., DiMascio, A. *et al.* (1979) The efficacy of drugs and psychotherapy in the treatment of acute depressive episodes. *American Journal of Psychiatry* **136(4B)**: 555–8.

Wells, K.B., Sherbourne, C.D., Schoenbaum, M. *et al.* (2000) Impact of disseminating quality improvement programs for depression in primary care: a randomized controlled trial. *Journal of the American Medical Association* **283(2)**: 212–20.

Wetzler, S. (1989) *Measuring Mental Illness.* Washington DC: American Psychiatry Press.

Whittle, P. (in press) Experimental psychology and psychoanalysis: what we can learn from a century of misunderstanding. *Neuro-psychoanalysis* **2**.

Widdershoven, G.A.M. (1999) Cognitive psychology and hermeneutics: two approaches to meaning and mental disorder. Feature article with peer commentaries. *Philosophy, Psychology and Psychiatry* **6**: 245–70.

Wiersma, D. (1996) Measuring social disabilities in mental health. In *Mental Health Outcome Measures*, G. Thornicroft and M. Tansella (eds). Heidelberg: Springer Verlag, pp. 110–22.

Wiersma, D., Kluiter, H., Nienhuis, F.J., Ruphan, M. and Giel, R. (1991) Costs and benefits of day treatment with community care for schizophrenic patients. *Schizophrenia Bulletin* **3**: 411–9.

Wilkin, D., Hallam, L. and Doggett, M.A. (1992) *Measures of Need and Outcome for Primary Health Care*. Oxford: Oxford University Press.

Williams, B. (1994) Patient satisfaction: a valid concept? *Social Science and Medicine* **38(4)**: 509–16.

Williams, B. (1995) *The Role of the 'Person' in Person-centered Mental Health Care*. Bangor: University of Bangor.

Williams, B. and Grant, G. (1998) Defining 'people-centredness': making the implicit explicit. *Health and Social Care in the Community* **6(2)**: 84–94.

Williams, B., Coyle, J. and Healy, D. (1998) The meaning of patient satisfaction: an explanation of high reported levels. *Social Science and Medicine* **47(9)**: 1351–60.

Williams, R. (1981) Logical analysis as a qualitative method. *Sociology of Health and Illness* **3**: 141–87.

Wilson, B.A. (1991) Behavior therapy in the treatment of neurologically impaired adults. In *Handbook of Behavior Therapy and Psychological Science: an Integrative Approach*, P.R. Martin (ed.). New York: Pergamon Press.

Wilson, B.A., Alderman, N., Burgess, P.W., Emslie, H. and Evans, J.J. (1996) *Behavioural Assessment of the Dysexecutive Syndrome*. Bury St Edmunds: Thames Valley Test Company.

Wilson, G.T. and Fairburn, C.G. (1993) Cognitive treatments for eating disorders. *Journal of Consulting and Clinical Psychology* **61(2)**: 261–9.

Wing, J. (1996) SCAN (Schedule for Clinical Assessment in Neuropsychiatry and the PSE (Present State Examination) tradition. In *Mental Health Outcome Measures*, G. Thornicroft and M. Tansella (eds). Heidelberg: Springer Verlag, pp. 123–30.

Winston, A., Pollack, J., McCullough, L. *et al.* (1991) Brief psychotherapy of personality disorders. *Journal of Nervous and Mental Disorders* **179(4)**: 188–93.

Winston, A., Laikin, M., Pollack, J. *et al.* (1994) Short-term psychotherapy of personality disorders. *American Journal of Psychiatry* **151(2)**: 190–4.

Wittchen, U. and Nelson, C.B. (1996) The Composite International Diagnostic Interview: an instrument for measuring mental health outcome? In *Mental Health Outcome Measures*, G. Thornicroft and M. Tansella (eds). Heidelberg: Springer Verlag, pp. 179–87.

Wood, R.L. (1987) *Brain Injury Rehabilitation: a Neurobehavioural Approach*. London: Croom Helm.

Woody, G.E., McLellan, A.T., Luborsky, L. and O'Brien, C.P. (1995) Psychotherapy in community methadone programs: a validation study. *American Journal of Psychiatry* **192**: 1302–8.

Woolgar, S. (1988) *Science: The Very Idea*. Chichester: Ellis Horwood Limited.

World Health Organisation (1973) *International Pilot Study of Schizophrenia*. Geneva: WHO.

World Health Organisation (1980) *International Classification of Impairments, Disabilities and Handicaps*. Geneva: WHO.

World Health Organisation (1992) *The ICD-10 Classification of Mental and Behavioural Disorders*. Geneva: WHO.

Yap, P.M. (1965) Koro – a culture bound depersonalisation syndrome. *British Journal of Psychiatry* **111**: 43–50.

Young, J. (1990) *Cognitive Therapy for Personality Disorder: A Scheme-focussed Approach*. Sarasota, FL: Professional Resources Exchange.

Youngson, H.A. and Alderman, N. (1994) Fear of incontinence and its effects on a community based rehabilitation programme after severe brain injury: successful remediation of escape behaviour using behaviour modification. *Brain Injury* **8**: 23–36.

Yuen, H.K. (1993) Self-feeding system for an adult with head injury and severe ataxia. *American Journal of Occupational Therapy* **47**: 444–51.

Zarin, D.A., Pincus, H.A. and McIntyre, J.S. (1993) Practice guidelines (editorial). *American Journal of Psychiatry* **150**: 175–7.

Zucker, K. (1928) Experimentelles über Sinnestäuschungen. *Archiv für Psychiatrie und Nervenkrankheiten* **83**: 706–54.

Zucker, K. and Zador, J. (1930) Zur Analyse der Meskalin-Wirkung am Normalen. *Deutsche Zeitschrift für Nervenheilkunde* **127**: 15–29.